Assessment of Aphasia

Assessment
of
Aphasia

OTFRIED SPREEN
ANTHONY H. RISSER

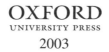

OXFORD
UNIVERSITY PRESS
2003

OXFORD
UNIVERSITY PRESS

Oxford   New York
Auckland   Bangkok   Buenos Aires   Cape Town   Chennai
Dar es Salaam   Delhi   Hong Kong   Istanbul   Karachi   Kolkata
Kuala Lumpur   Madrid   Melbourne   Mexico City   Mumbai
Nairobi   São Paulo   Shanghai   Taipei   Tokyo   Toronto

Published by Oxford University Press, Inc.
198 Madison Avenue, New York, New York 10016
http://www.oup-usa.org

Oxford is a registered trademark of Oxford University Press

Library of Congress Cataloging-in-Publication Data
Spreen, Otfried.
Assessment of aphasia / Otfried Spreen, Anthony H. Risser.
p. ; cm.
Includes bibliographical references and index.
ISBN 0-19-514075-3
1. Aphasia—Diagnosis.   I. Risser, Anthony H.   II. Title.
[DNLM: 1. Aphasia—diagnosis.   WL 340.5 S768a 2003]
RC425 .S675 2003
616.85'52075—dc21   2002066802

2 4 6 8 9 7 5 3 1

Printed in the United States of America
on acid-free paper

Preface

This book is addressed to the practicing speech clinician and neuro-psychologist dealing with aphasic adults and children, as well as with children who have delayed or disordered language development. It is also written as a primary or ancillary text in graduate courses dealing with the assessment of speech and language problems. To view the development of assessment methods in context, a brief historical introduction is necessary. In addition, we attempt to establish a frame of reference for reviewing available methods by describing key requirements for an acceptable testing method in general and for the examination of brain-damaged populations in particular.

The main content of this book deals with contemporary methods of assessment, ranging from basic screening for aphasia to detailed comprehensive methods. Each test is described in some detail, including ordering information and price, but particularly the method of testing. We then review the strengths and weaknesses of each test, including those designed for children from infancy to school age. Information on test procedures, psychometric properties, available norms, the theoretical positions of test authors, and the most appropriate areas of use and corresponding research are described to provide the clinician with sufficient information to choose tests suitable for the individual patient. Other tests that have found little use in published studies are listed only briefly. The last part of the book provides a discussion of contemporary clinical practice, with special reference to widely differing problems, ranging from purely research-oriented questions to questions of measuring day-to-day improvement during therapy and assessing communicative ability in the home or occupational setting.

In preparing this book, we note that during the last two decades there has been particular interest and active research in the testing of aging patients, in dementia, in the psycholinguistic approach to language disorders, and in the development of scales for functional communication as a more pragmatic, ecologically valid method of assessing day-to-day living abilities.

We are grateful to helpful colleagues in speech/language pathology, particularly to Dr. Martha Taylor Sarno at New York University who suggested the preparation of this book and for her valuable assistance over the course of writing it. Thanks also to Dr. Harold Goodglass of Boston and Sonya E. Bates, M.Sc., in Adelaide, Australia, for valuable comments on the manuscript. Carol Stach, M.A. at the Houston (TX) Veterans Administration Medical Center and Ruth Fink, M.A. at Moss Rehabilitation Research Institute in Philadelphia are thanked for making available their testing resources for examination on a number of occasions. Finally, we thank our editor, Fiona Stevens, for her patience and guidance.

Victoria, British Columbia   O.S.
Houston, Texas   A.H.R.

Contents

Acronyms

AAPS   Arizona Articulation Proficiency Scale—Revised (Barker-Fudala, 1998)

AAT   Aachen Aphasia Test (Huber et al., 1984); English version (N. Miller et al., 1998)

ACTS   Auditory Comprehension Test for Sentences, (Shewan, 1980)

ADP   Aphasia Diagnostic Profiles (Helm-Estabrooks, 1992)

ALFA   Assessment of Language-Related Functional Activities (Baines et al., 1999)

ALPS   Aphasia Language Performance Scale (Keenan and Brassell, 1975)

ANELT   Amsterdam-Nijmegen Everyday Language Test (Blomert, 1990)

APPLS   Assessment Protocol of Pragmatic Linguistic Skills (Gerber and Gurland, 1989)

ASHA-FACS   American Speech Language-Hearing Association Functional Assessment of Communication Skills for Adults (Frattali et al., 1995)

AST   Aphasia Screening Test (Reitan, 1991)

BASA   Boston Assessment of Severe Aphasia (Helm-Estabrooks et al., 1989)

BDAE, BDAE-R, BDAE-3   Boston Diagnostic Aphasia Examination (Goodglass et al., 2000)

BEST, BEST-2   Bedside Evaluation Screening Test, 2nd ed. (West et al., 1998)

BNT   Boston Naming Test (Goodglass et al., 2000)

BVAT   Bilingual Verbal Ability Tests (Munoz-Sandoval et al., 1998)

CAAST   Children's Acquired Aphasia Screening Test (Whurr, 1996)

CADL, CADL-2   Communication Abilities of Daily Living-2 (Holland et al., 1998)

CELF-3   Clinical Evaluation of Language Fundamentals, 3rd ed. (Wiig et al., 1992)

CETI   Communicative Effectiveness Index (Lomas et al., 1989)

CIU   Correct Information Unit (L. Nicholas and Brookshire, 1993)

COWA   Controlled Oral Word Association (Word Fluency subtest of the MAE; Benton et al., 1994)

CREVT   Comprehensive Receptive and Expressive Vocabulary Test (Wallace and Hammill, 1994)

DCT   Discourse Comprehension Test (Brookshire and Nicholas, 1997)

DDST   Denver Developmental Screening Test (Franenburg and Dodds, 1990)

D-KEFS   Delis-Kaplan Executive Function System (Delis et al., 2001)

EFA-3   Examining for Aphasia, 3rd ed. (Eisenson, 1993)

F-A-S   Word Fluency subtest of the NCCEA (Spreen and Benton, 1977)

FAST   Frenchay Aphasia Screening Test (Enderby et al., 1987a,b)

FCP   Functional Communication Profile (Sarno, 1969)

FIM   Functional Independence Measure

HRNB   Halstead-Reitan Neuropsychological Battery (Reitan and Wolfson, 1985)

ITPA, ITPA-3   Illinois Test of Psycholinguistic Ability (Hammill et al., 2002)

LNNB   Luria-Nebraska Neuropsychological Battery (Golden et al., 1980)

MAE   Multilingual Aphasia Examination (Benton et al., 1994)

MAE-S   Multilingual Aphasia Examination—Spanish (Rey et al., 1999)

MTDDA   Minnesota Test for Differential Diagnosis of Aphasia (Schuell, 1973)

NCCEA   Neurosensory Center Comprehensve Examination for Aphasia (Spreen and Benton, 1977)

NEPSY   Neuropsychological Developmental Assessment (Korkman et al., 1997).

OWLS   Oral and Written Language Scales (Carrow-Woolfolk, 1996)

PALPA   Psycholinguistic Assessment of Language Processing in Aphasia (Kay et al., 1992)

PICA   Porch Index of Communicative Ability (Porch, 1967)

PICAC   Porch Index of Communicative Ability in Children (Porch, 1981)

PLAI   Preschool Language Assessment Instrument (Blank et al., 1978)

PLASTER-R   Pediatric Language Acquisition Screening Tool for Early Referral—Revised (Shulman and Sherman, 1996)

PLS-3   Preschool Language Scale-3 (Zimmerman et al., 1992)

PP   Pragmatic Protocol (Prutting and Kirchner, 1987)

PPVT, PPVT-3   Peabody Picture Vocabulary Test—III (Dunn and Dunn, 1997)

RCBA, RCBA-2   Reading Comprehension Battery for Aphasia-2 (LaPointe and Horner, 1999)

RHLB   Right Hemisphere Language Battery (Bryan, 1995)

SAS   Sklar Aphasia Scale (Sklar, 1983)

SLES   Speech and Language Evaluation Scale (Fressola et al., 1990)

SRT   Sentence Repetition Test (Spreen and Strauss, 1998)

STAL   Screening Test for Adolescent Language (Prather et al., 2000)

STDAS-2   Screening Test for Developmental Apraxia of Speech, 2nd ed. (Blakeley, 2000)

TACL-3   Test for Auditory Comprehension of Language, 3rd ed. (Carrow, 1998)

TOAL-3   Test of Adolescent and Adult Language, 3rd ed. (Hammill et al., 1994)

TOLA   Test of Oral and Limb Apraxia (Helm-Estabrooks, 1992)

TONI-3   Test of Nonverbal Intelligence, 3rd ed. (L. Brown et al., 1998)

TONI-C   Test of Nonverbal Intelligence, Computer Version (Hammill et al., 1996)

TOPA   Test of Phonological Awareness (Torgesen and Bryant, 1994)

TOPL   Test of Pragmatic Language (Phelps-Terasaki and Phelps-Gunn, 1994)

TOWL-3   Test of Written Language, 3rd ed. (Hammill and Larsen, 1996)

TT   Token Test (De Renzi and Vignolo, 1962)

WAB   Western Aphasia Battery (Kertesz, 1982)

WAIS, WAIS-R, WAIS-III   Wechsler Adult Intelligence Scale, 3rd ed. (Wechsler, 1991)

WAST   Whurr Aphasia Screening Test (Whurr, 1996)

WISC, WISC-R, WISC-III   Wechsler Intelligence Scale for Children, 3rd ed. (Wechsler, 1996)

Test Sources

(Note that some tests are also available for distribution by Pro-Ed, PAR, and Psychological Corporation.)

Academic Therapy Publications, 20 Commercial Blvd., Novato, CA 94949.
  Canadian distributor: Institute of Psychological Research, 34 Fleury St.,
  Montreal, P.Q., Canada H3L 1S9.
American Guidance Service, 4201 Woodland Rd., P.O. Box 99, Circle Pines, MN
  55014-1796.
Applied Symbolics, 16 W. Eary St., Suite 300, Chicago, IL 00000 (now Pro-Ed)
Communication Skill Builders, 555 Academic Ct., San Antonio, TX 78205-2498.
Consulting Psychologists Press, Palo Alto, CA.
Denver Developmental Materials, Inc., P.O. Box 6919, Denver, CO 80210-0919.
Hawthorne Educational Services, Inc., 800 Gray Oak Dr., Columbia, MO 65201.
Lippincott Williams & Wilkins, 600 Washington Sq., Philadelphia, PA 19106.
Multi-Health Systems, Inc., 3770 Victoria Park Ave., Toronto, Ont., Canada
  M2H 3H6.
NFER-Nelson Publishing Co. Ltd., Windsor, England. E-mail: baeni.mackin@nfer-
  nelson.co.uk
PAR—Psychological Assessment Resources, Inc., P.O. Box 998, Odessa, FL
  33556 (1-800-331-8378).
Pro-Ed Inc., 8700 Shoal Creek Blvd., Austin, TX 78757-6897.
Psycan, P.O. Box 290, Station U, Toronto, Ont., Canada H6R 3A5.
Psychological Corporation, 555 Academic Ct., San Antonio, TX 78204-2498.
  Canadian source: 55 Horner Ave., Toronto, Ont., Canada M8Z 4X6.
Psychology Clinic, University of Victoria, Victoria, B.C., Canada V8W 3P5.
Riverside Publishing, 425 Spring Lake Dr., Itasca, IL 60143-2079.
Sopris West, 4093 Specialty Pl., Longmont, CO 80504.
Stoelting Co., 1350 Kostner Ave., Chicago, IL 60623.
Thames Valley Test Company, 7-9 The Green, Bury St.Edmunds, Suffolk IP28
  6EL, UK.
University of Minnesota Press, 75 East River Rd., Elliott Hall, Minneapolis, MN
  55455.

Western Psychological Services, 12031 Wilshire Blvd., Los Angeles, CA 90025-1251.

Wide Range Inc., 15 Ashley Pl., Suite 1A, Wilmington, DE 19804-1314.

Whurr Publishers Ltd., 19b Compton Terrace, London N1 2UN, UK; US: Taylor & Francis, 7625 Empire Dr., Florence, KY 41042.

I

INTRODUCTION

1

Introduction to Aphasia Assessment

Aphasia is defined as "the loss or deterioration of verbal communication due to an acquired lesion of the nervous system involving one or more aspects of the processes of comprehending and producing verbal messages" (Basso and Cubelli, 1999). Related disorders of articulation, reading, and writing are usually included in the description of aphasia. Though primarily occurring in adulthood, acquired aphasia due to cerebral disorders may also occur in children, although it is more common for children to show developmental dysphasia or other developmental language disorders due to congenital causes.

Different conceptualizations of the nature of aphasia underlie the design of its assessment. Test construction is directly influenced by whether we see aphasia as a specific disorder of selected abilities or as a pervasive disturbance of communication, and whether we conceive of aphasia as unitary in nature or as consisting of many "subtypes." Benton (1967) pointed out that the choice of a model of language functioning determines what kind of test we construct or use. He indicated that the problem is similar to the one posed by the conceptualization of intelligence; it is similar also in the sense that no common agreement exists. Although Benton at that time still expressed some hope for the possibility of achieving a consensus, the development of research in aphasia (and in test construction) would seem to suggest that we have reached an impasse similar to that reached in the conceptualization (and testing) of intelligence. As a result, two approaches to test construction should be recognized as equally reasonable at this time:

1. To construct tests on the basis of one of the currently accepted conceptions of aphasia. This "taxonomic" or diagnostic approach en-

3

sures that the test measures all aspects viewed as important in a specific theoretical approach but makes it probable that it will not be widely used as long as different conceptualizations of aphasia are held by other workers in the field.

2. To approach the problem pragmatically, avoid specific conceptualizations, and construct a test that contains a variety of probes of all abilities described by researchers of widely differing theoretical viewpoints. This pragmatic approach, quite commonly used in the field of intelligence testing, will not be fully satisfactory to any of the prevailing schools but may gain wider acceptance if the test instrument is otherwise well constructed and of demonstrated use in clinical practice. One drawback of this empirical approach to test construction is the possibility of including redundant or highly specific material that may be irrelevant to the assessment of aphasia. This problem can be solved by future factor analytic investigations as long as the range of material is sufficiently wide to allow such solutions.

Both approaches have been applied in the construction of currently used tests. Whether evaluation proceeds from an objective psychometric or from a theoretically based framework is a topic that has also been discussed by Kertesz (1994). In the description of individual tests, we attempt to make specific reference to the conceptual framework used in each for the information of the reader unfamiliar with a given instrument.

Even within these two approaches, specific assessment instruments will show a good deal of variability. Matching the assessment to any given patient requires that the clinician maintain a flexible and knowledgeable manner of dealing with the task of examining aphasia. This manner of examination is core to what it means to work as a clinician, rather than testing patients as a technician or as a gatherer of research data (e.g., Matarazzo, 1990). In order to meet a full range of expectations, speech clinicians will base their examination approaches upon the needs created by the patient, the referral issue, the context in which the examination will take place, and the availability of other information about the patient. Also, clinicians will tailor the assessment to include data useful for providing subsequent treatment, and one's preferred approach to treatment will also have an impact on the assessment process. The best way to operate at this level of clinical service requires two things of the clinician: first, that one learns as much information as possible about the test instruments currently available; second, that this learning process will be continuous, as the clinician's level of personal knowledge responds to changes over time, as new tests, approaches, or normative standards become available, and as older tests perhaps lose (or retain) their value in a steadily accumulating clinical research literature.

A further distinction to be made in aphasia assessment is whether the effort has its foundation in either the clinical-neuroanatomical or the psycholinguistic approach to understanding the language problems found in aphasia. The traditional clinical approach to aphasia assessment dates back to the discoveries of Wernicke. It relies on defining subtypes on the basis of clinical data and neuroanatomical substrates, that is the area of brain lesion presumed to be responsible for the form of aphasia presented in a given patient. In contrast, the psycholinguistic approach relies on theoretical conceptions of language processing. Although this approach was recognized earlier by students of aphasia like Arnold Pick (1913; Spreen 1973), and Joseph Wepman (1951; Wepman et al., 1973), it has found wider application only in recent decades. The psycholinguistic approach uses theoretical models of language processing: the various forms of aphasia are viewed in the context of these models. Because of their importance for assessment, we describe both approaches briefly in this introductory chapter.

Clinical-Neuroanatomical Approach to Aphasia

In clinical practice, a distinction between fluent and nonfluent aphasia, depending on the characteristics of the patient's speech, is usually accepted. Studies of acquired aphasia in children have shown that aphasic syndromes found in adults are also found in children, with identical lesion sites (Cranberg et al., 1987; Martins and Ferro, 1991, 1992, 1993; Martins, 1997). Authors disagree in the further breakdown of types of aphasia.

Nonfluent aphasia

Global aphasia represents the loss of both comprehension and speech, involving larger lesions of the left fronto-temporal-parietal areas.

Broca's aphasia is characterized by poor speech production, agrammatism, anomia, and verbal paraphasias, with relative comprehension, involving mainly the left frontal areas. Lesions in the lower 50% of the prerolandic gyrus (lower motor cortex) also produce a form of Broca's aphasia (sometimes described as aphemia) in which articulation and prosody are affected. This condition can also be due to damage to the subcortical outflow of the lower motor cortex, and occasionally results in a "foreign language syndrome" (M. Alexander, 1997). Broca's aphasia is often accompanied by right hemiparesis, buccofacial apraxia (i.e., the inability to make purposeful movements of the speech musculature with intact motor innervation), and ideomotor apraxia of the left arm.

Transcortical (extrasylvian) motor aphasia (TMA) presents with severely impaired spontaneous speech output, but adequate ability to comprehend and repeat even complex sentences, and involves lesions in the premotor frontal areas, but occasionally only white matter lesions. Benson and Ardila (1996) distinguish this form from TMA-II, which shows the same symptomatology but is based on lesions caused by anterior cerebral artery occlusion, affecting primarily the supplementary motor cortex. These cases are characterized by paralysis and sensory loss of the lower extremities, and some dysarthria. Some cases show frequent initiation blocks, reduction in phrase length, and simplification of grammatical form (M. Alexander, 1997; Berthier, 1999). Some cases appear to be mute initially and cannot repeat. Mixed transcortical aphasia results from lesions combining those of transcortical motor aphasia and transcortical sensory aphasia.

Fluent aphasia

Wernicke's aphasia is characterized as abundant, even logorrheic, but incomprehensible speech, with phonemic and neologistic jargon, involving the posterior part of the superior gyrus of the left temporal lobe (i.e., Wernicke's area).

Conduction aphasia is characterized by fluent speech with frequent self-corrections, paraphasias, and severely impaired repetition. It is due to lesions in the supramarginal gyrus and adjacent white matter as well as the auditory and insular cortex. Initially, limb ideomotor apraxia is frequently found. Partial recovery is usually expected (Kertesz, 1979).

Transcortical (extrasylvian) sensory aphasia presents with good repetition without understanding the meaning of what is spoken, frequent paraphasias, circumlocutions and filler words, due to lesions of the posterior language area—the middle and inferior temporal gyrus, but sparing Wernicke's area.

Amnesic or anomic aphasia involves word-finding difficulties, with the individual often producing filler words or circumlocutions. It occurs frequently as the lasting residual feature of an earlier and more severe aphasia, and localization varies dependent on the original deficit. Word-finding ability has been associated specifically with activation of the left temporal lobe in positron emission studies (Beauregard et al., 1997). It has been suggested that with anterior temporal lobe damage word-finding difficulties for nouns are more pronounced than for verbs (Damasio and Tranel, 1993; Glosser and Donofrio, 2001). The term *anomia* is sometimes used synonymously with word-finding problems, in the absence of aphasia per se. This can sometimes cause confusion in understanding whether a patient is (or was) actually aphasic.

Figure 1–1 (H. Damasio, 1991, p. 47) shows the brain areas corresponding to most of these syndromes. It should be noted, however, that only about 20% to 30% of patients can be reliably classified (Albert et al., 1981; Prins et al., 1978). One reason for this is that lesions are frequently larger, overlapping several regions.

In addition, rare cases of *subcortical aphasia* (good repetition and comprehension, poor production, frequent anomia, due to left thalamic lesions) have been described (Basso and Cubelli, 1999). Recently, Marien et al. (2001) proposed the notion of a "lateralized linguistic cerebellum" that is reciprocally connected to frontal areas via the pons and the thalamus. Spinella (personal communication, 2002) provided a case report of dense Wernicke's aphasia, and Silveri et al. (1994) report a case of agrammatic speech following a right cerebellar lesion.

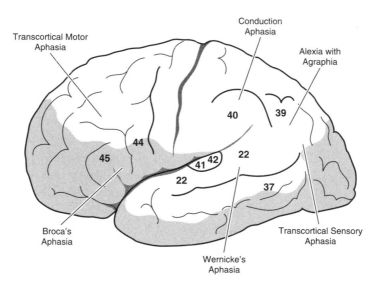

Figure 1–1. Diagrammatic representation of the major loci of lesions in the principal types of aphasia. Brodmann's areas 44 and 45 correspond to the classic Broca's area; area 22 to Wernicke's area; areas 41 and 42 to the primary auditory cortex, located deep in the sylvian fissure; area 40 is the supramarginal gyrus, and area 39 the angular gyrus; area 37 is located in the posterior portion of the second and third temporal gyrus (H. Damasio, 1991, p. 47, with permission of Academic Press).

The term *primary progressive aphasia* (PPA) is used for a rare form of aphasia in patients with neurodegenerative processes initially confined to the perisylvian or opercular regions (Mesulam and Weintraub, 1992; Karbe et al., 1993). Mesulam (2001) has proposed a set of diagnostic criteria for PPA, which includes onset, progression, associated cognitive functioning, and needed differential diagnosis (e.g., CVA, brain tumor) as ascertained by radiological studies. This form of aphasia can be expressive or receptive, often accompanied by alexia (Parkin, 1993, though see Westbury and Bub, 1997), and occurs in the absence of global dementia typically in the 50s or 60s, but may occur at other ages and even in childhood. "PPA-Plus" syndromes also may be observed, with additional deficits observed in visual recognition and in executive (i.e., so-called frontal lobe) functioning (Mesulam, 2001).

Crossed aphasia in right-handers refers to unexpected aphasia after lesions of the right hemisphere, suggesting atypical language lateralization. However, in some instances mild aphasias occur after large lesions that would usually cause severe aphasia. It has been speculated that in such cases discrepant localization of phonologic and semantic processing exists (M. Alexander and Annett, 1998). Aphasia in left-handers occurs only in a small proportion (30%) as a result of a right-hemisphere lesion. Hecaen (1981) calculated that, in addition, about 15% of left-handers would probably be aphasic after lesion to either hemisphere because of bilateral language representation.

Right hemisphere lesions in right-handers tend to show disorders of the affective aspects of language and aprosodia. In addition, disturbances of higher levels of language processing can occur, for example, on semantic discrimination tasks, extracting main points of a story, and interpreting abstract or figurative language (proverbs, idioms, metaphors) (Pimental and Kingsbury, 1989a), which can result in functional communication problems. The comprehension of abstract word meaning has been shown to be more impaired than that for words referring to concrete objects (Franklin, et al., 1994). Additionally, detailed examination of discourse comprehension in nonaphasic patients with right hemisphere damage suggest that limitations in the suppression of inappropriate interpretations of sentence meaning can contribute to these individuals' communication limitations. Speech clinicians have increased the scope of their clinical services over the past decade by examining the impact on language and communication of nonaphasic cognitive deficits caused by right hemisphere lesions and providing treatment for these difficulties (Myers, 1999; Tompkins, 1995).

Finally, speech clinicians over the past decade have shown a dramatic increase of interest in neurological problems that reflect diffuse or multifocal brain disease, such as Alzheimer's disease and traumatic brain injury. While aphasia as a distinct syndrome may be observed in the picture of neurobehavioral syndromes, it is more common for patients with these conditions to experience nonaphasic problems in language function and in meeting the everyday demands of communicating with others.

Psycholinguistic Approach to Aphasia

While some of the testing methods based on the clinical–neuroanatomical approach make use of conversational speech in a natural setting with limited structure, a series of studies have attempted to analyze the language of aphasic patients from a linguistic rather than a clinical point of view. This approach makes use of the patient's natural speech in a setting that makes no specific demands on the patient. Ideally, one could record a patient's utterances in the course of a day in the hospital or at home on audio- or videotape. The main goal of such studies is not, however, a direct assessment of communicative abilities but a more detailed study from a psycholinguistic point of view. Studies of use and abuse of syntax; grammar; word choice; frequency of word usage, pauses, and hesitations; speed of utterance, and so forth, can be conducted with such "free-speech" samples. The alternative approach is to focus on each aspect of psycholinguistic analysis individually and construct an experimental setting that allows an analysis of the types of errors produced by an aphasic patient.

This field of research has grown rapidly during the last 30 years and produced considerable insights into the mechanisms of normal and disordered language. Detailed reviews are presented by Caplan (1987, 1992) and Gernsbacher (1994).

More recently, the deterioration of language in aphasics has generated insights into the rules and processes of language and support for linguistic models of language comprehension and production (Fig. 1–2, Kay et al., 1996). The contrast between clinical and linguistic approaches is apparent in the detailed surveys of aphasic phonology (Blumstein, 1998; Denes et al., 1999), lexical-semantic problems (Rapp and Caramazza, 1998; Semenza, 1999), and grammar (Berndt, 1998; Miceli, 1999). These lines of research attempt to analyze pathological disorganization of language without recourse to disciplines outside of

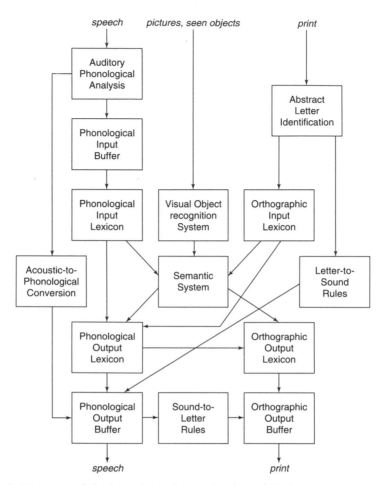

Figure 1–2. Diagram of the hypothetical organization of the language processing system, ranging from speech, visually perceived objects, and print (input), through processing systems of lexicon, phonological conversion, recognition, and semantic systems to output lexicon and speech and print output (Kay et al., 1996, with permission from Psychology Press).

linguistics, such as neuroanatomy or neurophysiology. They make use of the analysis of longer samples (e.g., 100 words) of discourse, "naturally occurring language that extends beyond the sentence level or across sentences" (Ehrlich, 1994), developed detailed scoring methods for speech samples, for example, the description of the Cookie-Theft picture of the BDAE. The term *normative approach*, used in the context of these studies only, refers to comparison with discourse production in normal adults, not psychometrically established norms. For this reason, the results are strictly descriptive—few if any group results (with very few subjects, usually 10 or less) are presented (Haravon et al., 1994). In fact, it is often argued that single case studies provide more information than group studies because specific deficits (e.g., selective sparing or loss ["dissociation"] of names for geographical terms, or for body parts, or selective comprehension deficits for colors or "indoor objects" [Semenza, 1999]) may not be recognizable in group studies. Single case studies are of particular interest if progress during therapy is being charted (see Kearns, 2000).

However, recent studies have successfully used discourse analysis in group studies, and related the results to those of psychological tests. For example, B. Brookshire et al. (2000) examined the retelling of a story ("The Lobster and the Crab") in 68 eight- to-seventeen-year old children with severe head injury and 23 with mild head injury at least 3 years postinjury. Children with severe head injury produced reduced content and information, showed impaired organization and difficulty in expressing the story's essential meanings and main ideas, and used fewer words and less complex sentences. Measures of core and gist information and number of dependent clauses were related to the results of the MAE-COWA and the Wisconsin Card Sorting Test, that is, measures of general verbal ability and verbal fluency as well as problem solving and working memory. Chapman and her colleagues have provided additional comprehensive studies in the use of discourse analysis (Chapman et al., 1992; 1998). Mann et al. (1994) developed a linguistic communication measure (LCM) that allows the analysis of narratives for amount of information, proportion of informative and noninformative words, and grammaticality of the expression. The analyses in other discourse studies involve a variety of these and other parameters of both the macrostructure (cognitive structure, global semantic meaning of a text, including organization, cohesive ties, reduction of complex information, topic adherence and topic shifting, etc.) (Ulatowska et al., 1992; Ulatowska and Chapman, 1994) and microstructure (morphology, syntax, and pragmatics) (Haravon et al., 1994), but the coverage of linguistic parameters and the method of scoring varies from study to study. Very detailed coding like that used by Haravon et al. is designed for a specific study only, and should not be confused with that used in formal tests of aphasia. The Discourse Analysis Test and the PALPA show that specific tasks can be created to approach the requirements of a formal test.

Figure 1–3 (Bloom, 1994, p. 89) shows a "synergistic" model of discourse production, synergistic because the "components are autonomous and exist independently of each other." It stresses the difference between contributions from the left and the right hemisphere, using a

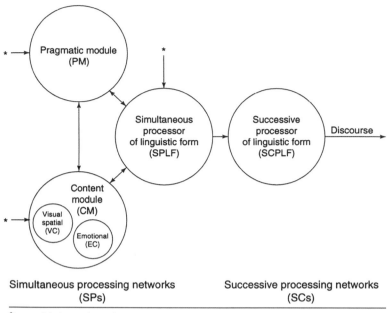

Figure 1–3. Synergistic model of simultaneous and successive processing in discourse production (Bloom, 1994, with permission from Lawrence Erlbaum).

successive versus simultaneous processing model based on Luria (1966) and Das et al. (1979) without acknowledging these sources. "A unit of discourse is generated on the basis of input to any of the simultaneous processors. The pragmatic component implements the verbal pragmatic rules that describe what a speaker needs to do in order to convey a message to the listener ... The simultaneous processor of linguistic forms may serve as input if the speaker has heard the story before" (p. 88).

Bloom's review suggests that the discourse of left hemisphere brain-damaged patients reflects the cognitive style of the unimpaired right hemisphere, that is, "they are able to take advantage of emotional content, emphasize their messages, and generate internal representation of story structure" (p. 87), while the right hemisphere brain-damaged patient's production "reflects the unimpaired linguistic capacities of the left hemisphere, but shows deficits in the particular cognitive style of the right hemisphere." This is based mainly on Bloom's and a few other studies mentioned in her review, using picture story techniques with emotional, visuospatial and neutral content for left and right brain-damaged patients. The studies showed that all brain-damaged patients were impaired relative to judgments of conciseness, relevancy, etc.; that left brain-damaged patients were pragmatically impaired, that is, produced less content in visuospatial and neutral, while right brain-damaged patients showed pragmatic impairment in the neutral condition (Bloom et al., 1993). This finding was in part independently confirmed by a study of picture descriptions of 17 right-handed, right-hemisphere stroke patients (Mackenzie et al., 1997), which found that, compared to matched control subjects, these patients were weaker in comprehension of metaphors and inferences, used fewer words, produced less information, and spoke for a shorter period of time during picture descriptions; they also showed limited facial expression, less eye contact, and monotonous intonation patterns.

Boles (1998) used conversational discourse analysis (CDA) as a means of evaluating progress during a 7-week therapy program of a single patient with Broca's aphasia. Progress was found in word repair, utterance production, and relative frequencies of words spoken by the patient and the conversation partner, parallel with improvement on standardized tests such as WAB, CADL, and measures of psychosocial well-being and communication readiness. Although the author acknowledges the practical limitations of CDA (especially that it is very time-consuming), he emphasizes that CDA tapped aspects of language that are not evident from standard language testing.

Another analysis of "procedural discourse" was performed by Ulatowska et al. (1992, 1994), who demonstrated that in a role-playing situation to elicit discourse, aphasics showed reduction in complexity and amount of speech but not in terms of sentential grammar, discourse grammar, and subjective rating of content and clarity. Additional studies (Glosser and Deser, 1990) have continued to analyze free speech samples, comparing three types of patients with fluent language disorders (i.e., left hemisphere stroke, head injury, and Alzheimer's disease) on measures of microlinguistic (syntactic and lexical errors) and macrolinguistic (thematic coherence) measures. Hartley and Jensen (1992) used retelling of a story and creating a story out of a cartoon sequence to analyze measures of productivity (e.g., speech rate), content (clarity, accuracy), and cohesion in patients with head injury and controls; they found three profiles, (a) confused, (b) impoverished, and (c) inefficient, of which only the first scored in the aphasic range of the WAB. Chapman et al. (1998) compared 10 normal adults with 10 mild to moderate aphasics and 10 patients with early to moderate stage Alzheimer's disease on tasks of retelling, gist statements, and lessons to be learned from verbal and written presentations of fables and proverbs, and viewing a Norman Rockwell painting. A five-point rating of each item was made on linguistic formulation, communicative intention, and drawing inferences. On virtually all linguistic measures, aphasics performed more poorly than Alzheimer's disease patients, while normals showed the best performance. Errors were found mostly in hesitations, revisions, circumlocutions, paraphasias, and ambiguous pronouns, disrupting the coherence of the text. Alzheimer's disease patients had more problems drawing inferences, the pragmatic domain of the responses, although there was considerable variability within each patient group. Similar significant findings were reported in a study of naming (Le Dorze and Durocher, 1992); stimulus length was an additional factor in this study. In eleven 9–17-year-old children with severe head injury, compared to a matched control group, Jordan et al. (1997) found not only poor confrontation naming, but also specific linguistic impairment, including specific disruptions (e.g., interjection of stereotypic phrases such as "you know," repeated use of starters such as "and then," overuse of indefinitives such as 'something', circumlocutory descriptions), that is, strategies to "buy time," silent pauses and pause strings, suggesting name-finding difficulties in the absence of frank aphasia.

A considerable amount of research has focused on finding confirmation for the existence of a semantic and an orthographic system and their interdependence.

As a somewhat oversimplified view of the systems involved in language (shown in Fig. 1–3), one can visualize how a new stimulus like "dog," perceived visually or heard, can stimulate the semantic representations, also called *lemmas*, consisting of already existing stimulus traces, such as animal, mammal, domestic, four legs, barks, etc. In order to name such a stimulus, the phonetic system, in turn, must search for appropriate associations and produce the correct name. If weakened, both systems may produce only an approximation of the proper name although recognition of the stimulus is fully realized ("tip of the tongue" phenomenon); hesitation, apparent memory failure, and the production of circumlocutions may be the result of such weakening. Goodglass et al. (1999) describe an ingenious experiment in which 21 elderly as compared to 21 young adults were required to give speeded judgment of whether a pictured object matches a named category, a named physical attribute, or a rhyming cue. The measured latencies for young adults were fastest for category judgment, and slowest for rhyming; in contrast, latencies for the elderly were equal for category and rhyming judgments. These results seem to support a two-stage model of name retrieval in which semantic processing precedes and mediates access to phonology. In addition, the cognitive processing system ("thinking") is closely interwoven with the semantic and the phonological systems, but adds organizing information from other systems as well, and leads to structuring, sorting, decision making, etc.

Unfortunately, each of these authors developed a somewhat different model of language processing and different methods of analysis appropriate to the model. This makes it difficult to compare studies, especially since the methods are usually developed without considering psychometric properties. Additionally, it makes it difficult for speech clinicians to decide whether and how to apply these findings in planning assessments and interventions for individual patients. The development of the PALPA (Kay et al., 1996) as a psycholinguistic assessment instrument promised a more widely acceptable solution to psycholinguistic methods of assessment. However, it also brought problems with limited psychometric investigation into focus (Wertz, 1996, see PALPA, Chapter 9).

2

History of Aphasia Assessment

Aphasia has fascinated brain researchers for centuries because it may appear without other neurological symptoms and because of the oft-heated debate over the relatively specific localization of language skills in the brain. Benton and Anderson (1998) offer an outline of the history of medical interest in aphasia (for a history reader, also see Eling, 1994), and the first volume of Henry Head's (1926) two-volume work on aphasia and related disorders provides a thorough review of explorations of aphasia through the nineteenth century and the first decades of the twentieth century. A new history of aphasia, ranging from prehistoric writings to contemporary schools of thought was compiled by Tesak (2001). Even very early records of medical knowledge make reference to language disorders after brain damage (Benton, 1964). Accounts of simple clinical examinations were often included in such reports, but it was not until the second half of the nineteenth century (specifically after the publications of Broca; Joynt, 1964) that aphasia was explored more systematically. Case reports by Wernicke (1874/1908) and contemporaries contained detailed descriptions of examination procedures for individual patients. Whereas some of these examinations were probably standard procedure in certain hospitals, others were invented on the spot to explore individual features of a specific syndrome of aphasia. Understandably, these reports focused on the patient's specific disorder rather than on the examination procedure.

The clinical examination as developed in the late nineteenth century has been modified and augmented, but remained the essential tool of the clinical neurologist throughout the twentieth century. Such examinations are exemplified in the writings of Hughlings Jackson (1915) and

Pick (1913). The standard repertoire of many clinical examinations still includes such routine procedures as the Paper Test of Pierre Marie (1883), the Hand-Eye-Ear Test of Henry Head (1926), and Geschwind's (1971) "no ifs, ands, or buts" repetition as simple tasks with high multiple demands on the patient's understanding, processing, and repeating abilities.

The clinical examination has a number of disadvantages, which gradually led to the development of formal screening tests and more generally applicable and standardized comprehensive assessment instruments. The earliest attempts to construct an objective aphasia battery, such as Rieger's test set published in 1888, did not catch on (Weisenburg and McBride, 1935). Subsequent attempts to produce a standardized aphasia examination were more successful, specifically one published by Head (1926), who insisted on a detailed "clinical protocol." Indeed, Weisenburg and McBride (1935) credited Head as "the first to direct general attention to the development of test methods exclusively for aphasia" (p. 2). Head's protocol was designed to be administered in a straightforward and replicable manner, with emphasis placed on a set of measures to be given in a specific sequence, that had enough trials to permit some consistency in allowing a valid deficit to be observed, and that followed a graduated level of difficulty within a task to allow the clinician a sense as to the severity of a failure to perform a specific task demand. Tasks included object and color naming, a clock test, repetition, reading, writing, and the Hand-Eye-Ear test noted before. Another examination published during that time period was by Froeschels et al. (1932).

The first comprehensive battery of psychological and educational achievement tests for the assessment of aphasia was used by Weisenburg and McBride (1935) in their 5-year study of 60 aphasic patients. Schuell et al. (1964) called this study a landmark because it was the first to use control subjects, to compare aphasic with nonaphasic brain-damaged subjects, and to use a standardized methodology. Noting the lack of tests constructed for specific use with adults, they borrowed a number of tests designed for use with children. Their battery included automatic word sequences, naming, word repetition, understanding spoken language (including Head's Hand-Eye-Ear Test), reading (using an early version of the Gates reading test), writing, sentence completion, analogies, opposites, digit and letter sequences, and sound recognition. Subtests from the Stanford-Binet test and the Stanford Academic Achievement test were used. Supplementary tests included a series of tests with less of a linguistic basis to them, such as formboards, digit-symbol substitution, drawing a chair from a model, and the Goodenough Draw-a-Man task. Speech clinicians in practice today would clearly recognize most of the task demands present in this effort from the early 1930s as not being dramatically different from subtests found on contemporary diagnostic batteries, such as the BDAE-3.

Several other batteries were developed in the 1950s by Wepman (1951, 1961), Eisenson (1954, 1993), and Schuell (1957), partly as a result of intensive treatment efforts with World War II veterans. Benton (1964) reviewed the development of assessment procedures and noted the work done in various centers, criticizing that none of these procedures had been published in "usable form" for others outside of the immediate locations of test authors and their proximate colleagues. The descriptions of procedures were insufficient, no standardization information was presented, and neither exact criteria for scoring nor detailed guides for interpretation were included. He compared the state of the art of aphasia testing with the "pre-Binet stage" in intelligence testing: "We are today where intelligence testing was in 1900" (p. 263). This comparison meant that clinicians and academics were without a generally agreed upon approach and a specific and shareable test instrument for assessing a phenomenon of notable interest and clinical concern.

Turning now to the history of psycholinguistic studies, both the open-ended free-speech and the experimental approach have been used extensively in aphasia research (Goodglass and Blumstein, 1973; Spreen, 1968). These studies represent experiments rather than attempts to assess the aphasic patient's deficit, and have been mentioned in the previous section. However, some of these studies have led to conclusions about the nature of the deficit in specific types of aphasia and perhaps can be translated into suitable methods of assessment. We briefly describe these studies and point out their potential application in the development of assessment techniques.

The first comprehensive studies of a psycholinguistic nature were conducted by Wepman and collaborators (Spiegel et al., 1965; Wepman et al., 1956; Wepman and Jones, 1964). Part of this work was based on stories told by 50 aphasic speakers on the Thematic Apperception Test (Morgan and Murray, 1943), a test requiring individuals to make up stories about each of a set of pictures. Various linguistic parameters were calculated, including grammatical form class usage, grammatical correctness, intelligibility, and word-finding problems (the latter three problems correspond to the syntactic, semantic, and pragmatic types of aphasia in Wepman's terminology). The studies involved subjecting collected data to complex calculations as well as to judgments by linguistically trained researchers; the results cannot be readily translated into more directly accessible forms of assessment.

The second major research program was conducted by Howes and collaborators (Howes, 1964, 1966, 1967; Howes and Geschwind, 1964) and involved the detailed analysis of conversational speech of 5000 words of each of more than 80 aphasic and nonaphasic speakers. The analyses concentrated on lexical diversity (i.e., the frequency of word usage in aphasic versus nonaphasic speakers) and also distinguished between "fluent" and "nonfluent" speakers (who were viewed as being similar to Wernicke's and anomic aphasics, and to Broca's aphasics, respectively). Benson (1967) developed a simplified and clinically useful rating scale system based on the information from Howes's study and included additional rating dimensions. The ratings used a three-point scale and involved rate of speaking, prosody, pronunciation, phrase length, effort, pauses, press of speech, perseveration, word choice, paraphasia, and verbal stereotypes. These 11 characteristics were related to brain scan localization. It was found that anterior lesions tended to produce speech with low verbal output, dysprosody, dysarthria, considerable effort, and predominant use of substantive nouns, whereas posterior lesions produced speech that was normal or near-normal on all these features but showed paraphasic errors, press of speech, and lack of substantive words.

A third study using a comprehensive analysis of conversational speech with a minimum of 1000 words from 50 aphasic and 50 normal speakers was conducted by Spreen and Wachal (1973; Wachal and Spreen, 1973) in a computer-scored interaction analysis of psycholinguistic aspects of spoken language. Crockett (1972, 1976) designed five-point rating scales for 17 characteristics of speech—including rate of speech, prosody, pronunciation, hesitation, false starts, phrase length, effort, pauses, press of speech, perseveration, word choice, paraphasia, communication, naming, grammar, use of interstitial connectives, understanding of spoken language, uses of inflection, tense or gender, and neologisms—in an attempt to translate psycholinguistic speech characteristics into basic rating scale dimensions. Interrater agreement among five judges was satisfactory after some training, and learning carefully worded descriptions of each characteristic.

Although Benson's (1967) and Crockett's (1972, 1976) ratings of psycholinguistic aspects of aphasic speech appeared to be quite successful within the limited scope of the research problems under investigation, further use of this approach has been limited. Three specific instruments that attempted to include these psycholinguistic applications are the BDAE and two analytical approaches. Several of the ratings were incorporated into the BDAE and its subsequent revisions. Shewan (1988) developed a system to describe and quantify aphasic subjects' connected language in describing pictures, using phonologic, semantic, and syntactic components as well as general parameters of output (e.g., number of utterances, time, length, articulation, repetition, paraphasias). The Shewan Spontaneous Language Analysis (SSLA) also received some psychometric support, indicating adequate intrajudge, interjudge, and test-retest reliability, and validity based on clinical judgment of severity of connected language impairment. L. Nicholas and Brookshire (1993, 1995) developed a Correct Information Unit (CIU) analysis of connected language. The CIU is a standardized, rule-based scoring system for which psychometric properties have been documented. However, Nicholas and Brookshire (1993) reported that the separation between aphasic and normal speakers was highly significant only for three of the calculated measures: words per minute, percentage CIU, and CIU per minute. Oelschlaeger and Thorn (1999) found that CIU measures, applied to naturally occurring conversations of aphasics could not be obtained reliably (with interrater reliability of 63% or less) owing to insufficiencies in the scoring rules and human error in the application of scoring rules.

Another detailed analysis of free conversational speech samples (Crockford and Lesser, 1994) stressed the analysis of editing elements (Schlenk et al., 1987) produced by the patient, amount and type of collaborative "repair" (Barnsley, 1987), and the proportion of conversational "load" (N. Miller, 1989) carried by the patient and the conversational partner, as well as the analysis of unfilled and filled pauses, unsolicited repetitions, phonemic approximations, circumlocutions, and neologisms. Crockford and Lesser (1994) found this type of analysis to be a more sensitive indicator of change or stability of language impairment as compared to rating scale schedules completed by relatives or an analysis of speech elicited by role playing (Amsterdam-Nijmegen Everyday Language Test, ANELT, Blomert, 1990; Blomert et al., 1987, 1994). Whitworth et al. (1997) developed the Conversation Analysis Profile for People with Aphasia (CAPPA; Singular Publishing; $125). In addition, Gerber and Gurland (1989) developed an Assessment Protocol of Pragmatic Linguistic Skills (APPLS), and Kay et al. (1992) published PALPA. Kerschensteiner et al. (1972) used a rating system for the study of conversational speech, and Voinescu et al. (1987) rated the communicative value of 27 stimuli in a standard interview to measure treatment progress.

These studies demonstrate clearly that the somewhat elusive aspects of speaking style can be translated into scales that are usable. Perhaps one reason for the infrequent use of such ratings has been that most have been developed in the context of relatively complex research rather than as part of the development of assessment tools. Another reason may be that psycholinguistic aspects of aphasic speech are rather complex in themselves and not readily understood without prior linguistic training; hence, the clinically oriented examiner tends to shy away from psycholinguistic evaluations and use relatively more concrete standard testing methods. Additionally, in looking at linguistic applications for understanding normal and abnormal language development in individuals, Carrow-Woolfolk (1988) noted that a limitation in clinical application is that it is not always clear whether assessment findings remain within the wide range of normal variability, rather than reflecting something of clinical importance. This may be less of a problem when the diagnosis of aphasia has clearly been made by other means, but, even then, use of a psycholinguistic assessment instrument still requires the speech clinician to remain cautious in assuming that poorer performances reflect truly defective changes in language. The SSLA, the PALPA, and the CIU, however, point toward first steps in offering systematic efforts to provide practical devices. Additionally, as will be discussed in a later chapter, a number of functional communication instruments and rating scales also attempt to at least be somewhat sensitive to often broadly defined pragmatic and psycholinguistic dimensions of communication. As Goodglass and Wingfield (1995) pointed out: "The enterprise of neurolinguistics is sufficiently vast that we cannot afford to reduce efforts that do not yet make contact with other disciplines. There is still much to be learned from examination of clinical-anatomic correlations using static lesion data, pre-cognitive-linguistic approaches, and animal models when appropriate" (p. 162).

3

Purposes of Assessment

It is important to consider the purpose for performing an examination when evaluating and choosing specific assessment instruments. Methods of assessment vary greatly, depending on the examiner's goal. Matching the examination to the patient and to the referral request requires a flexible and knowledgeable approach to assessment.

Six general types of evaluation purposes may be distinguished in aphasia assessment: (a) screening procedures; (b) diagnostic assessment; (c) descriptive testing in rehabilitation and counseling; (d) progress evaluation; (e) assessment of functional or pragmatic communication; and (f) assessment of related disorders. A balanced approach using any of the six types when appropriate is empirically and clinically sound but requires a commitment to thoughtful decision making by the practitioner. Though having explanatory value in introducing assessment instruments, these distinctions will often overlap and dissolve in daily practice, as clinicians pursue multiple goals to understand and manage language problems in individuals.

Screening Procedures

Screening refers to a brief and cursory examination to detect the presence of aphasia, often not exceeding 5 or 10 minutes. The procedure is best pursued when the clinician can identify in advance the implications of positive or negative results from the screening. Three types of screening procedures relevant to aphasia are (a) the bedside clinical examination; (b) screening tests per se; and (c) standardized tests limited to measuring a specific aspect of language functioning, but notably sensitive to the presence of aphasia.

The *bedside clinical examination* is a clinical evaluation in the tradition of classical neurology (e.g., Kirshner, 1995; Strub and Black, 1993). Historically, the bedside exam has been the primary method of assessing aphasia and it remains a standard tool for many attending physicians, neurologists, and speech clinicians. It permits a brief and practical evaluation of the language of inpatients during, for example, the acute stage of recovery from a stroke. The skilled clinician makes maximal use of communication with the patient to rule out aphasia, to establish a diagnosis, or to reach the decision that a more comprehensive diagnostic assessment is warranted. The breadth of these screens ranges from unstructured conversation with the patient to a structured set of items, such as pointing to a watch or listing the days of the week.

Screening tests, such as the one described for the Halstead-Reitan test battery (Reitan, 1991; Wheeler and Reitan, 1962) differ from bedside examinations in that they are usually constructed in some type of standardized fashion. They often reflect the once-popular application arising out of clinical psychology in the 1950s of screening for the presence of 'organicity' (a loose term referring to any form of damage to the nervous system affecting psychological functioning), particularly in high-risk groups and in conjunction with psychiatric evaluations. In relation to aphasia, some relatively brief and highly sensitive screening tests are available, but screening for the purpose of diagnosing 'organicity' has lost its attractiveness and usefulness since the 1950s. One reason is that the accuracy of screening devices is limited, usually around 80% (Spreen and Benton, 1965). Another reason is that in clinical practice such cursory 'detective work' is rarely necessary, since most patients are referred with an established clinical impression of aphasia from the bedside examination, a known organic etiology, and neuroradiological data. Finally, the information obtained from these tests offers poor specificity (i.e., there are many reasons why a nonaphasic patient might fail an aphasia screening test) and reveals little to indicate the severity of the detected aphasia. Thus, screening tests per se have been all but abandoned in favor of other approaches.

Finally, standardized *specific-function tests* may possess features that will allow their use for screening purposes. These tests are created and standardized in order to assess a specific facet of language in a detailed manner. Unlike a screening test, they usually include enough items to demonstrate a reasonable sampling of the behavior of interest and to do so with suitable levels of measured statistical reliability. Their use as aphasia screening devices derives from the understanding that they are measuring certain language problems that are highly sensitive to the presence of aphasia or—in broader fashion—nonaphasic language disorders that are due to impaired neurological functioning. They can easily be incorporated into a more comprehensive examination to "screen" (explore) the nature of language functioning to determine the need for additional testing. Additional testing may be required, because these very sensitive measures usually lack correspondingly high levels of specificity. The use of these types of tests for screening purposes has increased in areas of language assessment to search for or rule out "subtle," subclinical, or early-stage cognitive disorders (e.g., Crosson, 1996) and those that speech-language pathologists have come to refer to as "cognitive-communication impairments" (e.g., Myers, 1999). Such screening is also appropriate for disorders that are not traditionally associated with aphasia per se (i.e., the early stages of a neurodegenerative disease such as Alzheimer's disease, traumatic brain injury, or lesions of the nondominant hemisphere).

The Token Test (DeRenzi and Vignolo, 1962) has proven itself to be the most durable and broadly employed of these specific-function tests. Versions of the Boston Naming Test have also developed appeal as stand-alone screens for language, particularly in examining healthy elderly persons and individuals at higher-than-typical risk for degenerative brain diseases (e.g., Morris et al., 1989). Subtests of established aphasia batteries, such as the NCCEA Word Fluency (F-A-S) task and portions of the MAE, are also commonly employed in screening, particularly in the assessment of traumatic brain injury (e.g., Crosson, 1996).

Diagnostic Assessment

Diagnostic assessment refers to the thorough examination of a patient's language performance to arrive at both a diagnostic impression and a detailed description of areas of associated cognitive strengths and weaknesses. It is sometimes forgotten that comprehensive assessments of this type are also valuable for treatment purposes; for example, Kertesz (1988) likened treating an aphasic patient in the absence of diagnostic data as "trying to navigate an uncharted sea" (p. 316). Because of the comprehensive nature of this type of examination, it is suitable for patients who are medically stable in the later acute or postacute period of their recovery and for initial and follow-up evaluations of outpatients with subjective complaints of language and related problems. Diagnostic assessments tend to elicit samplings of performance in many different areas of cognitive function and may not necessarily be of immediate use to the speech clinician interested in a detailed exploration of a particular problem. When the evaluation is confined to performances on language and aphasia-related tasks, the diagnostic impression may either refer to the type and severity of aphasia or go beyond the description of the functional deficit and arrive at speculative conclusions about the nature and location of the underlying brain disorder. Impressions from a broader cognitive evaluation will include the type of aphasia as only one of a number of neurobehavioral syndromes, such as dementia, confusional states, amnestic syndrome, attentional disorder, and so forth, in order to determine the full spectrum of the patient's deficits (i.e., the process of differential diagnosis). In this manner, disorders that are related and that can co-occur with aphasia are usually explored within the context of the same examination. Broader diagnostic examinations allow the clinician to examine the impact of aphasia upon other aspects of cognitive functioning, such as attention and memorization, and to explore the impact of premorbid attributes (e.g., estimated intellectual functioning) upon test performances.

Aphasia test batteries are inevitable choices for clinicians looking for a comprehensive diagnostic instrument. There are a variety of these batteries available to clinicians. However, unless all subtests in a battery are required to score performance, clinicians pursuing a comprehensive assessment can usually pick and choose at the subtest level from many different tasks found in those comprehensive batteries. Some batteries, such as the third edition of the Boston Diagnostic Aphasia Examination (Goodglass et al., 2000), are structured so as to offer the clinician the choice of shorter or longer administration formats, in addition to a standard-length format.

For better or worse, diagnostic batteries reflect the particular school of thought of the test author. Most test authors advocate a particular package or battery of diagnostic tests that, in their view, will produce a comprehensive overview of significant aspects of language behavior in the aphasic patient. For this reason, becoming fully familiar with the theoretical position of test authors is imperative. J. Marshall (1986) pointed out that most aphasia batteries use classification schemes that rely on a Wernicke/Lichtheim model and that a large proportion of patients remain unclassified by such models. Marshall stated that in traditional taxonomic classification attempts with larger patient populations, only 59% (Benson, 1979a), 20% to 30% (Albert et al., 1981;

Prins et al., 1978), or 49% (Reinvang, 1985) could be placed into one of the traditional aphasic syndromes. It is important for the potential test user to understand what the diagnostic categories provided by any given test mean and whether they correspond sufficiently with the clinician's own conception of aphasia as applied in daily practice.

Descriptive Evaluation

For the direct purposes of rehabilitation and counseling, a descriptive assessment is usually the most sensible approach. A clinician may choose, when warranted, from a variety of assessment procedures, for example, subtests from a diagnostic battery, a functional communication scale, a number of rating and observational scales, and so on. Rehabilitation and counseling pose different questions than can be answered from a traditional diagnostic assessment. In particular, it is important to gain as much information as possible about areas of functional strength: what the person can do despite the presence of deficits. This allows better-reasoned advice on what treatment activities to pursue, what vocational options remain open to the patient, and the actual communication level at which the patient is interacting with others. As an example, the ability of patients to name objects in the evaluation setting is diagnostically relevant but far less important in one's everyday environment than the ability to communicate and to be understood. For these reasons, the assessment shifts from a strict testing situation to the observation of communication and nonverbal behaviors supporting the communicative interaction.

Descriptive assessment in the rehabilitation setting also involves (a) making predictions of recovery and of response to treatment; (b) measuring the ability to process, learn, and remember new material and, hence, to be able to actively participate in and benefit from individualized treatment programs; and (c) fine-tuning treatment tasks and tactics.

A bridging of test contexts is necessary in order to compare the relation between specific language deficits with the general ability to communicate. Though sometimes victim to the polemics of promoting one approach as better than another, this bridging can be a rich area of cross communication and cooperation between clinicians who are primarily diagnosticians and those who are primarily therapists.

Progress Evaluation

Progress evaluation is closely related to descriptive evaluation, but may serve several additional purposes. Progress evaluation permits an examination of spontaneous recovery when initial measures are repeated in follow-up fashion. Day-to-day or week-to-week progress can be charted in treatment settings when understanding the impact on intervention is considered to be an integral part of a plan of therapy. The clinician caring for the patient would like to be able to chart changes accurately over time rather than rely on subjective judgments or enthusiastic endorsements of the usefulness of therapy made by the patient or relatives. No formal tests have been developed specifically for this purpose, mainly because these assessments have to be tailor-made for each individual and her or his current level and range of deficit. In addition, criteria need to be established for what will qualify as significant progress, as this is likely to vary on a case-by-case basis depending on the patient's premorbid characteristics. Ad hoc assessments may be formulated for the entire domain of communicative functioning or for the modification of specific language behaviors.

Progress evaluation can also explore aspects of prognosis, as changes over time can be examined in terms of expectations about eventual outcome. The ability of patients to relearn or compensate for what they have lost can become a part of their progress evaluation. This evaluation is a neglected aspect of traditional aphasia assessment. Most tests merely measure the status quo but deliberately exclude any practicing or learning during the testing procedure. Providing cues to the patient during diagnostic evaluations is usually seen as contributing to measurement error, and hence should be avoided. If a test were to be designed to provide information on the relearning capacity of the patient, the approach would systematically include a variety of short learning trials with different kinds of cues in order to investigate whether the patient's language performance benefits, at least within the immediate testing situation. Obviously, the inclusion of such procedures in the assessment of aphasia would dramatically change the usual form of testing, affect test reliability, and, presumably, add to the length of the test. Yet it is our impression that the benefit of such tests will outweigh the additional problems of test construction and validation, and that such tests will be a major concern of test development in the future. Finally, changes over time can be employed to build up a set of data that explores the utility of interventions themselves as part of programwide evaluations (e.g., Frattali, 1998).

Functional and Pragmatic Assessment

Over the past 40 years, there has been a blossoming of rating scales and tests to explore the functional or pragmatic aspects of language, that is, how well one can communicate despite the presence of a language disorder. Over this time period, communicative assessment has coexisted alongside diagnostic aphasia batteries, and only recently have these descriptive scales reached equivalent levels of psychometric precision; also, diagnostic batteries have found room in their structure to include facets of functional communication. These functional methods vary from bedside observation, to rating scales, to formal tests (Manochiopinig et al., 1992). Some of these measures employ techniques that derive from psycholinguistic research, while others stem from traditional psychometric approaches to assessing behavior. Examples include the Pragmatic Protocol (Prutting and Kirchner, 1987, also reprinted in Ball et al., 1991), which uses a two-point scale; the Profile of Communicative Appropriateness (Penn, 1983, also reprinted in Ball et al., 1991), using a five-point scale; the Communication Activities of Daily Living, 2nd ed. (Holland et al., 1998), and the ASHA-FACS (Frattali et al., 1995).

Practical approaches sometimes go beyond the patients themselves to examine the effectiveness of communication in social settings, assessing patients and their family members or caregivers engaged in a communicative interaction (e.g., Florance, 1981; Holland, 1982).

Related Disorders

An examination of *articulation* is usually included in a full assessment of aphasia. However, articulation problems (dysarthria) are not necessarily part of the aphasic syndrome and are often caused by deficits of muscular control of the speech mechanism (phonation, respiration, resonance, articulation) due to damage to the central or the peripheral nervous system, or the cerebellum. Specific syndromes of flaccid, spastic, ataxic, hypokinetic, hyperkinetic (chorea, dystonia), and mixed (in amyotrophic lateral sclerosis and other disorders) speech have been identified. Since testing usually consists of repeating spoken or written test words, care should be taken that aphasic distortions, as they frequently occur in Wernicke's aphasia, not be mistaken as indications of dysarthria.

Aprosody of speech (lack of or inappropriate speech intonation) can be subdivided into affective (whether a spoken sentence is sad, happy, or angry) and nonaffective prosody (emphasis; whether the sentence is in the interrogative, declarative, or imperative form). E. Ross (1980), Heilman et al. (1984), and Grosjean and Hirt (1996) suggest that the latter is more affected by left hemisphere lesions, while affective prosody is more affected in patients with lesions of the right hemisphere. However, recent studies (e.g., Adolphs et al., 2001; S. Baum and Pell, 1997; Haveman, 1994; Pell, 1998) and a review (S. Baum and Pell, 1999) contradict this claim and suggest that patients with lesions in either hemisphere have difficulty in production and perception of affective speech prosody; in patients with left hemisphere lesions the nonaffective prosody is more often impaired, perhaps because of primary aphasic production and comprehension problems.

Apraxia of speech (Hall et al., 1993) is another articulatory disorder referring to the inability to program the position of the speech musculature and the sequencing of muscle movements for the volitional production of phonemes in the absence of significant weakness, slowness, or incoordination when used for automatic-reactive speech. The result is an effortful, groping speech output; phonemic omissions, substitutions, distortions, additions, and repetitions, both perseverative and anticipatory, are prominent, and are, in contrast to dysarthria, highly inconsistent, although they occur more often with initial rather than final sounds, and most frequently with fricatives, affricatives, and consonant clusters. Apraxia of speech may be due to lesions in parts of the left posterior frontal motor strip or due to lesions disconnecting this area to other parts of the brain. Prosodic changes may be associated with articulatory problems or perhaps in compensation for it. *Oral* (buccofacial) *apraxia* (execution of sequential movements with the mouth) and *limb apraxia* are often, but not always, observed with apraxia of speech.

Gestural communication is a significant contributor to the understanding of language (G. Beatty and Shovelton, 1999; reviews by Goldin-Meadow, 1999; Morford, 1996), dating back to ancient literature (Grieve and Campbell, 1999), and includes indicative (pointing, shrugging, nodding, head-shaking, indicating amount by numbers of fingers), representative (describing an activity or object by hand gestures, pantomime, for example, saw, axe, camera), and expressive-emblematic ("symbolic") signs; the latter are actual signals (e.g., raising the hand in greeting) that are generally understood within one cultural group, but not necessarily in others (e.g., in Italy, three short jabs with the edge of the hand in the stomach region indicates "I am hungry"). In addition, iconic gestures (creative gestures for which an existing gesture is not available) have been studied (Caldognetto and Poggi, 1995). Gestural communication is frequently impaired in aphasia ("asemesia"). Ducarne de Ribaucourt et al. (1982) reported that patients with Broca's aphasia can frequently use such signs, whereas patients with Wernicke's aphasia do not, but other authors report contradictory results (Peterson and Kirshner, 1981), and Benton et al. (1994b) report that 30% of 105 aphasic patients had near-perfect scores and an additional 30% performed within the normal range on a pantomime recognition test with most of the errors indicating semantically similar choices. Varney (1978) and Seron et al. (1979) found a close association between reading comprehension and pantomime recognition. Gestural communication may also be disturbed in aphasics because of cognitive or apraxic deficits (Borod et al., 1989; Caldognetto and Poggi, 1995; Moly, 1998) as well as in Alzheimer's disease (Glosser et al., 1998), and in autism (Buffington et al., 1998).

Gestural communication and both American Indian Gestural Code (Amerind) and American Sign Language (ASL) have been used in treatment, although success varied greatly from patient to patient (Feyereisen et al., 1988; Peterson and Kirshner, 1981). Even severe, global aphasics have been reported to acquire simple forms of gestural communication (H. Gardner et al., 1976). Drawing has also found limited use as an alternative to verbal communication and as a means to improve language skills in aphasic patients (Lyon and Helm-Estabrooks, 1987).

Certain language functions are likely to show severe deficits if the patient experiences loss or distortion of *visual perception, stereognosis, or hearing*. Patients are not likely to produce valid responses on tactile naming, for example, if impairment of motor functions or astereognosis is present. Similarly, unilateral visual neglect and hemi-inattention frequently occur in the contralateral visual field after unilateral cerebrovascular accident (CVA) and tends to interfere with reading as well as with responding to complex picture material in naming, visual multiple-choice, and similar tasks (Heilman et al., 1993; Lecours et al., 1987). A simple screening for neglect can be performed with a line-bisection task in which the patient is asked to mark the center of a horizontal line drawn on a sheet of paper. Patients with hemispatial neglect or inattention tend to place the bisection mark off-center favoring the non-impaired side of the visual field and neglect the impaired one. Similarly, when asked to cancel certain letters on a page, they tend to neglect those on the impaired side of vision. Screening for hearing loss should be carried out at 25 db at several frequencies. If the patient fails this screening, a full audiological evaluation is indicated.

Other deficits such as *finger agnosia* and *right–left disorientation* may frequently be found in aphasic patients. These disorders require specific assessment (e.g., with tests by Benton et. al., 1994) and may also affect the results of standard aphasia assessment. Finger agnosia, right–left disorientation, acalculia, and agraphia have been proposed to form a specific syndrome, the Gerstmann syndrome (Gerstmann, 1930), related to left parietal lobe lesions, although the existence of such a syndrome has been debated by Benton (1961). In children, a developmental Gerstmann syndrome has been described (Schwartz et al., 1981) that does not necessarily implicate left hemisphere dysfunction.

Disturbances of reading and writing often mirror the receptive and expressive problems of the aphasic patient. *Alexia*, the inability to read due to brain damage, and *agraphia*, the acquired inability to write, are related disorders that frequently accompany aphasia, and in some cases mirror the aphasic deficit (i.e., in reading and writing similar errors occur as in aphasia itself). However, LaBarge et al. (1992) did not find a strong relationship between agraphic errors and clinicians' assessment of aphasia on psychometric tests of language ability when testing healthy elderly and dementing patients. Both alexia and agraphia must be distinguished from *dyslexia*, the inability to read or write due to congenital causes, and from *illiteracy* due to lack of exposure to written material or schooling. Tests for reading and writing are included in many aphasia batteries, and numerous specific tests have been designed for learning-disabled children and adults. *Acalculia*, the inability to perform arithmetic operations, also requires special attention.

Comprehension may be impaired by *attentional losses* as well as by language deficits. Some authors of aphasia tests have built in supplementary tests for related functions, which are automatically administered if the patient fails on specific language tasks; in other tests, the clinician must ascertain the basic abilities of the patient without such guidance (requiring considerable training and experience). In multidisciplinary settings, clinical neuropsychologists provide comprehensive evaluations of cognitive status (Lezak, 1995; Spreen and Strauss, 1998) that may be interpreted in conjunction with results from aphasia tests. Regardless of the employed route, the description of the aphasic deficit will be more clearly understood if the examination is not restricted to features of linguistic performance, and if ancillary and pragmatic communication deficits are formally considered (e.g., Benton, 1982). The neuropsychological evaluation can also be employed to explore the presence of acquired deficits in new learning and memorization, and to appreciate the residual learning capacity of aphasic patients, features of considerable importance in treatment planning and community reentry.

4

Construction Principles of Aphasia Tests

Test instruments are essentially refinements and extensions of traditional clinical observation. For language and other aspects of cognition, tests and clinical observation explore the same areas of functioning and, by consequence, of disorder. The distinctions between tests and clinical observation lie in the quantification that is inherent to a test instrument and in the opportunity to compare these quantitative scores with reference norms for the instrument. Hence, a test could be considered to be a structured clinical observation that meets a number of additional psychometric requirements. Meeting these structural requirements increases the value of the test for the clinician, not the least of which is that it allows subtler distinctions between normal and defective performances to become measurable.

The following section describes the psychometric requirements that well-constructed tests need to meet and what potential test users will want to evaluate for any test they consider using. It should be stated beforehand, however, that few tests in aphasia assessment fully meet the stringent psychometric requirements recommended by psychometric specialists and by associations concerned with the standards of testing (American Psychological Association, 1985). A primary reason for this is that most tests in the field of aphasia have been developed in individual clinics in the context of ongoing clinical services and are not generally adopted by a large number of facilities and institutions. The collection of norms and the conduct of validity and reliability studies proceed slowly and are almost entirely dependent on the resources of test authors and their collaborators. The demand for such tests remains small as compared, for example, to tests of general intelligence and academic achievement. In other words, test development is demanding in terms of both time and money. Aphasia tests are not bestsellers; as a result, psychometric development has been less than optimal in many instances and neglected in others.

General Requirements for Tests

The most frequently stated requirements for tests of any kind are demonstrated standardization, reliability, and validity (Anastasi and Urbina, 1996; Gregory, 2000).

Standardization

Standardization is an arduous undertaking. Pilot studies and field studies are required to refine a test instrument and present it in published form. This process involves creating the structure of the test, how it is to be administered and scored, and the demonstration of its reliability and validity.

Standardization refers first to test structure and administration. A standardized test is one that remains uniform in its important parameters from patient to patient, and from one examiner to another. These parameters include aspects such as the face-to-face nature of presenting the stimuli, the suggested ambient environment, and the instructions for completing the tasks that compose the test. Rules as to how the test is to be given are explicitly described in a standardized instrument. If test administration and the conditions under which the test is performed are kept as constant as possible, measurement error can be kept to a minimum.

Minor variations in the use of a test are inevitable and must be accepted as practical and, probably, trivial. Whether an examiner wears blue-colored clothes or a white hospital coat would be essentially irrelevant to most test standardization rules. Deciding not to use the required time limit for a task in order to place a phone call while the patient is completing the task, though, would be a relevant deviation. Other deviations may be due to simple human-factors errors (e.g., Proctor and van Zandt, 1994), such as variability in orally presented stimuli by the test administrator or the use of a poorly designed scoring sheet. Many deviations are not due to poor decision making by the clinician or poor test design but are those that possess potential clinical value, such as allowing a patient to continue performing a task beyond the time limits imposed by the test in order to obtain information perhaps more useful for treatment than the fact that the task could not be completed in time. Regardless of such reasons, any notable deviation from a standard administration procedure will inevitably produce more variability in test scores and, hence, undesirable variance when the scores of patients or groups of patients are compared.

Three common areas where standardized procedures are important are when scoring requires judgment, how repetition may be used, and limit testing beyond task failures. A critical need for standardization exists for those tests (or components of tests) where scoring requires a certain amount of judgment on the part of the test administrator. For example, if the patient is asked to describe the use of a hairbrush, the response "for hair" may be judged to be unsatisfactory by one scorer and satisfactory by another. Another common instance occurs when the person provides an incorrect response but continues responding and ends up providing the correct response; one test administrator might end the trial upon the initial answer and move onto the next trial, while another might allow the patient to continue responding. In practice, interscorer differences in dealing with these types of situations can be reduced to a minimum if the test manual contains sufficient scoring instructions and examples of how a given response should be scored. The test manual for the CADL-2 (Holland et al., 1999) offers a lucid example as to how scorers can be given guidance for judgment-based scoring in order to promote consistent adherence to standardization.

Whether a test administrator is permitted to repeat instructions or re-present stimuli to a patient needs to be explicitly addressed by the test manual. Neither is inherently more correct than the other. Yet test norms created under conditions where repetition is permitted may differ from ones where it is not permitted. A final problematic area occurs as the clinician may often be tempted to use the test material to explore how much a patient may improve as a result of simple aids and cues. However valuable, it should be understood that test results achieved under such modified conditions are usually no longer comparable to the published norms; that is, they contain an undesirable degree of measurement error. Exploration of the impact of aids and cues on a nonstandard, ad hoc basis has often been referred to as "testing the limits," and is frequently used for descriptive rather than diagnostic purposes. Some manuals offer suggestions as to how to test limits, but will at the same time remind the user not to compare the obtained performances with the normative data.

Standardization also refers to the establishment of normative data against which the performance of an individual can be compared. A good test manual will offer a description of all relevant features of the standardization sample. The sample used to create normative data should be representative of the population for which the test is intended. In major test instruments, such as measures of intelligence and academic achievement, the normative sample includes several thousand individuals stratified according to national census information as representative as possible of the general population. The large majority of language tests are unable to meet such lofty goals. This limitation requires that the prospective test user review the standardization sample with thoroughness and care. For aphasia tests, the description of the standardization sample may include or fail to include information about *(a)* the age range of the sample; *(b)* whether the sample is limited to patients with cerebrovascular disease or includes a proportion of individuals who, for example, sustained traumatic brain injury; *(c)* whether the sample includes patients who learned English as a second language; and *(d)* whether the sample includes people at the extremes of educational achievement (e.g., high school dropouts, professional degrees).

For example, the CADL-2 test manual reports that the standardization sample comprised 175 adults with "neurogenically based communication disorders." Demographic information for the sample (i.e., race, ethnicity, gender, urban–rural residence, and geographic region) is included and compared to 1997 U.S. census data. All individuals spoke English as their primary language. The authors include sample data about medical diagnosis, level of care, hemispheric localization, and a mild-moderate-severe global rating of communication disorder based upon clinical observation. If, however, a potential test user felt that knowing the educational range for the CADL-2 sample was important in deciding whether to use the test, this information is not reported in the CADL-2 manual.

Another example is the Amsterdam-Nijmegen Everyday Language Test (ANELT), a measure of functional communication. This test has yet to publish English normative data to correspond to available Dutch and German standardization samples. Yet detailed information about the test and its standardization is available for review in the English-language literature (Blomert et al., 1994). The published information includes demographic information about the standardization sample, as well as a breakdown of the sample into traditional aphasia subtypes (based on the Aachen Aphasia Test) and information that aphasia-causing etiologies were limited to left hemispheric cerebrovascular etiologies. As an example of how even the best intentions may result in some inconsistency, Blomert et al.'s paper reported that this sample, limited to cerebrovascular etiologies, included several patients with traumatic brain trauma and tumors.

A potential test user serving a population of aphasics for whom English is not the primary language or someone who wants to use a test that offers separate norms for individuals with either fluent or nonfluent types of aphasia would be aware of the limitations of the CADL-2, based upon what is reported in the manual. A potential test user receiving the referral of a native Dutch-speaking immigrant who has sustained a left hemisphere stroke would, in turn, be aware of the benefits of the ANELT, based upon what is reported in the literature. If a test manual or related publication is not helpful in answering the questions that a potential test user might have, the test authors can be contacted directly for additional information.

Norms represent the set of scores obtained from the standardization sample, also known as the reference group. These data are often expressed in percentile ranks or in relation to a normal distribution score in terms of z-scores, t-scores, and so forth. Converted scores like these will indicate a patient's score in relation to the distribution of scores. For example, a score at the 90th percentile indicates a performance better than that of 90% of the reference population. If the test is constructed for a variety of populations, standardization needs to reflect this diversity. For example, if scores tend to vary greatly with age, sex, or educational level, separate norms have to be established. Often, additional norms can be avoided by using correction scores for these factors, but this may be impractical if more than two of these factors interact with each other.

Norms for speech/language pathology tests usually reflect the performance of a sample of healthy men and women without neurological impairment or aphasia, which allows the examiner to see where a given client's performance lies in the distribution of scores. Clinically, the examiner can determine whether a patient's performance is within normal limits, represents a borderline performance, or is defective (e.g., a performance less than the 1st or 5th percentile). Norms developed for neurologically intact individuals may not be sufficient for the evaluation of the aphasic patient; this issue is discussed later in the context of specific requirements for tests of aphasia.

Over time, a successful test instrument may be the source for additional normative studies by the original authors or others. It is an accepted psychometric phenomenon that norms "age" and their representativeness can "shift" or deteriorate over time (e.g., Strauss et al., 2000). While the presence of refined, updated, or expanded norms is generally welcome, an abundance of normative information can result in some confusion when a test score can mean one thing in one sample, but something else in another. Mitrushina et al. (1999) explored this issue for a number of psychological instruments, including the Boston Naming Test and measures of word fluency. In their review of the psychometric properties of popular aphasia tests, Jackson and Tompkins (1991) made the useful recommendation that test publishers add update sheets for the tests they sell to inform test purchasers about the results of psychometric studies performed after the publication date of tests.

Reliability

Reliability refers to the consistency, stability, and accuracy of a test's scores (Anastasi and Urbani, 1996). Three types of reliability are relevant for aphasia tests: the internal consistency of the test, test-retest stability, and the interrater reliability of the test when administered and scored by different examiners. Internal consistency can be demonstrated by giving an alternate form of the test during the same or at a subsequent session or by subdividing the items within a single form of a test. Test-retest reliability can be demonstrated on repeat administration after a reasonable time interval and under the same conditions. One method to assess interrater reliability is to give the test records to two or more independent scorers and compute a correlation between scorers. This type of reliability is highly desirable, since poor interrater reliability will obviously not only affect the general reliability of the test but also introduce measurement error into studies of validity and other psychometric properties.

Reliability statistics are correlation coefficients, denoted as a single number between -1.00 and $+1.00$ with 0 indicating no relationship. The closer to 1.00 a test's measure of reliability is, the better (e.g., Gregory, 2000). Many published aphasia tests are able to attain reliabilities above .80, at times above .90. The standard error of estimate (SEM) can also be employed to look at test reliability, especially when examining stability over time.

Generally, reliability is best demonstrated with normal, healthy subjects, since the measurement error in patient populations and the likelihood of change in performance due to changes in the patient's condition are high. Patient groups employed to assess reliability of aphasia tests typically comprised individuals who have recovered for a long enough period from the aphasia-causing event that their condition is stable and any deficits are of the type that are considered chronic or residual in nature.

Validity

Validity refers to the demonstration that a test actually measures what it claims to measure, and that inferences made about performance on that test are appropriate. It is probably the most crucial requirement of any test. Validity can be measured in a variety of ways; usually, a distinction is made between criterion (predictive or concurrent), construct, and content validity.

Of the three forms of validity, the demonstration that a test is a valid *criterion* of whether the patient is aphasic is the most popular, but of limited value in several ways. The demonstration of criterion validity relies entirely on the fact that the aphasic patient's performance can be discriminated from that of normal subjects on the basis of test results; in other words, the demonstration of validity comes close to the screening problem described earlier. Such a demonstration relies on the clinical judgment made for the aphasic group but neglects the fact that the discrimination between aphasics and normals could result from entirely irrelevant (for aphasia) or trivial test items. In the ideal case, other contrast groups in addition to healthy, normal subjects or brain-damaged patients without aphasia should be used. The question of validity for predicting membership in a specific subgroup of aphasics, for example, Broca's aphasia, is addressed later.

Construct validity is often demonstrated by investigating the correlation of a new test with another test of known validity. Since few tests in the field of aphasia have known validity, another form of validity examination—the demonstration of factorial construct validity—is frequently used. Factor-analytic statistical techniques are used to show whether the tests in a given battery all contribute to one or more major factors of common variance that represent language functions.

Content validity refers to the adequacy of sampling from the domain of behaviors to be measured. In the case of testing for aphasia, for example, it is generally agreed that measuring word fluency alone would not be sufficient, because it does not appear to sample the whole range of language behavior. In other words, test items should be based on sound reasoning, and should not be trivial or selectively biased. The content should also agree with the content areas as defined by other researchers. The range and diversity of the content of a test can also be explored by factor analysis.

A detailed example of how validity (as well as reliability and standardization) is assessed for a contemporary test instrument can be found by reviewing the documentation presented in the administration manual for the ASHA-FACS (Frattali et al., 1995).

Specific Requirements for Tests with Brain-Damaged and Aphasic Patients

In addition to the general requirements for the construction of tests, several specific issues exist in the design of tests for use with brain-damaged patients and specifically for those with aphasia. These issues arise in terms of the range of item difficulty, the need to clarify the nature of specific deficits revealed by the tests, the overlap of examinations for aphasia with measures of intelligence, and the usefulness of a test in conjunction with recovery and therapy.

Range of item difficulty

Range of item difficulty is usually determined by selecting from a range of "very easy" to "very difficult" items. In a well-constructed test, items should be homogeneously distributed; that is, the difficulty range (expressed in percentage of subjects passing each item) should rise in linear fashion from the first to the last item. The principle of homogeneity of item distribution is relatively easy to follow if we are dealing with a test for a normal population that is reasonably well defined (e.g., a stratified sample of U.S. school children, based upon census data). The principle can also be followed fairly well for a language test constructed to test normal adults. However, if aphasics were given such a language test, most items would be too difficult for a majority of the patients. As a result, most aphasics would have scores in the bottom range of the distribution (i.e., a "floor effect"). Consequently, aphasia tests must shift the difficulty of item distribution toward the lower, or "easy" end to make it possible to discriminate between mild, moderate, and severe levels of aphasia, and to determine aphasic subtypes. In other words, the range of item difficulty will have to be determined by the target population of aphasics, not by the general, healthy population. This shift inevitably produces a "ceiling effect" if the test is then applied to normal subjects, because they would likely score at or near the 100% correct range. Truncated ranges represented by floor and ceiling effects may have an impact on reducing the measured reliability for a test. It is, of course, possible to include items that are easy enough to discriminate between different degrees of aphasia as well as items difficult enough for a normal population. Such a test, however, runs the risk of being too lengthy and perhaps impractical. For a test to be adequate in discriminating between aphasics of different degrees, the notion that the test would also be useful in normally functioning populations often has to be abandoned.

In situations where more than a single test is available to measure a specific aspect of language, it is prudent to explore beforehand how the set of tests vary in terms of their difficulty. This information will help a clinician determine the best choice of test instrument to match the individual patient.

Clarification of defects

Clarification of defects observed on testing is necessary in many cases. For example, if the patient cannot provide the name of an object, we cannot automatically ascribe this failure to an aphasic disorder. The presence of any sensorimotor limitations is important to examine in order to clarify the test performance. Other related disorders are discussed in Chapter 3.

Obviously, hearing defects may affect the results on tests of verbal comprehension. Divenyi and Robinson (1989) used a number of psychophysiological measures and found that deficits in all pitch-related measures were related to marked deficits in the performance on BDAE, PICA, and Token Test for nonaphasic patients with right hemisphere lesions. Likewise, a patient might have difficulty recognizing visually presented objects, given defective acuity or other visual problems (Kempen et al., 1994). If a patient cannot name an object placed in his or her hand, it is possible that sensory loss, inadequate motoric ability to handle the object, or inadequate stereognostic recognition is responsible (Benton, 1967). Task demands that require verbal responses may be made more difficult by independent problems with the vocal apparatus, and those that require pointing or writing may be affected by independent defects in fine and gross motor control.

As discussed in more detail later, there are additional higher-order problems that may need to be addressed before a defective performance can be attributed with clarity to aphasia. These problems are cognitive, psychological, and neuropsychological in nature and include the presence of acute confusion, depression, and dementia (see Chapter 13).

In a clinical examination, alternative sensorimotor explanations are frequently obvious and quickly excluded by appropriate informal observations or specific tests. Neurobehavioral explanations may be less obvious and require formal testing. It is important, however, to systematically rule out these associated deficits, since the test profile produced at the end of standardized testing with many standard batteries may easily be misinterpreted if used in a "blind evaluation" or by an inexperienced examiner. Some aphasia batteries include supplementary tests for associated deficits, and clear rules have been developed as to when supplementary tests should be used. Such supplementary tests should also follow standard psychometric principles if they are to be used routinely. The inclusion of supplementary tests (see, e.g., Benton, 1967; 1969) may expand the field of examination far beyond the area of aphasia. A comprehensive neuropsychological evaluation may be necessary to provide such a broad-based examination of the aphasic patient.

Overlap with intelligence tests

The overlap of assessment of aphasia with measures of intelligence, such as the Wechsler Adult Intelligence Scale (WAIS-III), has often gone unnoticed. It deserves special consideration in the context of item selection and in the context of our discussion of other defects found in association with aphasia (see also Chapter 13).

It should be stressed that the demands on the general intellectual abilities of the patient should be kept to a minimum in the examination of aphasia. In addition, previously acquired knowledge of specific concepts and terms should influence the assessment of aphasia as little as possible.

The problem does not usually arise with the "easy" items used in aphasia tests. But when items for the "difficult" level are constructed, the separation of what is strictly language from what is intelligence becomes blurred. For example, naming tasks can be advanced to any level of difficulty by adding rare words and concepts that are likely to be found only in the vocabulary of the college-educated person of above-average intelligence. Language tasks that require definitions, for example, invariably tend to place higher value on abstract, elegant wording and penalize the less educated person of average or below-average intelligence. Tasks requiring oral arithmetic reasoning or the finding of superordinate concepts or similarities are, in fact, part of standard intelligence tests currently in use. For this reason, aphasia tests must be carefully scrutinized for content that exceeds the basic examination of language abilities. If such content cannot be avoided because of the range of item difficulty, the test must contain separate norms for patients of different ranges of intellectual and educational background or must apply adequate corrections for such factors.

Use in measuring recovery

Aphasia tests are usually performed in the broader clinical context of recovery and therapy and, as a result, pose two concerns. The first issue is essentially an additional validity problem, that is, whether the test is suitable for the measurement of change over time. Tests adequate for the measurement of recovery may be slightly different in content from tests that indicate the type or severity of aphasia, and may require more items in certain difficulty ranges to allow measurement of small steps in recovery. Tests that are structured to allow an assessment of change over time may present equivalent versions of tasks, so that the same stimuli are not presented a second time. This type of structure allows for baseline and follow-up comparisons. The MAE is an example of a test structured to meet the demands of this use, as is the Dutch- and German-language ANELT.

The second issue reflects the related questions of the ability of the test to predict recovery or predict response to therapy, which must be established independently or in addition to other validation procedures. Interpretation may be complicated if changes over time merely reflect the patient's learning of the test ("practice effect") or remembrance of it, rather than actually indicating any underlying recovery. A prospective test user would want to see evidence in a test's documentation as to whether these potentially confounding factors have been explored by the test authors and examine the literature to see if this exploration has been confirmed independently by other clinical researchers. One source of this information is the mean and standard deviation data obtained during test-retest reliability examination, if available.

II

CONTEMPORARY TESTS AND METHODS

5

Clinical Bedside Examination

The bedside examination evolved from the historical foundation of aphasia assessment as the primary method for the practicing clinician and as the basis from which formal and standardized tests developed. It remains a standard tool, especially for the neurologist, although speech/language pathologists or neuropsychologists may be called upon to provide a brief examination of the patient in primary care or in a nonambulatory condition.

Bedside testing of language is most commonly part of the mental status examination—a broader (but still brief) look at cognitive functioning that typically includes orientation, attention, memory, praxis, visuoperception, and abstract reasoning, along with language (Kirshner, 1986; Strub and Black, 1993). This has always been the case in neurology, but bedside examination is more of a concern now that medical treatments within the first several hours after the onset of nonhemorrhagic stroke increasingly make clinical assessment of mental status a part of emergency care, not limited to times when the patient is medically stabilized or in transition from medical to rehabilitative care.

Kirshner (1986) provided the succinct purpose for bedside questioning: "the most important point about the mental status exam is the necessity of performing it" (p. 3). Aspects of cognition (including language) might appear normal until the patient is challenged in some way (e.g., asked to name an object or respond to a multistep command). Additionally, cognitive deficits may be masked by general observations and conclusions made at bedside (e.g., "the patient appears alert and oriented"), unless specific clinical attention is paid to them.

The primary goal of the bedside testing of language function is simply to determine whether the patient is aphasic (Kirshner, 1995). The advantage of the clinical examination lies in its flexibility, brevity, and suitability for even severely physically impaired patients, because the examiner can conduct a cursory examination at the bedside, quickly skipping across areas of strength where there is no obvious impairment. Its ad hoc nature is consonant with the busy schedule of clinicians, mentally accompanying them from patient to patient, with only the need for a few simple props usually found in one's pockets or on the patient's bedside table. As G. Davis (1993) suggested, all that the clinician really needs is a concept of what should be assessed and a few common objects. Bedside testing furnishes clinicians with a method of examination that they can individually tailor to their own decision-making and hypothesis-generating mental skills and provides a mechanism for clinicians to organize the next steps in patient care: who will need more extensive examinations and specialist consultations, treatment planning and initiation, prognostic explorations, and the early steps in educating the patient's significant others who have a need to understand their loved one's condition.

The three most important limitations of clinical examinations are *(1)* they tend to vary from one place to another, both in content and in the way in which they are administered; *(2)* what is considered abnormal remains up to the subjective judgment of the clinician; and *(3)* they are difficult to replicate and compare. The utility of the bedside examination in the hands of a skilled, experienced clinician is eroded when attempted by less skilled clinicians. The consequences of decisions made as a result of the bedside examination rely upon the individual skills and training of the clinician performing it: poor skills and limited training will result in errors and these errors will lead to misdiagnoses and incorrect treatment choices. An overreliance upon ad hoc testing may lead even the experienced clinician into a "black-and-white" approach to diagnosis, without due attention to the gray areas between the extremes. R. Brookshire (1997) noted the commonly accepted limitations that derive from unsystematic bedside testing, such as being apt to miss less overt deficits and not accurately allowing for comparisons across patients or the performance of the same patient at different times. In her reevaluation of the Short Examination for Aphasia, Schuell (1966) carefully debated the merits of the clinical examination in comparison to the comprehensive test. She stressed that only a comprehensive test can assess all aspects of "aphasia, [which] deals with one of the most complex and perhaps the only unique function of the human brain" (p. 138).

Numerous versions of the bedside language examination have been recorded; we note three of them. First, Strub and Black (1993) describe an approach within their context of the broader mental status examination in neurology. Second, the core of aphasiologists from the Boston school provide a number of descriptions of a simple six-part bedside language examination (e.g., Albert et al., 1981; Benson and Ardila, 1996; Benson and Geschwind, 1982). Finally, R. Brookshire (1997) offers a formal, though nonstandardized, 10-to-20-minute bedside language protocol. Other examples can be found in the literature, such as those in the general neurological examination (Poeck, 1974; Weintraub and Mesulam, 1985), individual case descriptions (e.g., Geschwind and Kaplan, 1962), and Luria's (1966) detailed description of his clinical examination.

Clinical bedside exploration of aphasia commonly includes:

1. Spontaneous, conversational speech. The clinician listens to and interacts with the patient either during history taking or specifically to assess speech output. For example, "Tell me why you are in the hospital" can provide useful information on both fronts. "What did you eat for breakfast (lunch) today?" is a reasonably good starting point, when a more neutral question is desired. Noting the fluency of output, effort, articulation, phrase length, dysprosody, paraphasic errors, and tendency to omit words will help determine the presence of aphasic problems.

2. Repetition. Items here will usually begin with the repetition of single digits and build up to the repetition of multisyllabic words, sentences, and verbal sequences.

3. Comprehension of spoken language. The clinician will attempt to determine whether the patient's ability to understand language is defective to a nature and degree that would suggest aphasia. If speaking is impaired, it may be necessary to restrict the examination to questions that can be answered with "yes" or "no" responses or by having the patient point.

4. Word finding. Usually, the patient will be asked for the names of common objects on the clinician's person (e.g., watch, pen) or in the patient's room (e.g., chair, telephone). Naming of object parts can occur along with naming general objects, especially as this may elicit problems in persons with milder disorders (e.g., Albert et al., 1981). This can be attempted first without and then with prompting. Frequently, the initial phoneme is offered as a cue, or an open-ended statement is provided to allow the word to be produced in an appropriate embedding or context.

5. Reading, usually from a newspaper or magazine or any item found in the patient's room (e.g., lunch menu). Unless the clinician car-

ries reading material for routine use, this facet of the exam will show the most variability from patient to patient and from day to day.

6. Writing, starting with the patient's own name, and proceeding to dictated words or sentences (e.g., "Spell 'doctor'") and spontaneous writing (e.g., "Describe your job").

Strub and Black. The language portion of Strub and Black's (1993) approach to mental status testing takes a slightly different approach than the six areas noted above and described in the two approaches that follow. While noting the importance of examining spontaneous speech, comprehension, repetition, and naming, Strub and Black consider writing and reading to be somewhat redundant or supplementary if the patient appears aphasic; testing these two areas takes on more meaning only if the patient does not appear to be aphasic. They consider the use of one of the 60-second word-generating tests for assessing controlled verbal fluency (e.g., "Name as many words that you can think of that begin with F"; see Chapter 7) as part of exploring spontaneous speech. They recommend that naming be assessed using the four categories of colors, body parts, clothing and room objects, and object parts; the interested clinician only need to assure him or herself that colored objects are available, as the rest of the objects are commonly on them or in the patient's room. The colored tokens from the Token Test or table-game pieces would suffice.

Benson and the Boston School. Benson and Ardila (1996) find what they term the "simple bedside examination" to be flexible and informative and useful for quick diagnostic impressions, though not suitable for planning a rehabilitation program or for clinical research purposes. They examine the six basic domains reported above: expressive language in spontaneous or conversational verbalizations, repetition of spoken language (usually judged on a simple pass–fail basis), comprehension of spoken language, naming, reading, and writing. They report that comprehension of spoken language is usually the most problematic part of the bedside examination, particularly when motor problems are present. The authors warn that bedside testing by inexperienced clinicians can be misleading and that, even when performed by experienced clinicians, results can be interpreted in an inconsistent manner. Albert and colleagues (1981) note that when listening to the patient's repetitions, the clinician should look for the same production features that can be further explored during the patient's spontaneous and conversational speech.

Brookshire. R. Brookshire (1997) offers an intermediate version of bedside screening that is more extensive than language testing in its mental status context, but without becoming a standardized and normed screening test. His version of a bedside measure retains some degree of flexibility but does attempt to offer a more formalized approach.

The dimensions examined include the six described above. In addition, Brookshire's protocol examines orientation and memory, a distinction between auditory and reading comprehension providing for both to be examined, the inclusion of automatized sequences (e.g., days of the week), and specific rating scales for spontaneous speech. The protocol relies on pictures that the clinician needs to find (e.g., cut out from magazines) and carry along; as a result, the increase in consistency carries with it a decrease in ad hoc flexibility.

In general, clinicians might want to assure themselves that they can perform a valid ad hoc testing of the patient's language at the bedside, spontaneously and just using the bulk of the material from what might be readily available in a typical patient's hospital room (keeping in mind that some patients might be assessed in the ER or the ICU). Maintaining this mental skill and anticipating the range of performances that would encompass normal (negative) and abnormal (positive) responses can be considered part of the routine repertoire of the clinician, even one whose primary practice relies upon comprehensive and standardized testing instruments.

6

Screening Tests

Screening in aphasia assessment can be performed in two ways: the use of tests designed for screening, which is discussed in this chapter, and the use of tests of specific language functions that are accepted as being sensitive to the presence of aphasia and therefore also can be used for screening (discussed in the next chapter). Aphasia screening tests are intended to quickly explore the presence or absence of the disorder. They do not claim to provide a detailed description of the aphasic disorder (or of any single language skill) but are designed to check for and focus the direction on the problem if aphasia is detected or seems probable. Clinicians often use these types of tests during a first visit with the patient in the acute stages of recovery when a more comprehensive examination would make too many demands on the patient. Another potential use of aphasia screening tests is their administration by staff members who are not speech clinicians, such as nurses in inpatient medical settings where speech clinicians are not readily available. A Norwegian research group examined the Ullevaal Aphasia Screening test for this specific use (Thommessen et al., 1999). The Frenchay Aphasia Screening Test (FAST) is another instrument designed specifically for use by nonspeech clinicians.

Whether or not (and how) to use screening tests has been a contested issue in aphasia assessment, as well as in related domains such as neuropsychological assessment. We would argue that the best use of these tests is to allow the speech clinician to reach a decision as to whether or not a more detailed testing is required. Such an approach would allow more individuals to be assessed using objective test instruments (rather than simple bedside interaction) while assuring that fuller diagnostic procedures remain available to those individuals for whom a more comprehensive evaluation is needed. This approach also recognizes the increased time demands and the decreased reimbursement opportunities prevalent in contemporary service delivery by speech clinicians. While the presence or absence of aphasia often can be determined by screening tests, this decision usually depends upon the severity of the language problem: it would be fairly straightforward to distinguish the responses of individuals with moderate to severe aphasic disorders from those with intact, normal levels of language skills. In these cases, though, such a decision could have been reached during subjective interactions with patients, making the unique contribution of the screen, the objective nature of its determination unnecessary. In milder forms of aphasia— and at the lower end of normal language skills—the distinction between a positive and a negative finding on an aphasia screening test might be difficult to obtain and interpret, though this is exactly the type of scenario where an excellent screening instrument might allow a more reliable and valid assessment. As reported later, these types of instruments may fail to show clear distinctions between patients with right and left hemisphere lesions (where the incidence of aphasia obviously differs) and aphasic patients and patients with adequate language but with defects in their visual and visuoattentional fields—common challenges in clinical practice.

Neuropsychological test batteries that are self-contained sometimes include a screening test for aphasia, as, for example, the Aphasia Screening Test described below, which is part of the Halstead-Reitan Neuropsychological Test Battery (Reitan and Wolfson, 1985). It should be remembered, however, that most of these batteries allow no discrimination of different aphasia syndromes. For example, Ryan et al. (1988) reported that another packaged battery, the Luria-Nebraska Neuropsychological Battery (LNNB; Golden et al., 1980), failed to produce distinctly different profiles for seven Broca's and seven Wernicke's aphasics on the language scales found in that battery.

Screening tests exist for many other purposes than the presence of aphasia in neurology and in psychiatry. They also attempt to screen for the presence of a dementing process (e.g., Alzheimer's disease), such as the Mini-Mental State Examination (MMSE; Folstein et al., 1975), and will typically include individual items that challenge language function. They would not, of course, allow a determination of the presence of aphasia, but they do serve to assure that language functioning is part of the screening of cognitive function.

Aphasia Language Performance Scale

The Aphasia Language Performance Scale (ALPS) (Keenan and Brassell, 1975) was designed to address the following questions: "What is the patient's best level of performance in each language modality, and how can we best use this information to plan effective therapy?" (p. 3). The authors consider the ALPS to be a "significant departure" from psychometric objectivity in aphasia assessment. The endpoint of such a psychometric trend, according to the ALPS authors, is such that examiners "are encouraged, in short, to divest themselves of their own personality, to suppress their individual responses to each change of their environments, and to behave rather like machines" (p. 31).

The ALPS is composed of four 10-item scales: listening, talking, reading, and writing. Item arrangement in each scale is in terms of difficulty. For each scale, a correct response is defined as that which the tester might expect from a normal adult. A correct or self-corrected response is given full credit (1 point); a correct response that requires prompting is given half credit (1/2 point). The examiner is free to begin each scale at whichever level he or she feels the patient may be competent. A scale is terminated after two consecutive failures. Criteria for determining normal performance, the need for prompting, and the point in the subscale at which the patient will be competent are at the discretion of the examiner. The number of correctly completed items is used as a score for each section and is directly translated into a scale of impairment. The authors have provided an arbitrarily determined descriptive scale of impairment for each section, ranging from "profoundly impaired" for a score of 0–1 to "insignificant impairment" for a scale score of 9.5–10.

Normative data are not provided. Given the subjective nature of the ALPS administration, however, normative data would be, for all intents and purposes, of little value.

The ALPS would seem to fall into the gray area between clinical and psychometric screening assessment: Although systematized to a greater extent than many personal clinical examinations, the ALPS falls short of being a standard and comprehensive test instrument. The authors disclaim any psychometric intentions in creating the ALPS. Hence, the interested clinician would do well to weigh the positive and negative aspects of the ALPS against his or her own personal, informal clinical assessment rather than attempt, as the authors did, to contrast the ALPS with psychometrically established comprehensive aphasia examinations.

Aphasia Screening Test

The Reitan (1991; Reitan and Wolfson, 1985; Wheeler and Reitan, 1962) version of the Halstead-Wepman Aphasia Screening Test (AST) (Reitan and Wolfson, 1985, 2nd ed., Reitan Neuropsychological Laboratory, $29.95, also for young and older children, $39.95) is designed to determine whether the patient can perform such simple tasks as spelling a word or naming an object. The AST procedures are such that the clinician should elicit the patient's best performance. A broad array of language functions is briefly assessed by one or two items each. For example, the patient is required to draw a shape, name it, and spell it; to read (e.g., "See the black dog"); to do a single pencil-and-paper and a single "in-head" arithmetic problem; and to demonstrate object use and picture drawing.

The test takes approximately 20 minutes to complete. The test manual provides many illustrative examples of performances. As stated in the introduction of this chapter, screening tests of this type have seen little use recently because they provide very limited information and tend to show only limited accuracy. The test is usually given within the context of a complete neuropsychological test battery intended to assess the full range of psychological deficits after brain damage. Interrater reliability has been reported as high (Barth, 1984) and internal consistency was moderate when used with 334 nine-to-14-year-old children (Livingston et al., 1999). The screening efficiency of the test as a single measure (discrimination between aphasic and nonaphasic brain-damaged patients) has been reported as 80% correct (Krug, 1971). However, effectiveness of distinguishing between different presentations of brain damage can be questioned, given the results of a study by W. Snow (1987) in which only one of 33 AST items differentiated between left and right hemisphere lateralized tumor and stroke patients.

It should be noted that Barth (1984), G. Goldstein and Shelly (1984), and Werner et al. (1987) reported significant correlations between the AST and IQ as well as educational level in large neuropsychiatric populations. Baker (1995) used the test to discriminate between 82 learning-disabled, 72 low-achieving, and 90 normal-learning children and found significant differences between groups; errors occurred mainly on items requiring spelling, constructional praxis, reading, articulation, arithmetic, and body orientation. A factor analysis of the test by J. Williams and Shane (1986) reported the presence of a general language abilities factor and a "sensorimotor coordination" factor in a sample of 197 adults with brain damage. Ernst (1988) reported normative data for elderly subjects.

This test should not be mistaken for Whurr's Aphasia Screening Test (1996), a test battery which focuses on an input–output, multimodality model, similar to that used in the Children's Acquired Aphasia Screening Test by the same author described in the chapter on children's tests.

Bedside Evaluation Screening Test, 2nd Edition

The Bedside Evaluation Screening Test, 2nd ed. (BEST-2) (West et al., 1998; Pro-Ed, $139) is designed to be administered and scored within 30 minutes. It requires that the patient being examined be able to sit up in bed and maintain eye contact with the examiner. The test's name and its stated purpose point directly toward its use as an alternative to reaching decisions based just upon clinical interactions at "the bedside" (i.e., very early in a patient's medical recovery from an acute neurological event).

The second edition replaces the original 1987 instrument, and the test has been restandardized. One change is an attempt to make the test more portable, by replacing magnetized objects with object pictures in a wire-bound stimulus booklet. In both instances, the objects are common household items, like a nail, a key, and a stamp. Despite the change, both versions could be considered compact and easily handled. Other structural changes are minor.

The BEST-2 comprises seven subtests: Conversational Expression, Object Naming, Object Description, Sentence Repetition, Pointing to Objects, Pointing to Parts of a Picture, and Reading. For most subtests, a question-and-answer format is used to obtain responses, which may be verbal or gestural (pointing) depending upon the subtest. Performance on each subtest can range up to a raw score of 30, with lower scores indicating a more impaired performace. A Total Score represents the sum of scores across the subtest set. In a review of the test, Morales (2001) commented that the BEST-2 scoring system is "easy and well explained" and that its manual is "well organized."

The BEST-2 was standardized on a sample of 164 aphasic individuals and 30 neurologically intact adults. The standardization samples ranged in age from 21 to 95 years and English was their primary language. Neurological etiology was predominantly cerebrovascular accident (CVA), with a smaller percentage of traumatic brain injury and tumors. Reliability and validity examinations appear favorable (e.g., reliability coefficient alphas at and higher than .88 and group differentiation of the aphasic and healthy samples at a 1 standard deviation distinction) and are described in the test manual. Raw scores are convertible into standard scores and percentiles. Performance levels can be described by degree of impairment. Finally, a factor analysis found the BEST-2 items to load on one general factor.

The test authors can be commended for cautioning users not to over-interpret BEST-2 performances or treat the test as if it were a comprehensive diagnostic battery, although their suggestion that the test can distinguish aphasia subtypes has been criticized as being "not substantiated" (Mitchell-Person, 2001).

Frenchay Aphasia Screening Test

Developed in Britain, the Frenchay Aphasia Screening Test (FAST; Enderby et al., 1987a,b; NFER-Nelson, England, £25) is designed to be administered by the nonspecialist and takes only 3 to 10 minutes to complete. In addition to clinical use, it has found use in a number of clinical research applications.

The test has four sections: Comprehension, Verbal Expression, Reading, and Writing. An overall Total FAST Score provides a summary of performance. A picture card of a scene and of shapes and five additional cards with commands are the basic test stimuli. Comprehension is assessed by pointing to objects and shapes on the picture card. Expression is assessed by having the person describe the scene presented on the card and by an overall rating of performance on a 60-second animal fluency task. Performance levels are compared to cutoff scores at two levels: up to the age of 60 years and older than 60 years of age. In his review, Towne (1995a) found the cutoff-score procedure used on the FAST to be problematic and poorly explained by the test authors.

Standardization and normative data were established using a sample of 50 CVA patients (20 of whom with an aphasia diagnosis) and 123 neurologically intact adults. Though the reported cutoff scores identified all 20 aphasics, it misidentified 14 of the remaining 30 patients, reportedly due to visual neglect and inattention. The manual provides some assessment of reliability and validity issues.

The FAST correlates significantly with the MTDDA and the FCP (Enderby and Crow, 1996). However, its sensitivity is not fully established, and it includes tasks that are not necessarily sensitive to aphasia (e.g., naming shapes) (Al-Khawaja et al., 1996; Towne, 1995a). O'Neill and colleagues (1990) reported that while the FAST showed itself to be sensitive to aphasia in a sample of elderly adults between the ages of 69 and 90 years and in a second sample of individuals (65 to 96 years of age) assessed 1 and 7 days after an initial CVA, problems with specificity were noted and the test did not offer advantages over a clinical evaluation of these individuals. Sweeney et al. (1993) found that 73% of an elderly (65+ years) population admitted to the acute ward of a department of medicine screened positive on the FAST for the presence of speech and/or language disorders. Orgogozo (1999) used the test in a battery to measure improvement of aphasia in 927 patients after stroke; patients who received piracetam showed better improvement and fewer deaths compared to those who had received a placebo. The test was used as one of a set of measures to assess the relative clinical effectiveness of conventional inpatient care and an early discharge policy for stroke patients by having access to a community-based rehabilitation team (Rudd et al., 1997). The test was also used in the assessment of acute confusional states for a small sample of delirious hospice patients, with relatively poorer performances noted on the test's writing task, which requires the individual to write a description of the scene presented on the picture card (Macleod and Whitehead, 1997).

Gibson and colleagues (1991) included the FAST with other screening measures in creating a battery of instruments that could be completed by hospitalized stroke patients in about an hour's time. They noted that the presence of hemianopia compromised FAST performances, but that, overall, the FAST along with the other tests showed promise in monitoring progress during rehabilitation and in identifying problems that would benefit by consultation with specialists.

As with other aphasia tests, users of the FAST need to be cautious when using the test with individuals known or suspected of having visual field problems or more serious visual neglect/inattention, as these problems may result in false positive FAST results. For the assessment of such associated deficits see Chapter 4.

Sklar Aphasia Scale—Revised

The revised Sklar Aphasia Scale (SAS; Sklar, 1983; Western Psychological Services, $75) provides a brief assessment of the aphasic patient's abilities along four dimensions: Auditory Decoding, Visual Decoding, Oral Encoding, and Graphic Encoding. Each of the four subtests is represented by five items for each area. A total score summarizes SAS performance. The 1983 revision replaced an earlier 1973 version of the test. Part of the revision was the inclusion of an interview to allow the user to formulate hypotheses about the person being examined, but which is not part of the test's formal scoring. The SAS is constructed within a theoretical framework of an input (decode), process (transcode), and output (encode) model of language and its disabilities.

Each response on the SAS is scored on a five-point scale, from a correct response (0) to no response (4). An impairment score for each test is obtained by finding the mean value of the four subtest impairment scores (0 = no impairment, 100 = full impairment). The total impairment score may be used prognostically in terms of potential benefit of therapy if modified by both the recency of the impairment and the patient's overall state of health. However, psychometric evaluation of the prognostication has not yet been presented.

The 1973 SAS test items were standardized on a sample of only 20 adults ranging in age from 29 to 78 years—a small sample, particularly if the prognostic applications are of interest. Sklar reported high correlations between the 1973 SAS performance and performance on Eisenson's aphasia examination, Schuell's short version of the MTDDA, and the AST in a sample of 12 patients. Although reliability data are not presented, the author described five studies on the validity of the SAS as an instrument to assess language ability in aphasics. The 1983 revision showed somewhat improved attention to standardization, with new norms created from a sample of 69 aphasic speakers. However, the limited attention to psychometric properties was criticized by Crocker (1989) in her assessment of the revised SAS. She pointed toward the lack of any measurement of internal consistency and test-retest reliability evidence as being a "decided shortcoming" on the SAS. Turton (1989) was similarly critical in his review, noting that the revision failed to address critiques of earlier versions of the test.

The validity of the 1973 SAS was examined using a German version of the test by R. Cohen et al. (1977). The research group examined the SAS performances of fluent and nonfluent aphasics, nonaphasic brain-damaged patients, schizophrenics, and normal subjects. The aphasic and nonaphasic groups were generally discriminable based upon their SAS performances, but fluent and nonfluent aphasic individuals were not. A factor analysis of the SAS and other language variables showed that the SAS (along with a version of the Token Test) loaded mainly on a general factor, but not on any of the more specific ones.

Other Screening Tests

Additional aphasia screening tests have been developed by Lecours et al. (1988) specifically designed for illiterates; Still et al. (Mini-Object Test, 1983); and Orzeck (Orzeck Aphasia Evaluation, 1964; Inglis and

Lawson, 1981); but they have found only limited use. Examining for Aphasia (EFA-3; Eisenson, 1993; $159 for the complete kit, Pro-Ed) has a long history and is in its third edition. The test lacks data on reliability and validity and offers no norm-referenced data, but does offer a shortened version for screening purposes. Little research with this instrument has been published. Despite its drawbacks, Kitchens (1995) recommends it as a potential screening instrument.

Comprehensive aphasia batteries sometimes include shortened versions that may be used as screening devices, especially if the goal is to determine whether to administer the full battery. The shortened version of the MTDDA has enjoyed a good deal of popularity among speech clinicians. The new version of the BDAE also has a short form but may be too long to be considered as a screening test. Screening using the BDAE typically follows the procedure discussed in the next chapter, that is, the use of subtests that measure in some detail a specific language function. Finally, the BASA (though a comprehensive instrument) often serves a screening role, given that usually only the more severely impaired patients are administered the test, and additional testing needs to be deferred given the global impairments such patients typically present with.

7

Tests of Specific Aspects of Language Behavior

Growing interest in clinical work and research with aphasia has also led to the construction of several tests that measure a specific aspect of language in detail. Such tests make no claim to cover all aspects of language or of aphasia, but they do provide a relatively thorough assessment of the function in question. These language functions include object naming, verbal fluency, and comprehension and application of linguistic information. Because such specific functions are usually central to aphasic disorders, however, they may also provide a reasonable discrimination between aphasic and nonaphasic patients. For this reason, some of these tests have gained favor for use as screening devices, although this usage was not necessarily the intent of the authors. However, clinicians will frequently pick and choose from these tests to add to their overall evaluations of patients with aphasia or with nonaphasic patients who may have language and language-related deficits. A number of these tests are described below, yet many more are not included in this review because of their limited range of application and use in recent years.

Auditory Comprehension Test for Sentences

The Auditory Comprehension Test for Sentences (ACTS) (Shewan, 1980[1]) provides an examination of comprehension for sentence-length

---

[1] Shewan (personal communication, September 2001) indicated that the test is temporarily unavailable.

material. Patients must listen to a sentence spoken aloud by the examiner and then must point to one of four pictures to indicate which one correctly represents the meaning of the sentence. Four training trials are permitted, which also serve as a screening device to determine whether a patient is too impaired to perform the task. These trials are followed by 21 test items, which vary in terms of sentence length, difficulty level of the vocabulary, and syntactic complexity. Pass–fail scoring and qualitative error analysis are possible; the use of each scoring system is made easy by a clear and concise ACTS response sheet. The test manual states that an average of 10 to 15 minutes is required to complete the ACTS.

A score of 18 of 21 (i.e., approximately 2 SD below the mean) is considered to be the lower bound of normal limits for adults with at least an elementary-school education. Shewan (1980) reported an internal consistency coefficient of .82, as well as test-retest reliability of .87. Flanagan and Jackson (1997) confirmed the test-retest stability of the measure in a sample of neurologically intact 50-to-76-year-old individuals. Two measures of validity are provided in the manual. First, a correlation of .80 was obtained between the ACTS and an eight-point clinical rating of functional auditory-verbal comprehension. Second, when compared with established tests, correlations of .52 between the ACTS and the BDAE auditory comprehension section, and of .89 with the WAB comprehension section were obtained. The lower ACTS-BDAE correlation was attributed to the wider range of abilities assessed by the BDAE compared to the ACTS.

Information about the ACTS standardization sample of 150 aphasics and 30 normal controls is provided in the manual. The aphasic sample comprised 134 CVA cases, 10 traumatic brain injury cases, and 6 postsurgical cases. Means and SDs of the performance of aphasic patients broken down by clinically diagnosed subtype also are provided. As might be expected, patients with Wernicke's aphasia performed poorest, followed in turn by those with Broca's aphasia, aphasics with anomia, and normal controls. Qualitative features of subtype differences are discussed in the manual. The ACTS was used together with the WAB to examine recovery and the differential impact of treatment in a sample of 100 aphasic patients grouped by subtype (Shewan and Kertesz, 1984); improvements over time were similar for treated and untreated patients.

The ACTS is brief, easy to administer and score, and requires only simple nonverbal responses by the patient. The test has demonstrated reliability and validity and appears to be a reasonable test of comprehension for sentence-length material with systematic variations of sentence length, difficulty, and complexity. The manual contains cautions

about evaluating the obtained performance, such as differences between the ACTS standardization sample and the clinician's referral base, as well as about educational and cultural influences on test performance.

Boston Naming Test

The Boston Naming Test (BNT; Goodglass and Kaplan, 2000) has emerged as a popular test of visual confrontation naming. This popularity has transcended traditional aphasia settings to include dementia and geriatric psychology workups (see also Chapter 15). It is available separately and as part of the newly revised BDAE-3 from Lippincott Williams & Wilkins ($35; $150 for the complete BDAE). The current 60-item version has several variants: the original 85-item experimental form (Kaplan et al., 1978); the short 15-item version, which is part of the screening battery for dementia developed by the Consortium to Establish a Registry for Alzheimer's Disease (CERAD; Fillenbaum et al., 1998; Ganguli et al., 1991; Morris et al., 1989; Unverzagt et al., 1996; 1999; Welsh et al., 1994) and has also been used in foreign-language populations (e.g., Jamaican: Unverzagt et al., 1999; Nigerian: Guruje, 1995).

Mack et al. (1992) developed four 15-item short versions of the BNT for patients who may be so impaired that the 60-item version may be burdensome. A 15-item version was adopted by Goodglass, Kaplan, and Barresi for the BDAE-3 (4[2], house; 7, comb; 10, toothbrush; 13, octopus; 20, bench; 23, volcano; 26, canoe; 29, beaver; 36, cactus; 39, hammock; 42, stethoscope; 45, unicorn; 52, tripod; 55, sphinx; 58, palette). A Spanish adaptation with extensive norms for American and South American Spanish speakers (Allegri et al., 1997; Kohnert et al., 1998; Ponton et al., 1992; Taussig et al., 1988) is available. It also forms part of the Neuropsychological Screening Battery for Hispanics (Ponton et al., 2000). The BNT has been used in Dutch (Marien et al., 1998), Korean (Kim and Na, 1999), Norwegian (Hestad et al., 1998), and other languages. Morrison et al. (1996) used the test with normal French-speaking subjects in Quebec, Canada. The test may be suitable for children from age 4:0 to 17:11 (see Chapter 13).

The stimuli for the BNT are line drawings of objects with increasing difficulty, ranging from simple, high-frequency vocabulary ("tree") to rare words ("abacus"). The administration requires a spontaneous response within a 20-second period; if such a response is not made, two

---

[2] Numbers refer to the item numbers in the published 60-item BNT.

kinds of prompting cues (one phonemic, one semantic) may be given. Rules allow for discontinuation after six consecutive errors and for entry into the test at an advanced level, thus saving considerable time for subjects without obvious impairment. However, Ferman et al. (1998) reported that using a "lenient" discontinuation method (allowing phonemically correct responses) led to changes in scores up to 16 points in persons older than 80 years, although scores were changed in only 3% of the total population of 655 normal elderly, and in 31% of 140 Alzheimer's disease patients.

Scoring counts the number of spontaneously produced correct responses, the number of cues given, and the number of responses after phonemic cuing and after semantic cuing. For example, if the response given for mushroom is "umbrella," the patient is given the first (semantic) stimulus cue "something to eat." If the subject then correctly names the item within 20 seconds, a check is entered in the stimulus cue correct column. If the subject is unable to name the picture correctly within 20 seconds, a second (phonemic) cue (i.e., the underlined initial phoneme(s) of the name of the item, e.g., *m*) is offered. The response is recorded and entered in the appropriate column (phonemic cue correct, incorrect) but no credit is given. In addition, M. Nicholas et al. (1996) developed a rating system of BNT errors based on relatedness to the correct stimuli.

Azrin et al. (1996) reported that African American individuals living in the U.S. South may employ regionally recognized words that should be scored as correct. Examples include: "snake," "worm," "rope" (pretzel), "tomwalkers," "walkers," "walking sticks," "sticks" (stilts), "falseface" (mask), and "harp," "French harp," "Jew's harp," "mouth organ" (harmonica), although on average the inclusion of these responses as correct increased the total score by only .32 points. Tombaugh and Hubley (1997) also noted that "mouth organ" and other incorrect responses ("lock" or "bold" for latch, "dice" for dominoes, "toadstool" for mushroom) often occur, and suggested that in these and similar cases a follow-up question should be asked ("What is another name for this?"). A major new study of regional and dialectical differences with 1387 subjects (Goldstein and Pliskin, 2002) found that these regional synonyms listed above were used by only 13% of their sample, most frequently by elderly, poorly educated persons living in southern as opposed to midwestern U.S. states, although "mouth harp" and "mouth organ" also occurred in the Midwest, and patients with Alzheimer's disease also used more of these synonyms. Adjusting scores for these variants led to minimal changes, which, according to the authors, were

"unlikely to change quantitative interpretations"; however, they warn that clinicians should be careful to avoid labeling such synonyms as paraphasias. The quantitative scores were affected by age, education, race (African American individuals older than 49 years of age scored 4 points lower), and gender (males scored 3 points higher than females).

Studies by Fillenbaum et al. (1997) and by Welsh et al. (1995) found that African American adults with AD scored lower than Caucasian subjects even when age and education level were controlled for. Schmitter-Edgecombe et al. (2000) note that "old-old" individuals (75+ years of age) are better in naming four words (i.e., "yoke," "trellis," "palette," and "abacus") than "young-old" subjects (58 to 74 years of age) to the extent that this obscured actual differences between the two age groups; they warn that these may be obsolete terms that can distort test results. Worrall et al. (1995) found scores to be 2 to 5 points lower than U.S. norms in elderly Australian subjects, and warn that word-frequency differences between cultures should be taken into account when interpreting scores of non-American subjects. A similar caution was raised by Barker-Collo (2001), who found that New Zealand students made 60% more errors on the items pretzel and beaver. A recently modified Australian version of the BNT has been used successfully (Cruice et al., 2000).

The original norms accompanying the test are based on small groups of adults aged 18 to 59 years. No age-related changes or differences between adults with 12 years of schooling or less and those with more than 12 years of education were noted. Norms included in the BDAE-3 expand the upper age limit to 79. Although statistical interpretation is not provided, the mean scores show some decrement with age: 41 persons aged 70 to 79 years had a mean BNT score of 48.9 (SD = 6.3), 56 persons aged 60 to 69 years show a mean score of 53.3 (SD = 4.6), and 49 persons aged 50 to 59 years show a mean score of 55.2 (SD = 4.0).

Other BNT normative data (Mitrushina and Satz, 1989; van Gorp et al., 1986; Albert et al., 1988; T. Ross et al., 1995) show a significant effect of both age and education when older subjects are included. The major age effect (a decrease of approximately 5 points) is found in the 70-to-80-year-old group. These norms are almost identical with those presented by Ivnik et al. (1996), who also include data for older age groups from a major normative data collection. Neils et al. (1995) confirmed the age/education interaction on a sample of 323 subjects between the age of 65 and 97 years: BNT scores declined more with age for less educated subjects. In addition, subjects living in an institutional setting showed lower scores, while other forms of living environment did not show any difference. Tombaugh and Hubley (1997), however, found a much smaller age effect (70–74: 54.5, SD 4.4, $n = 20$; 75–79: 53.5, SD 4.7, $n = 24$; 80–85: 53.8, SD 4.7, $n = 33$) in community-dwelling volunteers in Ottawa, Ontario. Subjects with less than 8 years of education scored approximately 10 points lower, and subjects with 15 or more years of education about 3 points higher. Wilkins et al. (1996) warn that normative data should not be applied to subjects with a WAIS-R vocabulary standard score of 7 or less, because such subjects scored much lower than the norms provided in the manual.

The norms presented by Spreen and Strauss (1998) are very similar to those reported by Welch et al. (1996) for 60 to 80+ year olds. The norms are also consistent with those published by Russell and Starkey (1993) and Taussig et al. (1988) for the current version; the preliminary norms based on a French Canadian population (Morrison et al., 1996); by LaBarge et al. (1986) and by Montgomery (1983) for the 85-item version; and by Villardita et al. (1985), by Rich (1993), and by Lansing et al. (1999) for 15-item versions. Lichtenberg et al. (1994) report values for a small sample of 70 to 80+ year-old subjects with lower education level; similar norms for older adults were obtained by Schmitter-Edgecombe et al. (2000). Further norms for a sample of 531 60-to-80-year-old adults can be found in Heaton et al. (1999) and for 384 healthy 15-to-83-year-olds in Dikmen et al. (1999). T. Ross et al. (1995, 1998) warn that for elderly subjects, hospitalized for nonneurological disorders in a demographically diverse medical setting (mean education 10.6 years, 56% African Americans), considerably lower values and higher SDs can be expected. Some of these exceeded even the cutoff points suggested by Mitrushina and Satz (1989; cutoffs for ages 57–65 = 51 points or less; ages 66–70 = 47, ages 71–75 = 44, ages 76–86 = 37); subjects with education below grade 12 scored about 7 points lower than those with an education of grade 12 and better, a difference that expanded to 12 points in the highest age group. Finally, Hawkins et al. (1993) found that education corrections based on reading level are needed for the full adult range (18 to 68 years). They did not find a correlation with age within the age range sampled. Killgore and Adams (1999) attempted a score correction based on vocabulary knowledge, using the WAIS-R vocabulary subtest. As expected, Ferraro et al. (1998) found that speed of response to the BNT items depended on both lexical frequency of the words and familiarity of the stimulus pictures.

Welsh et al. (1996) found that 60-to-80+ year-old males scored about four points higher than females. However, this gender effect is still questionable, since L. Henderson et al. (1998) found no gender or race effects in 100 eighteen-to-59-year-olds, half of them female, half of them African American. However, degree of acculturation did affect the test results (Manly et al., 1998). Ferraro and Bercier (1996) also found no effect of ethnicity in a study of 22 elderly Native Americans.

Albert et al. (1988) and L. Nicholas et al. (1989) point out that errors in older subjects consist mainly of substitutions of semantically related associations and circumlocutions on object rather than action names. An error analysis by Goodglass et al. (1997) suggests that, on the other hand, success in naming by aphasics and normals is best predicted by phonetically correct initial responses. Hamberger and Seidel (2001) warn that subjective complaints of difficulty in name finding may not always be detected by tests of confrontation naming like the BNT, but can better be confirmed by tests of semantic fluency (see below: Oral Verbal Fluency).

Reliability has been assessed in a number of independent settings. V. Henderson et al. (1990) reported an 80% response consistency for both uncued and cued responses in AD patients after 6 months. Another study constructed an "odd-item" and "even-item" as well as an experimental version of the BNT, and found that all three short versions discriminated well between AD, other dementing diseases, and normal older (mean age 73.7 years) subjects (B. Williams et al., 1989). This result was confirmed by N. Fisher et al. (1999), who also used an odd/even version. Another 30-item version, developed for a Chinese population, showed a sensitivity between 56% and 80% and specificity between 54% and 70% in separating demented and nondemented subjects of low and high educational background (Salmon et al., 1995). Lansing et al. (1999) reviewed previously presented short forms and developed a gender-neutral short form empirically by stepwise discriminant analysis with discriminability comparable to the full-length 60-item test. Fisher et al. (1999) found that the odd/even numbered item short forms provided almost identical total scores of 27.13 in 30 healthy individuals between 61 and 84 years of age, and that both discriminated well from Alzheimer's disease patients matched for age and education.

Flanagan and Jackson (1997) reported that 31 non-brain-damaged adults between age 50 and 76 scored on repeat testing within 4% or less of the total score 68% of the time. A test-retest reliability of .94 was found by Sawrie et al. (1996) after 8 months in 51 adult intractable epileptics. Dikmen et al. (1999) found relatively good retest reliability and minimal practice effects on repeat testing after an average of 11 months. Huff et al. (1986) divided the original version of the test into two equivalent forms and obtained between-forms correlations of .81

in healthy control subjects, and of .97 in patients with AD. Thompson and Heaton (1989) compared the experimental 85-item version with the standard 60-item BNT and with the two nonoverlapping 42-item versions in 49 clinical patients. The correlations between the 85-, the 60-, and the 42-item versions ranged from .96 to .92, whereas the two nonoverlapping short forms correlated .84. The authors recommend the use of the short forms, especially since they may be more suitable if repeat testing is required.

Sandson and Albert (1987) found that aphasic patients made more perseverative errors than patients with right hemisphere lesions; also, perseverations were more frequent in patients with posterior rather than frontal lesions.

Knopman et al. (1984) reported good measurement of recovery of naming after strokes of small volume in the left posterior superior temporal, inferior parietal, and the insula-putamen areas. Axelrod et al. (1994) found that the BNT loaded on three major factors of intelligence in adults: verbal comprehension, perceptual organization, and freedom from distractibility. The test is sensitive to subcortical disease (e.g., multiple sclerosis and Parkinson's disease) even if global mental status is only mildly affected; in addition, responses were slower than in normal controls (W. Beatty and Monson, 1989; Lezak et al., 1990). Scores by 87 patients with temporal lobe epilepsy were impaired (mean = 42.4) compared to 719 normal controls (mean = 52.3), but better than for 325 patients with Alzheimer's disease (mean = 34.4) (Randolph et al., 1999). Welsh et al. (1995) found that semantic errors and circumlocutions in AD patients were associated with left mesial and lateral temporal lobe metabolism as measured by positron emission tomography (PET) and fluorodeoxyglucose (FDG) emission techniques. In addition, the left anterior temporal area has also been implicated (Tranel, 1992). However, Trenerry et al. (1995) reported that carefully limited anterior right or left temporal lobectomy in 31 left and 24 right lobectomy patients with left hemisphere language lateralization did not positively or negatively affect BNT performance. The BNT was also not sensitive to side of epileptic focus in a study of patients with idiopathic epilepsy (Haynes and Bennett, 1990) and in patients with anterior temporal lobectomy (Cherlow and Serafetinides, 1976). In contrast, Bell et al. (2000) reported that patients with left temporal lobectomy showed some loss of word finding, following the age of acquisition rule, that is, that words acquired early in childhood were less affected than words acquired later.

The BNT did not discriminate between 10 fluent aphasics and 10 speech-disordered schizophrenics (Landre et al., 1992). Individuals with depression (mean = 48.50, n = 14) as well as depressed individuals with reversible cognitive dysfunction (mean = 45.64, n = 11) did differ significantly from Alzheimer's disease patients (mean = 27.23, n = 13) (Hill et al., 1992). While mild and even moderate depression has little effect on the test performance of elderly subjects (Boone et al., 1995), poor naming performance in depression has been described as a poor prognostic sign in a 6-month treatment study (King et al., 1991). Depression in otherwise healthy elderly Native Americans has been shown to decrease BNT scores (Ferraro et al., 1997).

As with other tests relying on pictorial material (e.g., Peabody Picture Vocabulary Test, PPVT), the integrity of the visual system should be checked if performance is defective. Kaplan and Goodglass (1983) noted that, particularly in patients with right frontal damage, "fragmentation responses" may be made (e.g., the mouthpiece on a harmonica interpreted as a line of windows in a bus; Lezak, 1995).

Over the years, the BNT has proven to be one of the most popular, reliable, and valid instruments for the general assessment of naming problems. A large amount of research focuses not on aphasia, but on aging and performance by other clinical populations, especially AD. The 15-item short version can be considered useful for quick screening but does not replace the full-length version of the test. Either short or long versions can be given alone or as part of the BDAE-III aphasia battery. Collaborators of the BNT authors have created a verb-based version, called the Action Naming Test (Obler and Albert, 1982).

Discourse Comprehension Test

The Discourse Comprehension Test (DCT) (R. Brookshire and Nicholas, 1997; Communication Skill Builders, $65) arose out of psycholinguistic research findings that suggested that word and sentence comprehension tests are unlikely to predict comprehension of multiple-sentence messages, and cannot examine contextual aspects of such messages, that is, the ideas that are implicit across sentences (e.g., L. Nicholas and Brookshire, 1995). The authors also cite work by H. Brownell (1988) that suggests that word and sentence comprehension measures may underestimate comprehension problems in patients with right hemisphere lesions. In this respect, the DCT can be considered as a natural extension of the ACTS.

The DCT has a narrative format. Paragraph-length stories are played for the patient on audiotape. There are 2 practice stories and 10 scorable stories. All stories seek to depict situations (such as a hapless baseball fan's plight) in a humorous light. The patient is queried after each story with eight yes/no questions. These questions are divided as follows: two deal with the story's overt main ideas, two deal with implied main ideas, two with stated details, and two with implied details. The authors' research found that both normal individuals and those with aphasia score higher on main ideas than on details, and higher on stated than implied material. The 10 stories are divided into two equivalent sets of 5 stories each. The examiner is advised to consider the patient's hearing ability and basic comprehension to produce valid and consistent yes/no responses before beginning the test. After one or two practice stories, one 5-story set is administered; if performance is variable, the second set is given (or all 10 can be given, regardless).

DCT scores include an overall score and scores for each type of question. The test employs cutoff scores to denote defective performance, set at the 5th percentile of the normal sample.

Standardization was based on 40 normal adults who were 55 to 75 years of age and had a range of completed education from 8 through 18 years. Results with samples from 20 aphasics, 20 patients with right hemisphere lesions, and 20 patients with traumatic brain injury were also reported. DCT overall scores correlated minimally with age (.08) and mildly with education (.21), both statistically nonsignificant. Test-retest reliability after 2 to 3 weeks was reported as .87 for aphasics and .95 for patients with right hemisphere lesions. Considerations of content validity are reported in the manual. These included itemization of questions that were checked for consistency across 10 judges, statistical comparison of test wording with wording in normal adult communication, and a comparision of the narrative monologue found on the DCT to the dialogue approach (albeit highly structured) used for an earlier, experimental version of the test (Katsuki-Nakamura et al., 1988). Criterion-related validity was reported as ranging from .54 to .76 for the DCT with the BDAE Auditory Comprehension subtests and with the four-subtest short version of the PICA (DiSimoni et al., 1980).

The manual includes instructions for a silent-reading administration of the DCT, using the same stimuli. Also included is the authors' Sentence Comprehension Test, which is used to determine whether consistent yes/no responses can be elicited from the patient (alternatively, they suggest using the WAB Comprehension subtest).

Instructions for the test suggest that the user be guided by sentence comprehension tests as to whether or not the DCT is administered. A clinician might also be guided by ACTS performance. While this rule may be appropriate for patients with severe comprehension problems to the point that yes/no responding is close to random, strict adherence to the rule might truncate the range of valid defective performance in clinical use and psychometric research, and therefore hinder a fuller appreciation of narrative discourse measurement.

The DCT extends the assessment of comprehension to the level of narrative discourse. The authors report that results may generalize to the level of highly structured communicative dialogue, but that it remains unclear whether it can be generalized to less structured dialogue. In addition to helping describe the communicative skills of brain-damaged patients, the DCT offers a potentially useful research instrument at a level between concise measures of single word and sentence comprehension (e.g., the ACTS), on the one hand, and subjective functional communication rating scales, on the other. The test's breakdown of questions based upon the information required to answer them has been independently examined in a study of Parkinson's and Huntington's disease (Murray and Stout, 1999), with findings consistent to that reported for aphasic patients.

Although not cited by the authors, a developmental study (Newton, 1994) reported that with young children the use of a picture that depicts the initial circumstances of a narrative story helps children to maintain a functional mental model to supplement comprehension as the story progresses. The use of such pictures for the DCT might provide a useful treatment-oriented adjunct, as well as an opportunity to compare patient performance with and without such visual aids.

The question remains whether the length of the stimuli and the number of questions per story introduce an undesirable attentional-memory component into the test that may influence performance. For example, Tompkins et al. (1994) commented on the relationship between memory capacity and discourse passages that require a revision of their plot as the story unfolds.

The weakness of the DCT is the relatively small size of the standardization sample. It remains open whether the cutoff scores would remain stable with a larger sample of normal controls. Larger samples of both aphasic and control subjects would also have permitted a more refined percentile scoring system. As it stands, the test has practical treatment-oriented descriptive and testing-the-limit uses, but diagnostic use may need to await further psychometric studies.

Iowa-Group Tests

In addition to developing two comprehensive aphasia batteries, Benton and his colleagues at the University of Iowa have developed a number of specific-function tests for use in the evaluation of aphasic patients. Some of these tests are described briefly.

Sound Recognition Test

The Sound Recognition Test (Spreen and Benton, 1974; Spreen and Strauss, 1998; Department of Psychology, University of Victoria, $50), presented on audiotape, allows the examination of auditory object recognition (e.g., train whistle) by requiring the identification of familiar sounds. The original form of this test consisted of two equivalent forms of 13 items each. Three modes of administration are offered: verbal response, pointing to one of four multiple-choice names, and pointing to one of four multiple-choice line drawings. Varney (1980, 1984b) modified the format such that all 26 items are presented and multiple-choice line drawings are used as the response format. Scoring standards are detailed in Spreen and Strauss (1998). Spreen and Benton (1974) described norms for normal adults and children, and the performance of brain-damaged adults. Varney (1980) provided normative information for his modified test. Impairment of sound recognition is usually limited to aphasic patients and frequently associated with aural comprehension deficits. Aphasics with aural comprehension deficits during the acute stage of recovery from CVA but with normal sound recognition show rapid and near complete recovery of aural comprehension, whereas patients with acute aural comprehension and sound recognition deficits show a much poorer outcome (Varney, 1984b). Defects in sound recognition are associated with a number of lesion sites, none of which appears specific for the manifestation of the defect (Varney and Damasio, 1986).

Pantomime Recognition Test

The Pantomime Recognition Test (Benton et al., 1994b; PAR, $189), presented on videotape, shows a man pantomiming different activities (e.g., using a telephone). The patient is presented with four multiple-choice responses: one correct, one semantic error, one neutral error, and one odd error. Defective pantomime recognition is an infrequent finding, observed most often in aphasic patients, and appears to be related to associated defects in reading comprehension level. Demented patients may perform defectively on the task. Taking another approach, Records (1994) designed an experimental test, evaluating the impact of gestures on comprehension in aphasic patients.

Phoneme Discrimination Test

The Phoneme Discrimination Test (Benton et al., 1994b; PAR, $39) is a brief test of the discrimination of phonemic sounds. The test was developed to examine the relation between oral language comprehension in aphasic patients and the underlying factors that might be related to this level of comprehension, such as phonemic decoding and sequential sound perception. The test consists of 30 pairs of one- or two-syllable nonsense words on audiotape. The patient has to indicate whether the pair members are the same or different. Practice or pretraining is encouraged to determine if the patient can make same–different responses reliably. Normative data and samples of 100 aphasic left hemisphere damaged and 16 nonaphasic right hemisphere damaged patients are reported in the test manual. Comparisons of the performance of aphasic patients on the Phoneme Discrimination Test and on the MAE Aural Comprehension subtest are also reported (see also Varney and Benton, 1979). Varney (1984a) presented longitudinal data on the Phoneme Discrimination Test in the context of evaluating additional measures of comprehension.

Peabody Picture Vocabulary Test-III

The Peabody Picture Vocabulary Test-III (PPVT-III) (Forms A and B, 3rd ed., Dunn and Dunn, 1997; American Guidance Service, $146.95 for each form) assesses auditory comprehension of picture names. It was initially constructed as a test of hearing vocabulary in children but has since been standardized for adults and used with a variety of clinical populations. The test requires the subject to choose one of four items displayed on a page that depicts the word spoken by the examiner. After five training items, 204 items of increasing difficulty can be given, but usually only 35 to 45 items need to be administered if a suitable entry point (six consecutive correct) is chosen; the test is discontinued after consecutive failures on six out of eight items. The time required is about 10 to 20 minutes. A Spanish version is available. In the new edition, a number of items have been revised or added to correspond to the negatively accelerating growth curve of vocabulary with age.

The new edition has been standardized on a sample of 2725 subjects representative of the 1994 U.S. census estimate, ranging in age from 2:6 to 90 years. Canadian norms are available from the distributor (Psycan). Kamphaus and Lozano (1984) note that in 6-to-11-year-old children with Spanish surnames (about half of whom spoke Spanish at home), standard scores were about 12–13 points below the national norms, although they showed regular, expected increases with age. Sattler (1988) recommends special care in the interpretation of scores of ethnic minority children because their scores tend to be lower, reflecting their verbal and experiential differences rather than ability.

The score on this test is simply the number of items passed including the items prior to the entry point. The manual allows translation of these scores into "age equivalents" (previously called "mental age"), "standard score equivalents" (previously called "IQ"), stanines, and percentiles. The new terms are intended to discourage the use of the test as a measure of "verbal intelligence" (as claimed in the 1965 edition). The authors have added a "true confidence band," indicating the range of scores in which the subject's true score can fall 68 times out of 100.

Split-half reliability has been reported as ranging from .61 to .88 in children and adolescents, and as .82 in adults. The reliability of the alternate form ranged from .73 to .91 (Stoner, 1981; Tillinghast et al., 1983). Retest reliability with the alternate form after a minimum of 9 days showed a median correlation of .78. In children, retest stability over 11 months has been reported as .84 for the revised PPVT (Bracken and Murray, 1984), as .81 in retarded children over a period of 7 months (Naglieri and Pfeiffer, 1983), and as .71 in a mixed clinical neuropsychiatric population after 2½ years (S. Brown et al., 1989). Internal consistency ranged from .96 to .98 in 6-to-11-year-old children (Kamphaus and Lozano, 1984).

Construct validity of the test as a measure of scholastic aptitude is good (Hinton and Knights, 1971). Bracken and Murray (1984) report a predictive validity of .30 with spelling, .54 with reading recognition, .58 with reading comprehension, and .59 with the total Peabody Individual Achievement Test (PIAT) for the revised PPVT; similar values were reported for the first edition (Naglieri, 1981) and for mentally handicapped children with the revised edition (Naglieri and Pfeiffer, 1983). Concurrent validity with similar tests—the Bracken Basic Concept Scale, the preschool version of the Boehm Test of Basic Concepts and its revised version—were .68, .65, and .62, respectively (Zucker and Riordan, 1988). Predictive validity of the PPVT with the Kaufman Assessment Battery for Children (K-ABC) and the Metropolitan Readiness Test after 1 year was .55 and .51, respectively (Zucker and Riordan, 1990). Since vocabulary is a subtest of most intelligence tests usually highly correlated with overall performance level, the PPVT also correlates with the WISC-R, although the results of several studies are somewhat contradictory. Correlations with measures of Verbal (.87), Performance (.80), and Full Scale (.88) IQ have been reported (Crofoot and

Bennett, 1980). Similar results were obtained by Altepeter (1989), who stresses that this indicates that the test is a good screening instrument for general intellectual functioning but not an index of psycholinguistic functioning. Altepeter and Johnson (1989) found only modest correlations in healthy adults with the WAIS-R (.47 with Full Scale IQ) and warn that in this age range the test tends to overestimate IQ in the lower ability ranges and to underestimate IQ in the higher ability ranges; in a cross tabulation of IQs in 10-point steps, less than half of the clients were classified correctly. Price et al. (1990) reported similar discrepancies in adult psychiatric inpatients. The PPVT also correlates highly with the McCarthy Scales in children (Naglieri, 1981), the 1986 Stanford-Binet Intelligence Scale (Carvajal et al., 1987), and with the achievement scale of the Kaufman Assessment Battery for Children in a learning-disabled population (.78, D'Amato et al., 1987). However, Faust and Hollingsworth (1991) found only a correlation of .34 with the Wechsler Primary and Preschool Scale of Intelligence-Revised (WPPSI-R) Full-Scale IQ, and of .30 and .31 with the PIQ and VIQ, respectively, in normal preschoolers. A. Williams et al. (1977) warn that the PPVT is not an adequate measure of hearing vocabulary in mentally handicapped subjects because it is also closely related to visual decoding ability as measured with the Illinois Test of Psycholinguistic Ability (ITPA), and that the use of the PPVT as a measure of intelligence in mentally handicapped persons may be misleading.

Hollinger and Sarvis (1984) stress the role of perceptual-organizational ability in PPVT performance of school-age children, and Taylor (1975) reached the same conclusion for preschool children based on a factor analysis of the WPPSI and the ITPA as well as the PPVT. In a factor analysis of PIAT, WISC-R, and PPVT results with a sample of child psychiatry patients, however, the PPVT loaded mainly on the first factor (verbal comprehension), and only minimally on factors of verbal achievement, perceptual organization, and arithmetic (Culbert et al., 1989; also Zagar, 1983). Children with impaired oral language production (Rizzo and Stephens, 1981) and nonpsychotic, emotionally disturbed adolescents (Dean, 1980) tend to produce variable results. Elliott et al. (1990) found also that the PPVT results in children between 6 and 11 years of age with normal pure-tone hearing were strongly influenced by the ability to make fine-grained auditory discriminations with consonant–vowel stimuli varying in timing and place of articulation.

The test showed significant differences between 28 young adults with specific language impairment and 28 controls (mean values of 82.36 and 92.79, respectively) (Records et al., 1995). Das et al. (1995) demonstrated that the PPVT is sensitive to mental decline (dementia) in older (i.e., older than 50 years) Down syndrome patients, with results parallel to those in a dementia rating scale.

The test is relatively nonthreatening and requires little verbal interaction, since it allows also for gestural or pointing responses. The test is suitable for language-impaired as well as autistic or withdrawn individuals. In line with the warnings mentioned previously, the auditory and visual-perceptual integrity of the patient should be carefully considered in interpreting the results of this test. Quattrochi and Golden (1983) found only small correlations with the children's version of the Luria-Nebraska Battery. Stone et al. (1989) reported beta weights and multiple correlation coefficients of both the oral and the written (printed on cards) format of the PPVT with the WISC-R and tests selected from the Halstead-Reitan Neuropsychological Battery (HRNB) for 934 learning-disabled children, ranging from .001 for location on the Tactual Performance Test to .377 for the Speech Sound Perception Test; 43% of the PPVT variance could be explained by the HRNB-WISC-R combination. Whether this demonstrates that "much of the information offered by the PPVT may be attributed to neuropsychological constructs" (Stone et al., 1989, p. 65), remains questionable.

An earlier version of the test was incorporated into the Florida Kindergarten Screening Battery (Satz and Fletcher, 1982), a test used to explore reading readiness.

Considering the large amount of research with and the continuing revisions of the PPVT, it clearly is the preferred measure of vocabulary for children and can be employed validly with adult and geriatric populations.

Reading Comprehension Battery for Aphasia-2

The original 1979 version of the Reading Comprehension Battery for Aphasia (RCBA) was revised by LaPointe and Horner in 1999 (Pro-Ed, $159). The RCBA-2 is designed "to provide systematic evaluation of the nature and degree of reading impairment in adolescents and adults with aphasia" (p. 1). The test comprises 10 core subtests, each one containing 10 test items, and 7 supplemental subtests, each of variable length. The supplementary measures are new to the test's revised version and are provided for consideration of the underlying reasons for problems in core RCBA-2 performances. The core subtests require about 1 hour to administer. Items on all subtests are scored in terms of being correct or incorrect; the time to complete each subtest is recorded. As with the original RCBA, the authors suggest that clinicians who wish a more refined measurement should employ the multidimensional scoring system created by Porch for the PICA battery (Chapter 9).

The 10 core subtests include measures of single-word comprehension, functional reading of short passages, synonyms, sentence- and paragraph-length comprehension, and syntax. Supplementary tasks examine single-letter recognition, identification of real versus nonsense consonant-vowel-consonant trigrams, and oral reading of words and sentences.

The test is described by the authors as a criterion-referenced measure with no normative basis. The authors include a chapter outlining the basis for stimuli in each subtest and details about how to interpret performances without a normative data set. The authors suggest recording errors on a verbatim basis in order to more fully appreciate performance. Performances are interpreted in terms of severity (based on number correct) and quality of errors.

The test manual reports rudimentary psychometric findings from the original RCBA. Reliability and validity were assessed by van Demark et al. (1982). A small sample of 14 aphasic patients was retested between 1 and 2 days after initial administration, which yielded a test-retest correlation of .94. An internal consistency coefficient of .96 was found. van Demark and colleagues also reported correlations between the RCBA and both the Gates Silent Reading Test and the PICA reading comprehension subtests. The manual also cites unpublished data by Pasternack and LaPointe offering additional psychometric data. Flanagan and Jackson (1997) examined test-retest reliability of the original RCBA in a small sample of non-brain-damaged adults and reported reasonable levels of reliability. The largest collection of aphasic performances on the original RCBA can be found in the 1980s Veterans Administration Cooperative Study, which examined aphasia treatment modalities (e.g., Wertz et al., 1986).

Reporter's Test

De Renzi (1980; De Renzi and Ferrari, 1979) employed the stimuli and most of the commands from the Token Test (TT; see later) to construct the Reporter's Test, a test for expressive deficits in aphasics. Potential users are advised to examine these two primary references to see how the Token Test tokens and verbal stimuli are adapted for use as the Reporter's Test, as no additional material or manuals for the test are required. The Reporter's Test was designed to meet two specific goals:

to elicit organized speech, and to limit the range of what the patient is expected to say. Whereas picture description tasks (e.g., the BDAE Cookie-Theft card) adequately fulfill the first goal, they fail on the second. Other task-description tests have been used in nonaphasic clinical settings (e.g., the "dice game"; McDonald and Pearce, 1995), but lack the overt constraints offered by the Reporter's Test (i.e., the limited range of movements and visual stimuli that can be observed during a TT performance).

The patient is required to act as a "reporter" to perform the task, that is, she or he must report the actions of the tester to an imaginary third person. For example, if the examiner were to touch the large red circle, the patient must verbalize the relevant information necessary for a third person to reproduce the tester's actions ("Touch the large red circle"). The Reporter's Test begins with several sample items to acquaint the patient with the task. The test comprises five sections; the first four are taken from the TT. De Renzi recommended that it be used following the TT, so that the patient is familiar with the stimuli and the required commands.

De Renzi (1980) described initial findings for the Reporter's Test in discriminating 24 aphasic patients from 40 hospitalized, nonaphasic non-brain-damaged controls. In this study, an actual third person sat next to the patient and performed the instructions given by the patient. Years of education, but not age, were significantly related to performance; scores were corrected to account for education. Using a cutting score expected to produce 5% false positives, a 97% hit rate was obtained. Classification accuracy between aphasics and intact controls was higher for the Reporter's Test than for four other tests of verbal expression: visual naming, oral fluency, sentence repetition, and story telling.

De Renzi and Ferrari (1979) described aphasic performance employing the original pass–fail scoring, partial credit for correct performance after repetition, and a weighted scoring (1 point for each bit of information on a trial but without credit for repetition). Aphasic patients, nonaphasic left brain–damaged patients, and nonaphasic right brain–damaged patients were described. Using the weighted scoring system, a cutting score of 54 resulted in an 82% hit rate while yielding 15% false positives in the nonaphasic left brain–damaged group. The authors recommend the use of both scoring systems to offset the weaknesses of each: lower classification for the weighted system and overly severe evaluation using the pass–fail scoring. Hall and Jordan (1985, 1988) examined performance on the Reporter's Test and the TT in a sample of school-aged children with language disorders and provided normative information for 286 healthy children in kindergarten through ninth grade.

Unfortunately, the test has never been used as widely in clinical settings and psychometric research as has the TT, although it can easily be used as an adjunct to the TT.

Sentence Repetition Test

The Sentence Repetition Test (SRT) requires repeating sentences of increasing length, presented orally or on audiotape by the examiner. This is a simple, though perhaps somewhat artificial task demanding short-term memory, but is highly sensitive to aphasic disturbances. A stand-alone version of this test (SRT-Victoria) is available from the Psychology Clinic, University of Victoria (audiotape, manual, and scoring forms cost about $40 U.S.) or can be easily copied from Spreen and Strauss (1998). Alternative standardized sentence repetition tasks that can be used include the Sentence Repetition subtests of the MAE and the BDAE-3.

The SRT-Victoria takes 10 to 15 minutes to complete. The tape contains two equivalent forms (A and B) of 22 tape-recorded sentences, increasing in length from 1 ("Look") up to 26 syllables ("Riding his black horse, the general came to the scene of the battle and began shouting at his brave men"). To allow for sufficient material at low and high levels of performance, the length increases in one-syllable steps for the first 11 and for the last 8 sentences; sentences 12 to 19 increase in two-syllable steps. In this version, grammatical structure and vocabulary have been deliberately held to simple, declarative sentences. The SRT-Victoria is actually a subtest (i.e., Test 5) of the NCCEA battery (Spreen and Benton, 1969, 1977). Children's norms for ages 6 to 13 are available (Spreen and Strauss, 1998). If the SRT is given orally a score adjustment of −1 point is made because, generally, patients respond with better attention to the oral format. Scoring rules provide for omissions, alterations (substitution, change of tense or location), poor articulation, and age and education corrections.

Forms A and B of the SRT-Victoria appear equivalent in difficulty. Correlation between Forms A and B in an unselected group of 47 subjects in the normative sample was .79, and in a mentally retarded population ($n = 25$) .81 (Spreen and Benton, 1966). S. Brown et al. (1989) reported a test-retest correlation of .71 in 248 children (mean age 8 years) with a variety of diagnoses after an interval of 2½ years.

The test score can be entered onto the NCCEA profile sheet. Percentile ranks for nonaphasic brain-damaged patients and for an unselected group of aphasics have been established (Lawriw, 1976). In 353 school-age children, Sentence Repetition formed a separate factor in a factor analysis using the 20 subtests of the NCCEA, accounting for 81% of the total variance of this factor, and was relatively independent of digit repetition (Crockett, 1974). The test contributed to the discrimination of four empirically derived subtypes of aphasia in adults; impairment of sentence repetition was especially characteristic of individuals classed as "Type A" (good comprehension, poor attention, memory, and reproduction of speech) (Crockett, 1977).

As mentioned earlier, sentence repetition is a standard part of other aphasia batteries, for example, the MAE, the BDAE-3, and the WAB. The MAE uses two parallel forms of 14 items each and with varying grammatical complexity; the MAE-SRT loaded strongly on a basic language skills factor (Lincoln et al., 1994). The BDAE-3 version uses 10 sentences that are related to one another, as they reflect an underlying story. The WAB uses 15 items and allows for partial credit for phonemic errors. The SRT-Victoria correlates .88 with the repetition of words, phrases and sentences on the WAB (Shewan and Kertesz, 1980). The correlation in adults with digit repetition forward is .75, with digit repetition reversed .66, with Full Scale IQ (holding age constant) .62 (Lawriw, 1976).

The SRT-Victoria is sensitive to brain damage, particularly if accompanied by aphasic disturbances. In a study of 23 children and 33 adolescents with closed head injury, 33% of those with severe injury and 15% with mild injury were found to score below the 6th percentile for their age (Ewing-Cobbs et al., 1987); the z-score mean for mild closed head injury patients was 48.35 and for moderate and severe injury 36.36. Peck et al. (1992) reported "normative" data for 75 head-injured adults (mean age 36 years) and found a significant effect of severity of injury ($p < .05$); patients with mild injury scored at a mean of the 45th percentile, those with moderate severity at the 39th percentile, and those with severe injury at the 18th percentile. A comparison with patients 12 months postinjury did not show significantly different scores, although this may have been due to unusually large variability (SD). In brain-damaged adults between 20 and 79 years, Vargo and Black (1984) did not notice any significant decrease with age ($r = -.08$) but found significant correlations with IQ (.329) and the Memory Quotient (MQ) of the Wechsler Memory Scale (.377). The most severe impairment was found in patients with dementia and toxic exposure as well as with left hemisphere lesions after CVA and closed head injury. A comparison of aphasics, nonaphasic brain-damaged patients, and controls of low average intelligence (Lawriw, 1976), and for an aphasic population unselected as to type and severity from referral sources in New York, Iowa City, and Victoria (N = 208) showed means of 12.12 (SD = 3.15) for left brain–damaged patients (including aphasics) and of 15.75 (SD = 2.58) when aphasics were excluded. Fifty-six percent of the aphasics scored below the lowest score of normal controls with low average intelligence. Patients with right hemisphere lesions had a mean of 17.64 (SD = 2.12); patients with bilateral or undetermined location of brain damage had a mean of 16.84 (SD = 5.87), and moderately mentally handicapped patients had a mean of 11.88 (SD = 3.15). M. Sarno (1986) reported that among closed head injury patients those with aphasia scored at the 35th percentile for aphasics, those with subclinical aphasia and dysarthria at the 58th percentile, and those with subclinical aphasia at the 70th percentile. The test is especially sensitive in cases of transcortical sensory aphasia, conduction aphasia, and agrammatism (Berndt et al., 1987; Berthier et al., 1996; L. Davis et al., 1978; Kohn et al., 1990; Kostrin and Schwartz, 1986). A study of patients with Alzheimer's disease (Small et al., 2000) varied sentence complexity (syntactive, predicative, padding dimensions, and serial position), and found SRT scores significantly related to measures of working memory. Patients with Alzheimer's disease also showed moderately, but significantly lower scores compared to normal controls matched for age, sex, and educational level (Murdoch et al., 1987), although mild cases of AD performed well (Holland et al., 1986). Similar findings were reported for a small group of amnesic patients (Shapiro et al., 1992). The MAE-SRT showed significant differences between 28 young adults with specific language impairment (SLI) and 28 controls (Records et al., 1995). A study by Stothard et al. (1998) confirmed this finding for 5-year-olds; mild difficulties were still found at age 15.

Normative data and appropriate percentile ranks are available with the SRT-Victoria for students and for hospital and community volunteers. Forms A and B produce highly similar mean scores. Williams (1965) reported that the average adult can correctly repeat sentences of 24 to 25 syllables in length. However, the Benton et al. (1994a) normative sample of 85 nonneurological patients showed an average of only 20 correctly repeated syllables.

Updated normative data for the SRT were reported by Meyers et al. (2000). Rosselli et al. (2000) found equal performance of bilinguals (English-Spanish) and monolinguals. The usefulness of the SRT for testing bilingual children was stressed by Natalicio (1977). In older, healthy, and relatively well educated adults a small but significant decrease is noted after the age of 65 that justifies the correction for age (66 to 75 years, mean = 15.5, SD = 4.02; 76 to 89 years, mean = 15.0, SD = 4.49; Read and Spreen, 1986). The normative data also show a slightly better performance in older females compared to men (approximately 1 point at each age range). Meyers et al. (2000) found an education effect but not an age or gender effect in their sample of 104 individuals between the ages of 16 and 86 years and educational levels from 8 to 22 years.

SRT in children. Norms for normal school children merged from four different sources are presented by Spreen and Strauss (1998). No education corrections are made, since they would be misleading for children. If such corrections were made, adult level of performance would be reached by age 12.

The norms for children are comparable to those presented by Epstein (1982) for Swedish children (means of 13, 16, and 17 syllables for age 7, 8, and 9, respectively). The higher number of syllables repeated in that study was probably due to practice, since the children repeated five sentences at each one-syllable increment in length. Epstein also found that children whose native tongue was not Swedish but who were taught in Swedish schools were approximately 8 syllables behind native-speaking children at age 6, but that this deficit was reduced to 6 syllables at age 7, 5 at age 8, and 3 at age 9. This finding may have some implications for the testing of children with a mother tongue other than English. Epstein (1982) found that dyslexics lagged behind normal-reading classmates by about 4 syllables at age 7, by 3 at age 8, and by 2 at age 9. Rourke (1978), on the other hand, found that 16 dyslexic children had scores in the average range, but that syntactic comprehension was impaired. A study by Spreen (1988) showed that 10-year-old learning-disabled children with neurological signs were able to repeat 10.4 syllables, while those with minimal neurological signs repeated 11.3, and those without neurological signs 15.0 syllables. At age 25, these same subjects repeated 12.8, 13.9, and 14.0 syllables, respectively, while a matched control group showed a mean of 15.5.

Children with brain damage, epilepsy, or both (Hamsher, 1980) had mean scores on the MAE–SRT of 9.5 at age 6, 10 at age 7, 11 at age 8, 11.5 at age 9, 12.6 at age 10, 13.2 at age 11, 13.7 at age 12, and 14.0 at age 13.

In sum, the SRT-Victoria is a well-developed test of sentence memory sensitive to neurological insult, and aphasia especially. The same may be said for the MAE-SRT. The value of the BDAE-3 approach of relating the underlying theme or plot of the sentences might offer additional information about repetition variability, though that remains undetermined. Whether versions with increasing complexity of sentences contribute to its discriminant value remains to be explored.

Token Test

The original version of the Token Test (TT) was introduced 40 years ago by De Renzi and Vignolo (1962) and has become one of the most popular individual tests employed in aphasia assessment. The TT is a brief measure to examine subtle auditory comprehension deficits in aphasic patients by having patients respond gesturally to the tester's verbal command. Since its inception, the original TT has been used, modified by the authors (De Renzi, 1980; De Renzi and Faglioni, 1978), and included in different formats in some aphasia batteries (Benton et al., 1994a; Spreen and Benton, 1977). The original test has spawned many variants; short forms (Boller and Vignolo, 1966; Spellacy and Spreen, 1969; Van Harskamp and Van Dongen, 1977); a concrete-objects version (Martino et al., 1976); a format with both auditory and visual presentation of commands (Kiernan, 1986); the five-item revised TT (Arvedson et al., 1985; Park et al., 2000); a Token Test "battery" (R. Brookshire, 1978); and a version with an expanded linguistic examination (The Revised Token Test, or RTT; McNeil and Prescott, 1978). Computer-generated versions of the TT have been created for use during neurophysiological studies of language comprehension (e.g., event-related brain potentials, D'Arcy and Connolly, 1999; PET-based regional cerebral blood flow, Musso et al., 1999). The many versions have led to some confusion as to what a "Token Test" performance actually represents. Equivalent versions in several languages are available in, for example, Italian, German, Portuguese (Fontanari, 1989); and Kannada (Vena, 1982). A German adaptation by Orgass (1986) is both a stand-alone test and part of the Aachen Aphasia Test (AAT) (Huber et al., 1983).

The TT is a portable test that, in most versions, comprises 20 plastic token stimuli of two sizes (large and small), two shapes (square/rectangular and round), and five colors. The tokens are laid out in front of the patient, typically in a standard 4 × 5 matrix. The test comprises different sections that increase in sentence length and linguistic complexity (e.g., from "Point to a square" to "Pick up the small, green square" to "Put the small red square on the large blue circle"). The number of sections vary from version to version. The McNeil and Prescott (1978) RTT version provides the most complex commands.

The TT is often one of the tasks included in examining the effect of aphasia treatments. The TT also has become a part of batteries designed for purposes other than traditional aphasia assessment. The MAE version of the TT, for example, is part of the Traumatic Brain Injury Model Systems neuropsychology battery (Millis et al., 2001) and was one of the tests used to create the extended neuropsychological normative data set for elderly individuals used in the Mayo's Older Americans Normative Studies (MOANS) project (Ivnik et al., 1996).

Some authors have reported age (Emery, 1986) and level of education (De Renzi, 1980; De Renzi and Faglioni, 1978) differences on certain versions of the TT. Gallaher (1979) reported day-to-day retest reliabilities for one version of the TT and its subsections to be greater than .90. Validation studies have shown the TT to be a strong and accurate discriminator between the performance of aphasic patients and that of normal hospitalized adults (De Renzi, 1980), nonaphasic right hemisphere damaged adults (Boller and Vignolo, 1966; Swisher and Sarno, 1969), and nonaphasic diffuse and focal brain–damaged adults (Orgass and Poeck, 1966). Morley et al. (1979) found the TT to discriminate particularly well between normals and aphasics with high levels of ability in comparison with discriminations on the BDAE comprehension section and the PICA. Poeck et al. (1972) demonstrated independence of TT performance and the fluency–nonfluency dimension in aphasic patients.

R. Cohen et al. (1977; 1980) studied construct validity and other aspects of TT validity. The memory component of TT performance was examined by Lesser (1976), R. Cohen et al. (1987), and Gutbrod et al. (1985), who concluded that the test measures deficits in the short-term storage of highly specific information in aphasics. In contrast, Riedel and Studdert-Kennedy (1985) claimed that a general cognitive deficit is responsible for poor TT performance. In Alzheimer's disease patients, Swihart and Panisset (1989) found that a short version of the test correlated only weakly with other simple auditory–verbal comprehension tasks, but highly with the Mini-Mental State Examination because of strong perseverative tendencies found in that patient population. A modified version was used successfully as a screening test to discriminate between 37 normal and 53 language-delayed children (Cole and Fewell, 1983), and in a similar German study comparing normal, right hemisphere–damaged, and aphasic children (Gutbrod and Michel, 1986).

The TT has maintained consistent popularity as both a clinical and an investigative instrument, and has also been examined for use as a therapeutic tool (Holland and Sonderman, 1974; West, 1973). Two major compilations of work with the TT are available (Boller and Dennis, 1979; McNeil and Prescott, 1978). At least three English-language versions are commercially available (Benton et al., 1994; McNeil and Prescott, 1978; Spreen and Strauss, 1998).

The TT's advantages lie in sound discriminative validity, portability, and brief administration time. R. Brookshire's (1973) early advice remains valid, that is, that the clinician should keep in mind that, although it is a sensitive indicator of comprehension deficits, the TT relies on a limited stimulus array. Other tests of auditory comprehension (e.g., the ACTS) may be used to supplement the TT. Rao (1990) also points out that the test introduces a somewhat artificial test situation and therefore has less "eco-validity" than functional communication measures. Other comprehension tests include Lexical Understanding with Visual and Semantic Distractors (LUVS; Bishop and Byng, 1984), which focuses on semantic comprehension, and an object-manipulation test designed to measure syntactic comprehension (Caplan, 1987).

Verbal Fluency Measures

Verbal fluency tasks (also called controlled oral word association or, simply, COWA) require an individual to generate as many words as possible within a restricted domain of possible responses during a defined period of time. For example, an average, neurologically intact, mentally healthy adult should be able to generate a dozen or more words that begin with the letter *S* (phonemic restriction) or up to roughly 20 animal names (semantic restriction) in a trial that lasts 60 seconds. Usually, fewer words can be generated if the first letter is used as the restriction compared to using a category like animals. A normal performance would usually be completed without any repetitions or other errors; occasionally, an error or two might occur and—more often than not—the person will recognize that they have already used the word. A close look at the performance can reveal that the person employed a cognitive strategy that resulted in a very effective use of the task's limited time, that is, starting with pets, continuing with birds, farm animals, etc. While most people produce the majority of their responses at the beginning of the time allotted per trial and trail off over time, others who may be prone to some performance anxiety show a little flustering at the start but then produce the bulk of their responses. Unlike most other aphasia-relevant tests, verbal fluency tasks do not have low ceilings when used in neurologically intact populations; this has made them popular for use in general testing.

A small number of standardized verbal fluency measures is available for clinical use. These measures may be distinguished by whether they require written or oral responses and whether they have letter-based (i.e., phonemic) or category-based (i.e., semantic) performance constraints. The most common verbal fluency measures are letter-based. These can be found as subtests of aphasia batteries, though they are frequently used as stand-alone measures. The phonemic task requires the patient to say as many word associations as possible to a specific letter of the alphabet, in a limited time period (usually 60 seconds). Instructions usually exclude the use of proper names and the use of the same stem word with different suffixes. The first of these tests (using the letters *F-A-S*) was developed by Spreen and Benton (1969, 1977) and included as a subtest of the NCCEA battery. The other frequently used version was created in the 1970s by Benton and Hamsher as part of the MAE battery (Benton et al., 1994a).

The category-based constraint that is used most often is the listing of animals, a semantic task that is found in the Stanford-Binet intelligence test, and in the BDAE and WAB aphasia batteries. Other semantic measures include the listing of items in a supermarket, included in the Dementia Rating Scale (Mattis et al., 2001) and in versions used by both Monsch and colleagues (1992) and Troyer (2000); the Set Test, which includes trials for animal, color, fruit, and town-name categories (Abrahams et al., 2000; Isaacs and Kennie, 1973); and "action fluency" (Piatt et al., 1999a,b). A variant on semantic constraints is the "switch format," which requires the individual to alternate between categories, such as fruits and furniture (e.g., Baldo et al., 2001); this variant is consistent with increasing demands on executive functions.

Not all fluency tasks are verbal in nature. Other restricted fluency tasks include several forms of design (sometimes called "figural" or "nonverbal") fluency (e.g., Jones-Gotman and Milner, 1977; Regard et al., 1982), and an olfactory-based measure of "odor fluency," which asks individuals to name as many things they can think of that smell like a certain odorant that is provided to them (Bacon Moore et al., 1999).

Educational level exerts a significant influence on verbal fluency tasks. In one large-scale study, for example, healthy older individuals at the highest educational level (i.e., 13 or more years of education) produced more than twice as many words as those in the lowest educational level (i.e., 0 to 6 years) (Crossley et al., 1997). Age also can exert an influence on verbal fluency performance, with older individuals producing fewer words than younger individuals.

Verbal fluency tasks provide a fast, efficient assessment in aphasic patients. It is important to note that these tests do not measure the fluency of conversational speech, as used in dividing aphasia subtypes into "fluent" and "nonfluent" forms. Aphasics who perform poorly produce only a few correct responses on these tasks; they may produce fewer words in general or they may generate a number of words, including many errors. Paraphasic errors may be elicited by the nature of the task demands. Performance on these tasks can be compromised not only in aphasia but also in other neurobehavioral syndromes resulting from anterior pathology or from diffuse neurodegenerative disease processes. Patients with nonaphasic brain damage often produce performances that are intermediate between normal levels and the performances of individuals with aphasia. As will be noted later, in some etiologies (particularly AD), semantic fluency is notably more difficult to perform than letter-based fluency—a pattern opposite to what is commonly observed in healthy individuals.

Few areas related to aphasia assessment have seen as much purely neuropsychological research interest over the past decade than the measurement and the neuroanatomical bases of performances on these tasks. Several clinical and research reasons account for this expansion of interest. In particular, the use of verbal fluency measures has increased in relation to an expanded assessment of so-called executive functions, which is central for patients with known or presumed frontal lobe pathology, especially traumatic brain injury (e.g., Tranel et al., 1994). In these populations, performance on the test is examined as much for a look at fluency and maintenance of rule set as for actual linguistic output. Some studies have also used variations of verbal fluency testing to examine age-related changes in executive functioning (Bryan and Luszcz, 2000), making use of an excluded-letter verbal fluency methodology (e.g., saying as many words as possible that do not contain an A; Bryan et al., 1997). Performance in the verbal modality has also been contrasted with somewhat similar task demands employing a nonverbal modality—(nonverbal figural or design fluency). However, studies of a dissociation between left (verbal fluency) and right (nonverbal fluency) frontal lobes show a complex relationship: an association between left frontal lobe lesions and defective verbal fluency, but no lateralizing relationship with defective figural fluency (e.g., Tucha et al., 1999). Verbal (and nonverbal) fluency measures are now being employed as subtests in new standardized batteries of executive functioning, such as the

Delis-Kaplan Executive Function System (D-KEFS; Baldo et al., 2001; Delis et al., 2001).

In addition to the lexical demands of these controlled word association tasks that are sensitive to overall word knowledge, effective performance requires attention and memory resources, as well as the ability to process information rapidly under time pressure and a complex of so-called executive function demands, such as planning and monitoring performance and the ability to shift mental sets. The cognitive correlates of verbal fluency in a sample of normal adults was examined by Ruff et al. (1997), who concluded that a distinction should be made in interpreting performance on these tasks between *(a)* poor word fluency based upon poor general vocabulary level or impaired attention; and *(b)* defective word fluency performances associated with dominant prefrontal lobe involvement.

A factor analysis was performed including word fluency with the letters *F*, *A*, and *S*, and performance on other tests sensitive to abnormal frontal lobe function (Wisconsin Card Sorting Test, Stroop Test, and Auditory Consonant Test) and performances on a short-form of the WAIS-R, the Rey Complex Figure Test, and Wechsler Memory Scale subtests (Boone et al., 1998), using 138 psychiatric patients and 112 controls with a mean age of 55.5 years and average educational level of nearly 14 years. A three-factor solution emerged: all three factors were associated with one higher-order "frontal lobe" factor. These factors were labeled as "cognitive flexibility," "speeded processing," and "basic and divided attention and short-term memory." Word fluency loaded on the "speeded processing" factor alongside performance on the Stroop Test and the WAIS-R Digit Symbol subtest. The authors concluded that word fluency failure can have as much to do with an impairment in speed of information processing as with an impairment in the generation of lexical items. Crockett et al. (2001) analyzed the results of 1220 neuropsychological hospital referrals with a mean age of 43 years, mean education of 12.5 years, and a mean IQ of 94.5. They found that F-A-S loaded on a separate factor in a heterogeneous battery of tests as well as in a battery of oral-verbal tests. They concluded that word fluency reflected "an aspect of cognitive functioning that clearly differed from both general neuropsychological test scores as well as from scores on tests of specific verbal skills" (p. 2).

Perhaps the most sophisticated explorations of a brain–behavior relationship for this contrast in fluency performances have been offered by Stuss and colleagues (1998) and by Gourovitch and colleagues (2000). Both offer underlying neuroanatomical support for the behavioral findings like those reported previously by Ruff et al. (1997). Stuss and colleagues examined fluency performances in a sample of 74 adults with single brain lesions classified as: *(a)* left or right dorsolateral and/or striatal frontal lesions; *(b)* left, right, or bilaterally superior medial frontal lesions; *(c)* left, right, or bilaterally inferior medial frontal lesions, *(d)* left temporal lesions; *(e)* left parietal lesions; and *(f)* a broader right-sided nonfrontal-lesion group [all based upon computed tomography (CT) and magnetic resonance imaging (MRI) findings]. Those with lesions of the dorsolateral and/or striatal areas of the left frontal lobe were the most impaired. Superior medial frontal lobe regions of either hemisphere had only a moderate impact on performance. Left parietal lobe lesions also were associated with performance deficits. All these areas were associated with performance decrements regardless of whether the fluency task was phonemically or semantically constrained, lending support to an increasingly sophisticated neuroanatomical understanding that verbal fluency deficits may be most notable in regions traditionally associated with language functioning and expressive aphasic symptomatology, but are not limited to them or to any single neurobehavioral syndrome.

Gourovitch and colleagues examined PET-based regional cerebral blood flow patterns in a sample of 18 normal adult subjects under three conditions: phonemic fluency, semantic fluency, and a control (nonfluency) language task. So-called subtle differences in activation patterns for phonemic versus semantic fluency were discerned: relatively greater activation of left frontal cortex for phonemic fluency and relatively greater activation of left temporal cortex for semantic fluency.

Increased interest has focused on contrasting phonemic (i.e., letter-based) versus semantic (category-based) fluency. The different task demands have given rise to hypotheses about the nature of fluency performances per se, the underlying neuroanatomical bases of different types of verbal fluency, and performance differences attributable to etiologic differences in neurological disease processes. This facet has seen much interest in examining healthy elderly individuals and patients with dementing disorders.

In patients with dementia, category (semantic) fluency tends to be more affected than letter association (phonemic fluency) (Butters et al., 1987; Monsch et al., 1992, 1994). There have been a number of research efforts to explore this apparent semantic deficit and to better understand it, including A. Sherman and Massman's 1999 study that confirmed this discrepancy in the majority (66.8%) of their subjects with Alzheimer's disease, but also reported the presence of a sizable minority

of individuals where the opposite pattern was noted; these two group-
ings did not show any difference in their performance on other neuropsychological measures.

These hypotheses about differences in semantic versus phonemic processing in normal and diseased conditions have been addressed in an
accumulating number of different neurological etiologies, for example,
Parkinson's disease (Piatt et al., 1999; van Spaendonck et al., 1996), unilateral pallidotomy in Parkinson's disease (Rettig et al., 2000), Alzheimer's disease, and Huntington's disease (e.g., Epker et al., 1999; Suhr
and Jones, 1998), mild and moderate AD versus vascular dementia (Crossley et al., 1997), unilateral temporal lobe epilepsy before and after neu-
rosurgical intervention (R. Martin et al., 1990), amyotrophic lateral sclerosis (Abrahams et al., 2000), and traumatic brain injury (Jurado et al.,
2000). Robert and colleagues (1998) examined distinctions between the
tasks in a psychiatric population (schizophrenia) versus healthy adults. A
generally consistent finding among the studies that have examined diffuse
or multifocal neurodegenerative processes is to suggest the presence of
more notable semantic (relative to phonemic) deficits and to provide interpretations of these deficits as reflecting degradation in semantic knowledge and access to this knowledge, though the nature and severity of the
deficit does not necessarily allow a distinction between different disease
processes (e.g., Binetti et al., 1995; Crossley et al., 1997).

Verbal fluency measures have also been used for an expanded exploration of language function in the healthy elderly, such as the Canadian
Study of Health and Aging (1994) and in normative studies designed to
extend original norms into an older population (e.g., Ivnik et al., 1996).
In addition, these measures have been used as screening tests for cognitive decline and batteries to rule out dementia. For example, MAE
COWA was one of a set of three brief measures (together with temporal
orientation and the Benton Visual Retention Test) employed by Eslinger
et al. (1985) in their brief battery of neuropsychological tasks found to
be sensitive to mental decline in the elderly.

Finally, qualitative interests in more fully understanding verbal fluency have led to extensions of scoring beyond the number of correct
responses. The fullest exploration here has been the analysis of "clustering" and "switching" performances. This has been examined in normal adults (Troyer, 2000), brain-damaged patients (Troyer et al., 1997,
Poreh, 2000), in dementia and normal elderly (Epker et al., 1999; Tröster et al., 1998), and in schizophrenia (Robert et al., 1998). "Switching"
in performance is based upon what could be considered the optimal
approach to the task: the subject could mentally identify a subcategory

of words, exhaust it in performance, then "switch" to another sub-category, and so on. "Clustering" refers to the production of contiguous words that are within a subcategory, such as "*fa*cile . . . *fa*bulous . . . *fa*st . . . *fa*ng . . . *fa*cade . . . ," as "Fa" words or a set of zoo animals ("giraffe . . . rhino . . . elephant . . . lion . . . tiger . . .") in animal fluency. While clustering may have a clear language-related or lexical basis, switching is more closely associated with the so-called frontal or executive functions and—at least descriptively—has commonality with other neuropsychological measures like the Wisconsin Card Sorting Test. Troyer (2000) offered a proposed set of scoring rules in an appendix to her paper. An unresolved problem with this approach, though, is that the scoring depends upon the rules established by the researchers or clinicians, not by the person performing the task. For example, ". . . cats . . . dogs . . ." might not be scored as a cluster if the rules do not provide for "house pets" to be a cluster. Even if it did, however, the response set may have been broadened to include ". . . bee . . . cats . . . dogs . . . pig. . . ," that is, the person was clustering together all the popular expressions he knew that involved animals: ". . . as busy as a *bee*; it's raining *cats* and *dogs*; as messy as a *pig* sty. . . ." In this case, the test rules would not capture the real response-generating cluster that the patient was actually employing. An even more detailed ap-proach to verbal fluency scoring has been presented by Giovannetti and colleagues (Giovannetti et al., 2001; Giovannetti-Carew et al., 1997), who added an "Association Index" measure to the examination of se-mantic clustering of animal fluency responses across an objective listing of different attributes (e.g., animal size, habitat, native versus foreign location, and class [such as mammal, reptile, or fish]).

Written verbal fluency

Thurstone Word Fluency Test. The Thurstone test, created in the 1930s as part of the broader Primary Mental Abilities Test (Thurstone, 1938), was the first of the psychometrically based word fluency mea-sures used in examining brain-damaged individuals. It is a written-response, letter-constrained measure. The patient is first required to write as many words beginning with a specific letter (i.e., the letter *S*) in a period of 5 minutes. Next, the person is required to write as many four-letter words that begin with the letter *C* as possible during a 4-minute trial.

Aphasia assessment at bedside or clinically had included testing flu-ency before it, but the Thurstone word fluency test offered a greater degree of standardization in assessing performance on this type of task.

Because of the frequent presence of a dominant-side hemiparesis in poststroke aphasic patients, this written test has been used only infrequently in aphasia examinations. This limitation contributed to the development of the oral-response approach by Benton and colleagues, although the written test continued to see use in examining individuals with frontal lobe disease, for example, Milner's (1964) examination of patients with left and right, frontal and temporal lobectomies in which she reported the test's sensitivity to left frontal lobe involvement. The increased need to comprehensively examine individuals with traumatic brain injury (TBI) has resulted in renewed interest in the Thurstone test.

Pendleton and colleagues (1982) examined Thurstone performances in a sample of 203 brain-damaged and 134 normal individuals. Patients were categorized by a set of focal lesion localizations or placed in a diffuse lesion category. In the normal sample, test performance correlated .46 with education and −.22 with age, a pattern also observed in the patient sample (.31 and −.16, respectively). The authors reported that test performance was sensitive to cerebral involvement in general and that individuals with focal frontal lobe involvement performed more poorly than those with focal nonfrontal lesions.

A new set of analyses of Thurstone performance has been provided by M. Cohen and Stanczak (2000). Reliability and validity were reported for 70 normal adult students aged 18 to 60 years and from archival data of 296 brain-damaged patients (etiologies predominantly TBI, CVA, seizure disorders, and neurodegenerative disorders) and 188 normal controls. A 6-week retest of 70 adult students resulted in a reliability coefficient of .79, in the context of a notable practice effect of an average eight-word gain on the second administration. Interrater reliability in this sample was .98. Thurstone performance correlated .81 with the F-A-S and .72 with the MAE COWA (using the letters CFL or PRW) test in these healthy adults. Archival results from the brain-damaged and the neurologically intact subjects showed that these two groups could be discriminated from each other, but that Thurstone performance did not clearly delineate left versus right, anterior versus posterior, and focal versus diffuse lesions. Education was noted to be related to task performance, but age was not; no definite conclusions were reached about the role of gender. A relationship between measured intellectual functioning and the component tasks of the test was noted: the letter C test was the best discriminator for the presence of brain damage in the low- (less than or equal to 89) and average-level (90 to 109) Wechsler VIQ groups, while the total score was best for those in the high-level (110 or higher) VIQ group.

Oral verbal fluency

NCCEA Word Fluency Subtest. Spreen and Benton's NCCEA version of the Word Fluency Subtest (also known as The F-A-S test or, simply, F-A-S) from the 1960s was the first of the modern measures of verbal fluency. It requires the patient to say as many words as possible that begin with the letters *F*, *A*, and *S* within 60-second time periods for each letter. Proper names and words that differ only in suffix are not acceptable; this information is provided to the individual as part of the test's instructions. Performance is gauged in terms of the sum of admissible words across all three trials. Spreen and Strauss (1998) provide formal administration and scoring rules for the F-A-S test.

Normative data from the test authors, along with corrections for age and level of education, are available (Spreen and Benton, 1977; Spreen and Strauss, 1998), as are additional normative studies that revised and extended the original norms (Tombaugh et al., 1999; summarized in their Table 2 on page 171 of the citation).

The Tombaugh et al. norms are based upon the performance of 1300 healthy individuals with English as their primary language (895 community-dwelling healthy individuals aged from 16 to 85 years, with an average educational level of 12.9 years, and 405 participants in the Canadian Study of Health and Aging; age 65 to 95 years, mean education 10.5 years), all of whom had a consensus diagnosis of "no cognitive impairment."

Performance on the F-A-S test is influenced by demographic factors. Individuals with higher levels of education tend to produce more correct words than those with fewer years of education. Older individuals tend to produce fewer words than younger individuals. However, level of education is related to performance to a stronger degree than is age. Gender has not been consistently noted to have a significant relation to task performance. Yeudall et al. (1986) reported a correlation of .32 with education and .19 with age. Tombaugh et al. (1999) performed a regression analysis using education, age, and gender. Education accounted for 18.6% of the variability in task performance and age accounted for 11.0%.

The letters employed in the NCCEA version are of the "easy" level. Borkowski et al. (1967) examined the number of associations by normal adult females for the letters of the alphabet. The number of associations was related to the difficulty, as defined both by the Thorndike-Lorge (1944) word count (.80) and the number of words per letter in *Webster's New Collegiate Dictionary* (.74). The authors also reported that a heterogeneous sample of brain-damaged patients performed less well than normal adults at all levels of severity, lending validity to the testing method. Patients with low IQ scores were better differentiated with easy-level letters, whereas patients with high IQ scores were better distinguished with more difficult letters.

Tombaugh et al. (1999) reported good internal consistency between the three letters of the test, with a coefficient of .83. Interscorer reliability on the F-A-S test is near perfect. One-year test-retest reliability has been reported as .70 (Snow and Tierney, 1988). Surprisingly, test-retest reliability after an interval of more than 5 years remains at an equivalent level, that is, .74 (Tombaugh et al., 1999).

F-A-S test performance shows modest levels of correlation with measures of intellectual functioning. Tombaugh et al. (1999) reported a correlation of .25 between the task and the WAIS-R Vocabulary subtest. Correlation with WAIS-R Verbal IQ was .14, and with Performance IQ .29 (Yeudall et al., 1986).

Adults with traumatic brain injuries had mean scores of less than 28 (M. Sarno et al., 1986), similar to means found by Spreen and Benton (1977) for nonaphasic brain-damaged patients, whereas aphasics ranged from 0 to 46 with a mean of 11.5 words (Spreen and Benton, 1977). Alzheimer's disease and Huntington's disease patients did not show reduced performance levels, but did produce more intrusion errors (wrong letters), perseverations, and variations (fish, fishy, fishing) (Adams, personal communication, 1988). E. Miller and Hague (1975) and Murdoch et al. (1987), however, did find reduced verbal fluency in AD patients, whereas patients with depression mimicking dementia showed little change compared to normals (Kronfol et al., 1978). The F-A-S was also part of the computerized AD Assessment Battery (Branconnier, 1986) and discriminated well between AD and normal control subjects. Consistent with clinical–anatomic expectations, F-A-S performance correlated with glucose metabolic rates in left prefrontal regions in poststroke aphasic patients (Karbe et al., 1995).

Variations on the test may be found in the literature. For example, Tucha et al. (1999) report using just the letter S from the F-A-S test and proceeding with that letter for a trial duration of 3 minutes, while Jurado and colleagues (2000) used all three letters, but expanded trial length to 90 seconds for each letter.

MAE Controlled Oral Word Association Subtest. Benton et al.'s (1994) version, the MAE Controlled Oral Word Association subtest (COWA), differs from the NCCEA in using three letters of progressively increasing associative difficulty; otherwise the testing is quite similar. Two equivalent versions (*C-F-L* and *P-R-W*) are available, allowing for repeated or follow-up administrations. Normative information, validation data, and age and level of education corrections are provided in the MAE manual.

The test was subjected to a normative updating by Ruff et al. (1996), who reported that test scores in their sample were generally higher than those shown in the original Benton et al. norms. The authors followed the standard MAE procedures for the task. They examined performance in 360 normal native-English speakers ranging in age from 16 to 70 years and in education from 7 to 22 years. The authors noted that this sample had a generally higher level of education than the sample of Benton et al. and that this may have contributed to differences between the original and updated norms. The subjects resided in predominantly urban and suburban settings in California, Michigan, and the U.S. East Coast, again somewhat different than the more rural original normative sample.

Ruff and colleagues reported that the internal consistency of the test was .83. Test-retest stability was examined in 120 subjects with an interval of 6 months. A significant correlation of .74 was reported, although there was an average gain of three words on the second administration. More years of education was related to a greater number of words generated on the test. Somewhat at odds to other findings, the authors reported that age was not related to word fluency performance and that a modest gender effect (i.e., well-educated females performing better than similarly educated males) was present. Normative tables are provided in the citation.

The COWA was one of the tests used to create the extended neuropsychological normative data set for healthy older individuals in the Mayo's Older Americans Normative Studies (MOANS) project (Ivnik et al., 1996). MOANS subjects were normal adults above the age of 54 years and living independently; age ranged into the upper 90s. The sample was predominantly Caucasian. The MOANS data have their own age- and education-corrected scaled scores that are defined in the citation. Seven hundred forty-three individuals completed the COWA. Correlations between COWA and education, age, and gender were .38, −.15, and .12,[3] respectively.

---

[3] It is not clear from the primary reference whether the very modest correlation between gender and performance reflected better male or female performances.

The C-F-L version of the COWA was employed by Iverson et al. (1999) to develop normative information for individuals following traumatic brain injury. They examined performances in a sample of 669 individuals with an average age of 36.1 years and an average educational level of 12.0 years. The sample was categorized into three levels of head trauma: mild, moderate, and severe. Individuals were tested in the acute stage of recovery (usually within the first week postinjury), that is, when Galveston Orientation and Amnesia Test (GOAT) scores exceeded 75. The task was sensitive to reduced verbal fluency in all groups, and performance showed a clear relation to severity. The MAE COWA is a part of the Traumatic Brain Injury Model Systems neuropsychology battery, used to collect standardized, longitudinal testing data from brain-damaged patients at a number of U.S. settings (e.g., Kreutzer et al., 1993). Model Systems patients are at least 16 years of age at the time of injury, had brain injuries that required admission to hospital and subsequent inpatient rehabilitation, and had brain injuries documented by loss of consciousness, posttraumatic amnesia, or objective neurological findings. Millis and colleagues (2001) reported 5-year Model Systems neuropsychological outcome data, including verbal fluency performance. COWA task performance in a sample of 176 patients indicated that mean performance at 5 years postinjury was a score of approximately 30 words, using MAE education and age corrections. Performances at a level less than the 3rd percentile were observed in 17.6% of the sample.

Wertz version. Wertz's (1979) format employs easy-level letters (i.e., S, T, P, and C). In contrast to the F-A-S and the MAE COWA, proper names are permitted. Age and level of education corrections are not employed for this task. Normative data have been provided by Wertz and Lemme (1974). Standardized instructions for Wertz's format are available in the protocol manual of the Veteran's Administration project (Wertz and Lemme, 1974). Wertz and collaborators reported correlations of COWA performance with PICA overall and verbal dimensions, and with performance on the last section of the version of the TT used in their study.

Animal name fluency. Animal naming is the most popular of the oral-response, semantic-constraint fluency tasks available for clinical use. The animal category has a tradition of use in child-evaluation settings as a subtest of the Stanford-Binet intelligence test. The most popular adult version of animal fluency was used in the original version and first revision of the BDAE battery (Goodglass and Kaplan, 1983). However, the subtest was removed by the authors from the most recent edition of the battery (i.e., BDAE-3; Goodglass et al., 2000). Instead, it has been included in the new Delis-Kaplan Executive Function Scale (D-KEFS, Delis et al., 2001). Individuals are instructed to say as many different animal names as possible. An example is provided, which the individual may use in their performance. A 90-second recording period is allowed, with responses recorded in 15-second blocks. The best 60-second period (usually the first 60 seconds) is scored. In addition to the norms accompanying the test, normative data for this task were obtained by Tombaugh et al. (1999) together with norms for the F-A-S test. Tombaugh et al. used the instructions reported by Rosen (1980) having the subject say as many animal names as possible during a 60-second trial. Task performance was found to be related to educational level and age. To a very modest degree, performance was related to gender (i.e., males produced, on average, one more name than females). Regardless of age, persons with eight or fewer years of education produced an average of approximately 14 animal names, persons completing 12 years of education produced an average of approximately 17 animal names, and persons completing 16 years of education produced an average of 19 animal names. From the ages of 16 through 59, average performances were in the range of 20 to 22 animal names, decreasing with age higher than 59 years. Animal and F-A-S fluency performances correlated at a level of .52. The correlation with WAIS-R Vocabulary performance was .17. Using the same format, Kempler and colleagues (1998) explored the effects of ethnicity on animal fluency performances in a sample of 317 healthy individuals between 54 and 99 years of age. They found a striking difference between Hispanic and Vietnamese immigrants, which they attributed to the predominance of one-syllable animal names in Vietnamese and multisyllable animal names in Spanish. This study also included scores for Chinese immigrants, Caucasians, and African Americans. The authors reported education and age effects consistent with those reported by Tombaugh and colleagues.

Another version of Animal Fluency can be found in the WAB (Kertesz, 1982), which also uses a straight 60-second trial. Other variations include the version used by P. Roberts and Le Dorze (1998) to explore bilingual verbal fluency performances in both neurologically intact and aphasic individuals; it allows for 2-minute performance trials. Animal Fluency is also a subtest of the CERAD (Consortium for the Establishment of a Registry for Alzheimer's Disease) dementia battery (Morris et al., 1989).

One procedural and interpretative problem with the use of Animal Fluency, especially in comparison with letter fluency is that performance is typically based upon a single trial, while letter fluency tasks proceed through several trials. This problem can be avoided if several trials for different categories are used. The Set Test discussed earlier provides for multiple performance trials. The D-KEFS measure of category fluency mentioned earlier includes trials for both animals and boys' names. The Category Fluency Test described by Acevedo and colleagues (2000) includes three trials: animals, vegetables, and fruits. The authors provide normative data for this measure from a sample of 424 English-speaking and 278 Spanish-speaking healthy adults living in Florida, aged 50 to 90 years.

Summary of verbal fluency tests

Tests of verbal fluency are quick and simple and do not require any test material except a timer. Their reliability and validity have been firmly established and reported by both the original test authors and by external researchers. These tests may not be very sensitive in discrimination of subjects at lower levels of ability, but they are capable of screening for the presence of less severe defects. The use of these tasks in aphasia assessment is well established. The extension of these tests into the examination of executive functions has been found to have utility. One factor analysis shows that performance on these types of tasks represents a different neuropsychological factor than other so-called frontal lobe measures, suggesting that even a simple screening for executive function deficits needs to involve more than a single test and that performance on a measure of verbal fluency offers a unique facet in that screening. These tasks have found a place in geriatric assessments as well.

Clinicians have a choice of several types of fluency measures. The clinical examination will help determine whether it would be worthwhile to explore performance under both phonemic and semantic constraints. However, having access to both formats in one's set of available test instruments is clearly practical. The F-A-S and the MAE COWA both have had a contemporary normative updating in large groups of individuals. Both tests examine performance over several (i.e., three) trials, unlike the more common measures of semantic fluency, which usually rely upon a single trial. Although measures of verbal fluency generally show reasonably good test-retest reliability, research examining day-to-day changes do report a good deal of performance variability (Boyle et al., 1991).

Using standardized semantic fluency tasks that have more than a single trial may also be prudent for diagnostic use. The animal fluency task offers two features that are relatively unique and that might be useful to explore in letter-based measures: dividing performance into 15-second blocks and using the best 60-second run in a 90-second trial. The first might be useful in aphasia testing, as some findings point to changes over time in the quality of responding on these tasks (Adams et al., 1989). The second might prove useful in general practice, as it is our observation that fluency tasks may be sensitive to levels of performance anxiety in a small subset of patients and in normal individuals who require a little bit longer than average to 'warm up' to the task demands. Finally, the development of scoring systems such as the analysis of clustering-and-switching has been based on nonaphasic samples. Though such a system might be inappropriate in moderate to severe aphasias, useful clinical variability and suggestions for treatment might be gleaned from looking at these measures in the performance of mildly impaired aphasics or those with a residual anomic deficit.

8

Functional Communication

How a patient performs on a diagnostic measure of acquired aphasia does not automatically predict how he or she communicates in the everyday environment. A diagnostic instrument will be useful to discern the nature and severity of the deficit, but the functional impairment in daily living caused by the deficit must be treated as a separate variable. Many speech clinicians have employed the 1980 World Health Organization (WHO) classification system—which offers operationalizations of deficit, impairment, and handicap—to help develop these distinctions in understanding language disorders (e.g., Murray and Chapey, 2001). Communication has at its core the basic language skills sampled in diagnostically oriented measures as discussed in earlier chapters, but it also includes a diverse set of nonlinguistic components. If one views communication as the functional goal of language, then tests of functional communication assess a much broader domain that is not limited to language. The social-communication demands placed on an aphasic patient are not limited to the improvement of deficits in core language skills. While communicating in everyday life may allow one to interact without the artificial rules and boundaries of a test, rules exist nonetheless: communication requires a relatively rapid and subtle give and take between speaker and listener or listeners. While some listeners may have the patience to take on a larger-than-typical conversational burden, others may not be willing to allocate the aphasic any needed additional time, and still others may be impulsive or disorganized themselves in their own communication. On the other hand, the artificially structured demands of a testing laboratory may actually provide support to some patients with associated cognitive and executive function problems.

These issues transcend the traditional diagnosis of aphasia. Speech pathologists such as Martha Taylor Sarno and Audrey Holland were early proponents in the 1960s and 1970s for examining the ability of aphasic patients to function in their communicative environments, regardless of how they perform on standard diagnostic instruments. They proposed that placing functional communication alongside diagnostic results would provide a fuller picture of the person who had acquired an aphasic disorder. Sarno's Functional Communication Profile (Taylor, 1965) was the first attempt to standardize the rating of the functional usefulness of language abilities in the everyday life of the patient. The Communicative Abilities of Daily Living test (Holland, 1980) was the first psychometric instrument to index the degree of disability faced by the patient in attempting to communicate in daily life, using observations of actual interactions. Diagnosticians have always been aware of these aspects of communication; Hildred Schuell—who developed the first version of her comprehensive diagnostic battery in the 1940s—included real-life functional tasks (e.g., making change) in her assessment, as well as consideration of how well a person's message was communicated, and the coherence, intelligibility, and relevance of the message.

A distinction between the selective language samples that are elicited in the typically structured test setting and a patient's ability to communicate in his or her everyday environment has intuitive value to the speech clinician in contemporary daily practice. Developing this test modality has been one of the primary assessment trends in examining language disorders over the past several decades. Among the reasons for this has been the sense that simply assessing the deficits an individual has acquired as the result of brain injury or stroke does not fully convey the problems that the individual may confront in communicating in a social world and also conveys little of the success an individual might have in his or her attempts to convey information and interact with others despite these deficits. Additional reasons include the expansion of speech and language services, particularly the provision of services to patients with head injuries (e.g., Larkins et al., 2000), and public policy and other practical reasons such as far stricter third-party reimbursement rules for clinical services (e.g., Frattali, 2000). Through the 1980s, such instruments may have been viewed as simply an option to supplement diagnostic batteries, but contemporary use approaches a regular balance between them and traditional diagnostic tests.

As Sarno and Holland promoted a functional approach, there was also increased attention given to that component of basic psycholinguistic applications that addressed the social or interactive nature of discourse aspects of the pragmatics of language (an early example being Prutting and Kirchner's [1987] Pragmatic Protocol). It is not always easy to draw a distinction between functional and pragmatic communication, nor is such a distinction necessary for the use of these tests in daily practice. However, these instruments have established themselves alongside traditional diagnostic batteries toward either of two extremes of a spectrum of pragmatic communication: "macro," or global communicative effectiveness at one end, and measures with a foundation in "micro," or psycholinguistic aspects of discourse, on the other. Regardless of these anchors on the spectrum, functional features relate as much to a psychosocial model of aphasia and language disorders as a medical one. Conversation, authentic and relevant contexts, turn-taking, discourse, and adaptive psychosocial consequences all form features in this pragmatic communication approach (e.g., Simmons-Mackie, 2000). This chapter places most of its emphasis on "macro" instruments but also discusses "micro" ones as well, such as the Pragmatic Protocol.

A third area of increased clinical attention over this time period has been the elaboration of rating scales beyond their more traditional uses. These traditional uses included ratings to offer summary judgments of the severity of any symptom or syndrome (e.g., in disability and worker's compensation assessments of percentage loss of ability from premorbid levels). Traditional use also included the rating of specific aspects of a patient's behavior that would not be amenable to quantitative scoring, such as the Activities of Daily Living, or ADL, scales that gained popularity in the 1960s with physical rehabilitation therapists as ways to track rehabilitation progress (e.g., Katz et al., 1963). These traditional uses of rating scales developed into more functionally oriented uses, such as providing Quality of Life (QOL) ratings and to represent entire classes of function, as seen most fully in the Functional Independent Measures (FIMs) that became commonplace in rehabilitation therapy settings during the 1990s (e.g., State University of New York, 1993).

Quality of Life ratings have become an important aspect of measuring the success of rehabilitation (M. Sarno, 1997). In this context, QOL addresses the question of how a person experiences aphasia, how its meaning influences behavior and interaction—the human response to an unexpected and unwanted life event (Sarno, 1997), and includes psychosocial factors such as loneliness, difficulty making friends, lowered self-esteem, and depression. Specific instruments have been designed to measure QOL. These instruments include the Caregiver Burden Interview (Zarit et al., 1980), the Functional Life Scale (J. Sarno et al., 1973), the Geriatric Evaluation of Relative's Rating Instrument (Schwartz, 1983), and the Community Dependency Index (Ward et al., 1998). We do not examine QOL rating scales in the current work; readers interested in them can read, among other sources, a review by Crewe and Dijkers (1995).

Coincident with the measures examined in this chapter is the increasing use of functional independence measures, or FIMs (B. Hamilton et al., 1987; Frattali, 1993), in rehabilitation units, which include items ranging from sphincter control and feeding to communication. A large number of FIMs have been developed. Some of these scales can also be employed in self-ratings. For example, Hachisuka et al. (1997) report that self-ratings in 171 stroke patients without severe aphasia or dementia with the so-called Barthel Index—Motor Score showed a retest reliability of .90, and concurrent validity with 12 ADL items was .83. Sensitivity can be improved by expanding the number of categories in each ADL function to obtain reliable ratings of progress during rehabilitation (Shah et al., 1989), although Beckers et al. (1999) warn that such scales may have critical ceilings beyond which improvement can no longer be documented. Herrmann et al. (1995) found that patients with aphasia and their relatives show significantly more severe professional and social changes than those without aphasia. Progress in aphasia rehabilitation is now frequently defined as progress in functional communication, although Crockford and Lesser (1994) stated that the actual use of such scales by practicing clinicians seems to be limited. FIM instruments sometimes attempt to reduce entire cognitive domains, such as communication, to a single scale of independence and various levels of dependence. It should be noted that single FIMs representing entire domains such as "Language Functioning" or "Memory Functioning" would seem to be of questionable value and validity.

Given that rating scales are not a substitute for psychometric testing and run the risk of reflecting the subjective biases and experience limitations of the raters themselves, any proposed rating scale should be subjected to careful interrater reliability studies, and possible users of these scales should examine the results from these studies. The ASHA-FACS (discussed later) is an example of a scale where these types of reliability studies have been performed and are key to appreciating the value of the instrument.

The trend toward the use of rating scales of functional communication, particularly for program evaluation, has been criticized by Sacchett and Marshall (1992). They argue that material that has been "squeezed" out of a patient by role playing or verbal prompts does not reflect natural conversational abilities and that ratings of functional communication or QOL for the sake of justifying speech therapy costs may lead to forms of intervention that merely promote abilities in those areas of speech that are subject to rating. Instead, they advocate a case study approach along psycholinguistic lines, arguing that this will "repair" or improve language processing, generalizing to the overall language use.

The rating of functional language and verbal processing skills in daily living has also become a common feature in many geriatric rating scales (see review by DeBettignies and Mahurin, 1989) and is available as separate language ratings (Patient Functional Communication Screening Instrument, FCS; Toner et al., 1984; 1990) or in mental competence batteries (e.g., the Cognitive Competency Battery; Wang et al., 1986), but these omnibus measures for use with the elderly often lack suitable standardization and item range for use with aphasic patients. Le Dorze et al. (1994) reported on the development of a scale for use with long-term-care patients, including those with aphasia, dementia, or both, based on 196 statements about communicative acts in daily living.

The 1990s saw a rapid development of all instruments addressing functional communication, some of which are presented in more detail below. Manochiopinig et al. (1992) provided a detailed overview of where the field stood at the start of that decade. This new wave of measures included: the Communicative Effectiveness Index (CETI; Lomas et al., 1989), which utilized ratings from family members; the American Speech-Language-Hearing Association-Functional Assessment of Communication Skills for Adults (ASHA-FACS; Frattali et al., 1995), which returned to an observational approach in measurement; the 1999 revision of the CADL (CADL-2) by Holland et al.; and the Assessment of Language Related Functional Activities (ALFA; Baines et al.), also published in 1999, which offered normative data for individual discrete functional tasks. The end of the 1990s saw publication of a detailed review about the assessment and treatment-utilization of functional communication (Worrall and Frattali, 2000).

There are a number of other, less frequently used instruments. Some are not easily found or commercially available. Others are in the public domain, but have not found much use, such as the Communicative Competence Evaluation Instrument by Houghton and colleagues (1982). A British instrument, the Assessment of Communicative Effectiveness in Severe Aphasia (Cunningham et al., 1995), uses standard open-ended conversational questions, objects, and pictures, but has so far only been examined for interrater and test-retest reliability with 10 aphasic and 10 normal speakers. A Dutch test, the Amsterdam-Nijmegen Everyday Language Test (ANELT; Blomert et al., 1994), uses everyday scenarios (e.g., communicating with neighbors and dealing with salespersons) to rate the adequacy of the information that the patient communicates. It does so by examining how understandable the communicated message is and how intelligible the specific verbal utterance is. The test has two equivalent versions, promoting easy test-retest applications. ANELT psychometric properties have been examined in Dutch and German standardization samples and the test is commercially available in those languages; a commercial version of the test providing English normative data appears to have been pending for a number of years but is not yet available. The Edinburgh Functional Communication Profile (EFCP) was released and subsequently revised (Wirz et al., 1990). A commercial version of the EFCP had been available at an earlier time but now seems to be out of print. The Australian La Trobe Communication Questionnaire has been used in a program of research examining communicative effectiveness in adults with traumatic brain injury (Douglas et al., 2000).

Although varied in their format, functional measures are alike in that they avoid obtaining pure, isolated samples of specific language behaviors in favor of simulated communication settings, general ratings, and consideration of complex and multifaceted real-life tasks—such as the ability to communicate on the telephone, handle money, read newspapers and product labels, and ask for, correct, and impart significant information to and from others. Because of this attempt to simulate what is going to be confronted by the patient in everyday experience, the information gauged on these profiles is a unique contribution to the overall assessment of the aphasic patient. This contribution provides the clinician with descriptive information about the communicative status of the individual, which can be considered as a second dimension of information not directly obtained from diagnostic testing procedures (M. Sarno, 1984a).

ASHA Functional Assessment of Communication Skills for Adults

The American Speech-Language-Hearing Association Functional Assessment of Communication Skills for Adults (ASHA-FACS) (Frattali et al., 1995; available from the American Speech-Language-Hearing Association, cost $149) is probably the one measure most written about while it was being developed. Unlike many tests that develop in relative isolation in a single setting or between a small group of collaborators, the

FACS "grew up" in public (e.g., American Speech-Language-Hearing Association, 1990; Frattali, 1992; Frattali and Lynch, 1989; Worrall, 1992). The authors speak of this instrument as "a measure of basic functional skills that are common to the majority of individuals regardless of age, gender, socioeconomic status, education/vocational status, or cultural diversity" (Fratelli et al., 1995, p. 2). As such, the authors note that the instrument is designed to meet both clinical and policy goals. They also note that the FACS is not designed to replace diagnostic tests, as it does not identify impairments but provides information about the effects of these impairments.

The scale rates 43 items on a seven-point scale. The ratings are based on the observation of the therapist, but may include observations reported by others. The authors suggest that it takes about 20 minutes on average to complete the rating scale and that using the computerized version and increased experience with the scale should further reduce the time requirement.

Four communication domains are identified: Social Communication (21 items; e.g., refers to familiar people by name, understands facial expressions and tones of voice); Communication of Basic Needs (7 items; e.g., recognizes familiar faces and voices, makes needs to eat or to rest known); Reading, Writing, and Number Concepts (10 items; e.g., makes basic money transactions, fills out short forms, writes messages); and Daily Planning (5 items; e.g., tells time, uses a telephone, keeps scheduled appointments).

Individual items are rated on a seven-point scale (from "Does Not" to "Does," with intermediate levels of needed assistance). These items are used to derive Scales of Communication Independence for each domain and one overall score averaging all ratings across domains.

In addition, each domain is rated on five-point Scales of Qualitative Dimensions of Communication for the following: Adequacy (understanding of message and gets point across), Appropriateness (communication is relevant and done under the right circumstances), Promptness (responds without delay and in an efficient manner), and Communication Sharing (extent of burden to a communication partner). The range of points for the first three dimensions reflect the frequency with which the dimension is demonstrated during communication (from "never" to "always") and the range for the last dimension rates the burden on the person communicating with the patient from "all" to "equal."

A combined communication independence score can be calculated. The ratings for each domain of communication independence and for the qualitative dimensions may be entered into profiles that facilitate plotting of a patient's progress during therapy. Computer entry of each rating allows computerized scoring and profile preparation.

The development and standardization of the FACS has been well documented in the administration manual. The primary FACS field study involved 45 examiners at 12 sites who rated 131 adult aphasic patients with left hemisphere stroke and 54 adults with traumatic brain injury (TBI) related cognitive impairments of communication. Premorbidly all subjects were fluent English-speaking adults with basic reading and writing abilities. They showed adequate hearing and ability to see large print, based either on clinical report or screening. One hundred thirty-three of the 185 subjects were male, 116 were Caucasian, and 176 were right-handed. Forty-nine had attained neither a high-school diploma nor a GED degree. Aphasia severity was based upon WAB performances for the stroke sample (50 severe, 46 moderate, and 35 mild), and the severity of "cognitive-communication impairment" (11 severe, 26 moderate, and 17 mild) for the head-injured group was based upon performance on the Scales of Cognitive Ability for Traumatic Brain Injury (Adamovich and Henderson, 1992). Of the total sample, 136 were living with family, 28 were living on their own, 7 were living with friends, and 14 were living in institutional settings.

Each rating point is well defined, as reflected in an interrater reliability between .88 and .92 for communication independence scores (total .95) and quality of communication (.72 to .84, total .88). Intrarater reliability ranged from .94 to .99. Internal consistency averaged .82 within domains, and .78 between items and overall score.

The external validity of the Overall Communication Independence Score for the aphasic group was .73, measured against the WAB Aphasia Quotient, and ranged from .61 to .83 against the Functional Independence Measure (FIM; State University of New York, 1993). The external validity of the Overall Qualitative Dimension Score for the aphasic group was .78, measured against the WAB Aphasia Quotient, and ranged from .59 to .85 against the FIM. Similar values were found for the TBI group. Construct validity, measured with a principal component factor analysis, resulted in one major factor, with minor factors representing the four domain scores. Overall ratings of functional communication by clinicians and family members correlated with FACS scores at a level between .58 and .63.

The authors do not provide percentile or other derived scores, stating that normative data would not be appropriate for the FACS, as a client with normal language would obtain perfect scores on all ratings. Mean performance levels for the aphasic and the TBI groups are given, but, of course, they rely on the range of severity of language impairment in these specific populations. However, they do show the sensitivity of the FACS. This is further documented by an account of the discrimination of the scores between groups of patients with different levels of severity of impairment. K. Ross and Wertz (2001) reported a correlational analysis between several demographic features (age, gender, and educational level) and FACS performance in samples of adult aphasics and normal subjects. Correlations within the aphasic group were not significant; educational level and FACS Overall Communication Independence score were significantly correlated ($r = .56$) in the normal sample.

Perhaps in keeping with the increased time demands and decreased reimbursement opportunities in the speech therapy community, the FACS is designed to be completed by a clinician based upon his or her previous interactions with a patient. The clinician need not meet face-to-face with a patient specifically to complete the measure, but can rely upon treatment-based interactions. Indeed, if the clinician has not had exposure to that specific item of behavior, he or she may make use of third-party (e.g., family members or other members of a treatment team) commentary or may leave the item blank. The authors report that there can be some tolerance for incompleteness, while still allowing for domain and other scores to be determined. It is incumbent upon the clinician to rely only upon direct observations of the patient who has been using any required sensory acuity aids (e.g., hearing aids, eyeglasses).

Assessment of Language-Related Functional Activities

The Assessment of Language-Related Functional Activities (ALFA) (Baines et al., 1999; Pro-Ed, $154) is designed to answer the question: "Despite the person's impairment, is he or she able to integrate skills adequately to perform selected functional daily activities?" The authors assess performance on 10 tasks, such as counting money, telling time, addressing an envelope, writing a check and rebalancing a checkbook as a result of that check, using a calendar, understanding medication labels, using a telephone, and writing down a telephone message. Performance on task items is scored either "1" for correct or "0" for incorrect, no response, or "I don't know" responses.

The test appears designed to appeal to busy speech clinicians who might want to bring assessment into ongoing treatment services. Giving the entire ALFA is reported to take between 30 minutes and 2 hours. The authors indicate, though, that there is no need to complete the test in one sitting. Which tasks to attempt and in what order they are administered are at the discretion of the clinician. Stimuli are included in the test kit, including a movable-hand clock face, envelopes, and plastic medicine pills. Some "props" are required, such as a telephone and a local phone book, as well as some change and $1 and $5 bills.

The test was standardized on a sample of 495 adult patients and 150 normal adults in 32 U.S. states. Clinicians were solicited to use the instrument and submit their findings (unfortunately, details of their training and of standardization instructions are not reported in the test manual). In the patient sample, 54% were female, 91% were Caucasian, education was varied (18% did not complete high school, 34% were high school graduates, 23% obtained associate's or bachelor's degrees, and 8% had advanced degrees). Forty-three percent were 75 years of age or older. Cerebrovascular accidents were the most common medical etiology (with slightly more right than left hemisphere localization), followed by traumatic brain injury (5%) and dementia (4%). Twenty percent of the etiologies were simply noted as being "other." In the normal sample, 62% were female, 93% were Caucasian, education was varied (with slightly fewer less-than-high-school and slightly more advanced-degree members than in the patient sample). Thirty-two percent were 75 years of age or older.

Performance evaluation on the ALFA uses raw scores, categorized into three levels. Level 1 performance shows a high probability that a person can function independently on a task, with a lower cutoff of 1 standard deviation of the normal group's mean performance on the task. At the other end, Level 3 performance shows a high probability that a person cannot function independently on a task, with a cutoff representing the first quartile of the patient group's performance on the task. A Level 2 performance is intermediate between these two levels.

Reliability is reported in the test manual. Internal consistencies in the range of .80 to .88 were noted. Post hoc interrater reliability (i.e., only scoring previously completed profiles) for two raters and 30 profiles were reported to be .99. The test's authors claim that test-retest reliability would not be an appropriate measure of the ALFA's reliability; changes over time were assessed during acute recovery periods and showed improvements in the 9-to-14-day postevent period relative to performance in the first week after the neurological insult.

Validity was also addressed. Correlations between the ALFA and the Reading Comprehension Battery for Aphasia for 103 subjects ranged from .43 to .71. The test was reported to reflect group differences (rather ill defined) in treatment settings and to distinguish those with right-sided, left-sided, and multiple CVAs.

Communication Activities of Daily Living, 2nd Edition

The Communication Activities of Daily Living, 2nd ed. (CADL-2) (Holland et al., 1998; Pro-Ed, $177) is the revised version of the CADL (Holland, 1980). Italian (Pizzamiglio et al., 1984), Spanish (P. Martin et al., 1990), and Japanese (Watamori et al., 1987) versions of the original CADL are available. These instruments were "developed to assess the functional communication skills of adults with neurogenic disorders" (Holland et al., 1998, p. 9) using simulated daily-life activities. The original version of the test required patients to perform simulated daily activities, such as dealing with a receptionist, communicating with a doctor, driving, shopping, and making telephone calls; the CADL-2 retains this approach. The test manual outlines a deliberate effort to enhance the realistic nature of stimuli, by using photographs rather than line drawings and by using common, everyday reference materials. Some role-playing duties were required on the part of the clinician in the first version of the CADL. The revised version eliminates role playing. Given its inherent focus on communicative—rather than language—ability per se, "getting the message across" via oral, written, gestural, or any other modality is acknowledged as significant.

The CADL-2 has 50 items (reduced from 68 in the CADL), which are scored as "correct" (2 points), "adequate" (1 point), or "wrong" (0 points) in rating the patient's communication. For example, at one point the examiner asks the patient, "Your first name is _____, right?" (saying a fictitious name). If the person's response includes both a negative response ("No," headshake, written response, etc.), and his or her correct name, 2 points are given. If the patient replies with a negative response without further elaboration, the response is considered adequate, but not fully appropriate and is scored 1 point. If the patient responds affirmatively, perseverates, echoes the question, responds incoherently, or simply does not respond, no points are allotted. Requests for repetition are considered legitimate parts of communication and are not penalized. However, if the patient fails to respond within 5 seconds, the item is repeated and only partial credit (1 point) is allowed for a subsequent correct response. Though shorter in length and briefer in administration time than the CADL, its overall structure remains the same. Testing time for the CADL-2 ranges from 30 to 90 minutes, averaging approximately 45 minutes, 15 minutes less than for the original CADL.

The CADL test environment is deliberately informal and its administration is to be done in "a relaxed and friendly manner." Removing as many of the typical accoutrements of formal testing from the patient's view is desirable. CADL-2 items follow a self-described "natural" sequence to promote an experience closer to real life. These items fall into seven categories: *(1)* reading, writing, and using numbers; *(2)* sequential relationships in communication; *(3)* social interactions; *(4)* divergent communication (i.e., responding to misleading information or proverbs); *(5)* nonverbal communication (e.g., recognition of facial emotion); *(6)* contextual communication; *(7)* recognition of humor, absurdity, or metaphor. Some "props" are needed for the test: a pencil, a working telephone, four single dollar bills, and four quarters.

The CADL-2 total score is the sum of all points for the 50 items (maximum score = 100). There are no subtests, although the breakdown into the categories noted above can be used by clinicians as a qualitative guide to their interpretation of an individual performance. Scoring is aided by the test manual; the manual provides examples for 0-, 1-, and 2-point responses for each CADL-2 item. Total raw scores can be used to derive percentile and stanine scores. A performance interpretation approach that used demographically determined cutting scores has been eliminated from the revised edition.

The normative sample providing the reference percentile scores for the CADL-2 was a clinical one; a neurologically intact sample was not used. The standardization sample consisted of 175 adults with "neurogenic communication disorders" between the ages of 20 and 96 years (mean of 67 years) and drawn from 17 U.S. states. All subjects spoke English as their primary language. The primary medical etiology was a cerebrovascular event, though traumatic brain injury was also represented. The majority of patients were clinically judged to have mild or moderate communication disorders.

Reliability is described in the test manual. The internal consistency coefficient of CADL-2 performance in the standardization sample was .93. The standard error of measurement for raw scores was 9.72 and 1.04 for stanine scores at the 95th percent probability level. Test-retest performances for an unstated number of patients with chronic aphasia at a median retest interval of 2 months, 20 days was .89. Interrater reliability for stanine scores was reported to be .99, based upon rescoring of previously completed protocols.

Concurrent validity was explored by comparing CADL-2 performance with that on the WAB. Performances in a small sample of chronic aphasic patients showed a correlation of .66. Concurrent validity between the original CADL with the BDAE was .84, with the PICA .93, and with the FCP .87. Content validity was assessed by consensus among a group of speech-language pathologists and by item analysis. Construct validity was reported as group differences in performances of the standardization sample and a sample of 30 adults without neuro-logical damage. Group means differed by approximately 1 standard deviation and the intact group showed performances at the ceiling levels of the test (mean = 97.1, SD = 3.50). Construct validity was also assessed by correlating CADL-2 performances with pretest global ratings of communication disorder (mild, moderate, or severe), resulting in a moderate relation between the two.

The CADL was shown to correlate with the number of communicative exchanges initiated by aphasics (Linebaugh et al., 1982), but not with measures of dyadic nonverbal communication (Behrmann and Penn, 1984). Correlation between the severity of aphasia and the CADL score in Holland's original sample was .73. Criterion validity was established by comparing CADL performance with communicative behavior observed during a 4-hour period (coded for features such as the frequency and appropriateness of communications).

The distribution of scores for different types of aphasia follows the clinical impression of their severity. Global aphasics showed the poorest performance, with a mean of 44.25 (out of a possible 136 points on the original version). All groups but for two patients with transcortical sensory aphasia were statistically superior to the globally impaired group. Wernicke's and mixed aphasics performed more adequately than global aphasics, but less well than the Broca's aphasics. The anomic group had near-normal scores (mean = 127.21). Aphasics living at home consistently had higher scores than those living in institutional (group-living) settings. An Italian study (Pizzamiglio et al., 1984) showed somewhat different scores for the various types of aphasia, as well as generally lower scores. This may be the result of sample selection and classification criteria, but it also suggests that scores should be interpreted with caution.

Performance on the original CADL was also examined in a sample of 130 normal adults. These individuals were fluent English speakers without a history of mental disorder, brain damage, and visual or hearing impairment. The original CADL test manual presented mean performance levels by occupation and gender: performance levels were not significantly different. However, some statistically significant decline was noted with individuals over 65 years of age. K. Ross and Wertz (2001) examined the relationship between demographic variables and CADL-2 performance in samples of 18 aphasic patients and 18 normal adults, between the ages of 40 and 80 years. All were native English speakers. Hearing and visual acuities were screened. Age, education, and gender were not significantly related with CADL-2 performance in the aphasic group, but education was significantly related (r = .55) in the normal group. These researchers also included a measure of CADL-2 completion time. As before, aphasic-group demography was unrelated to the performance variable, and only education was significantly related to completion time (r = .63) in the normal group.

Fromm and Holland (1989) compared 26 patients with Wernicke's aphasia with 26 normal controls, 48 patients with Alzheimer's disease (AD), and 15 depressed patients. Aphasics had markedly different profiles compared to AD patients. Alzheimer's disease patients showed performances corresponding to disease severity. Depressed patients showed lower scores than controls, but also showed incomplete responses rather than the irrelevant, vague, or rambling responses more commonly seen in AD. Penn and Cleary (1988) included the CADL in their detailed examination of compensatory communication strategies in six adult males who had sustained traumatic brain injury. Half of the sample performed above their demographically appropriate cutoff (a score of 128). However, the authors reported that the test performed less well than the Pragmatic Protocol in revealing the communication difficulties of the sample, especially those functioning at a higher level. A group of 30 adult mentally retarded subjects with IQs between 50 and 80, living either at home or in group settings, and able to be employable in at least a sheltered setting obtained scores in the aphasic range (mean = 94.80); IQ and CADL correlated .72 (Holland, 1980). In contrast, a group of hearing-impaired subjects (with hearing aids) showed near-normal scores, with a mean performance of 128.6 (Holland, 1980).

The CADL-2, like the original test, is easy to add to diagnostic aphasia testing or to complete at some point during treatment, as it provides an estimate of the patient's communication ability in a standardized fashion. In their review, Skenes and McCauley (1985) considered the CADL as one of the few tests that met fairly stringent requirements for test construction. The revised version of the test removes the need for the examiner to engage in role playing, which appears reasonable, as the authors note that some examiners may be uncomfortable with acting, and role playing may not always be successful with patients who refuse or cannot enter into such simulated interactions.

Given the generally slowed psychomotor and information-processing speed that frequently accompanies acquired brain damage, one wonders whether the 5-second time restriction of the CADL and CADL-2 is overly strict and might violate one of the goals of the test, namely to document communication success regardless of transmission method. Additionally, this is a potential source of variability between clinicians.

The manual does not put forward a clear rule on how to monitor the 5-second limit: some administrators might use a stopwatch and maintain a strict adherence to timing, while others might count mentally or simply guess at the passage of time.

The CADL-2 test manual is not as comprehensive as the original one, though it does provide administrative and interpretative guidance. For example, the test authors clearly state that because of the employed standardization sample, the test should be used with caution if administered to milder and to more severely aphasic patients. The absence of a standardization sample of healthy and intact individuals in the revision also reduces some of the breadth of the test's potential applications. The authors offer some guidance (based upon a knowledge base in adult neurological disorders that has increased over the past 20 years) that their earlier comments about the relatively poor performance of institutionalized patients on the original CADL may need to be reconsidered —given that these patients were likely to have additional cognitive and underlying neurological disorders.

Communicative Effectiveness Index

The Communicative Effectiveness Index (CETI) (Lomas et al., 1989) uses a 16-item questionnaire focusing on the ability to interact with other people. Each question is concerned with an everyday situation and paired with a visual analog scale (a line marked "not at all" at one end, and "as able as before the stroke" on the other), which a relative or other caregiver has to mark. For example, one question asks about the patient's ability to participate in a conversation with a stranger. The full set of questions can be found in the original 1989 article and has also been reprinted in several publications, including Holland and Thompson (1998) and Murray and Chapey (2001). A template is used to convert each mark into a 10-point scale; this allows easy comparison of test-retest scores during therapy and recovery. This measure is designed to use very little of the therapist's time. The authors also applied the scale to 11 recovering (6 to 10 weeks postonset) and 11 stable (more than 15 months postonset) aphasics; the recovering group showed, with the exception of two patients, the same or more recovery as the WAB; with the exception of three patients, the CETI showed the same or less change compared to the WAB for the stable group. On the other hand, Sorin-Peters and Behrmann (1995) found that the CETI showed positive correlations with the CADL in only two of three patients, while for the third patient the correlation was negative. They ascribe these divergent findings to varying abilities of individual patients to self-assess and self-modify communicative behavior. Crockford and Lesser (1994) found that the scale has limited potential for planning appropriate intervention: in a follow-up of eight aphasics, retested after 3 months, the CETI was less effective as a measure of stability and change of communicative effectiveness.

The interrater reliability has been reported as .73 for the combined group and as .94 for the stable group only. Test-retest reliability was .94, and the difference between first and second testing for recovering aphasics was significant. Internal consistency was .90. Concurrent validity with the WAB Aphasia Quotient was only .61 on first testing, and .52 on second testing. Correlation with a global rating of aphasia severity by caregivers was .79 on first testing, and .62 on second testing. However, correlation with a speech questionnaire was only between .46 and .43 for speaking, and between .47 and .56 for understanding. The authors (Lomas et al., 1989) ascribe this finding to the emphasis on language in the speech questionnaire, whereas the CETI stresses functional communication. Penn et al. (1992) used the CETI with South African patients and found that the results corresponded to overall severity of aphasia but did not differentiate patients in terms of time since onset. It appeared to be relatively "culture-free" when translated into Afrikaans, Sotho, and Zulu.

Little further research with this questionnaire has been published. At this time, its usefulness in the assessment of the aphasic patient, as compared to other functional communication techniques or test batteries, remains limited. Holland and Thompson (1998) indicate that in their experience using the CETI is helpful in treatment centers that emphasize conversation groups as a key part of therapy. Murray and Chapey (2001) discuss the CETI as an aid to acquiring intake information at the onset of services.

Functional Communication Profile

The Functional Communication Profile (FCP) (M. Sarno, 1969; Taylor, 1965)[4] was the first instrument designed to measure natural language use in everyday communication by adults with neurological disorders. The FCP attempts to index the aphasic patient's ability to employ language in common situations, relative to the patient's estimated premorbid level of ability. "Normal" performance on the profile is defined by

---

[4] The FCP is currently out of print. Copies may be obtained from the author.

the clinician's estimation of the patient's previous language ability based on available evidence (e.g., education level, occupation, interviews with family members). The effectiveness of a clinician-based rating scale of this type is directly related to the experience and skill of the user; therefore, the FCP is not recommended for use by testing technicians, clinicians with limited experience, or in settings where few adult aphasics are likely to be seen. Its usefulness may also be limited in situations where little premorbid information is available.

The clinician's primary role is to create an informal rapport with the patient wherein the clinician can observe the patient's natural communicative behavior without resorting to formal testing. Forty-five behaviors are rated on a nine-point scale of current ability as a proportion of estimated former ability. The scale ranges from "normal" (100%) to "absent" (0%). Examples of functional abilities include reliably indicating "yes" and "no," reading newspaper headlines, and making change. The 45 behaviors are clustered into five categories: Movement, Speaking, Understanding, Reading, and Miscellaneous Abilities (e.g., calculating and writing). Overall cluster scores are obtained by determining the mean rating of the items in a cluster.

Despite the subjective clinical nature of the scoring system, M. Sarno (1969) reported interrater reliability coefficients larger than .87 for each of the five FCP categories. Reliability was determined for three judges using a sample of 20 right hemiplegic patients with language symptoms of at least 2 months duration.

Gains on psychometric testing do not automatically imply improved functional abilities, and, conversely, functional gains may not alter diagnostic classification. The distinction between functional ratings and psychometrically measured language functioning was examined by J. Sarno et al. (1973). Measurements of improvement were determined by comparing original and follow-up performances on the NCCEA Visual Naming and Identification by Sentence (i.e., Token Test) subtests and the FCP Speaking and Understanding subscales. Only a modest relationship was found between the original and follow-up scores on both speech measurements (i.e., NCCEA Visual Naming and FCP Speaking), and no correlation was found between score changes on the two comprehension measures (NCCEA Identification by Sentence and FCP Understanding). On the other hand, M. Sarno and Levita (1981) reported some concordance between NCCEA Token Test performance and FCP Understanding in the examination of global aphasics at 1-year follow-up. Differences between male and female patients with closed head injury and stroke (with similar postonset times) were found to be minimal (M. Sarno et al., 1985; 1987).

The information obtained by the FCP is not designed to replace a comprehensive examination of the aphasic patient's language abilities and disabilities. Rather, its goal is to provide information about natural communication capacity (M. Sarno, 1984a). The information yielded by a properly administered FCP may well translate more easily into a description of the patient's everyday capabilities than the information provided by a standard comprehensive examination. The FCP is not a diagnostic test: for example, M. Sarno et al. (1987) found that scores for fluent (Wernicke's) and nonfluent (Broca's) aphasics on the FCP were highly similar after age, education, and time of onset had been controlled. When properly used, the FCP may provide information on the functional consequences of the patient's aphasic condition that is not otherwise available. Studies examining the accuracy of medical personnel and family members in estimating or predicting the aphasic patient's performance levels (e.g., McClenahan et al., 1992) indicate the potential educational value of the results of the FCP and similar measures in counseling the family and fine-tuning therapist and nursing communicative interactions with the patient. Repeated FCP administration may provide information on the recovery process of functionally relevant communicative abilities (Sands et al., 1969; M. Sarno et al., 1985; M. Sarno and Levita, 1979).

Pragmatic Protocol

First designed by Prutting in 1982, Prutting and Kirchner's (1987) Pragmatic Protocol (PP) is a rating scale that is in the public domain; it is provided as an appendix to their paper. The PP is a descriptive taxonomy of those aspects of language that relate to verbal, paralinguistic, and nonverbal aspects of communication. Prutting and Kirchner (1987) state that the instrument "appears to be suitable as an index of the extent to which clinical deficits affect communicative competence" (p. 115). Examples of verbal aspects of communication that are rated in the PP are how the language-disordered patient can take turns in the communicative act and how topics become part of the act. Paralinguistics involve the intelligibility and prosody of communication. Nonverbal facets include use of gestures, eye gaze, and physical proximity.

Clinicians observe patients engaged in spontaneous and unstructured conversation with a partner for a minimum of 15 minutes. The conversation can be rated live or from videotaped recording. Each of 30 facets are rated as "appropriate" or "inappropriate" (or "no opportunity to observe").

The 1987 paper reports results from 10 normal adults, 42 normal children, 11 adults with left hemisphere damage, 10 adults with right hemisphere damage, and 88 language-disordered children.

The test authors stress that the PP offers the opportunity to explore the presence of specific performance profiles that might be used to develop treatment strategies and clearly distinguish it from a diagnostic instrument. The distinction between pragmatic behavior and language impairment is not always clear and is likely to be influenced by factors that have yet to be fully elucidated (e.g., Avent et al., 1998).

Murray and Chapey (2001) conclude that the PP and similar rating scales can offer unique information that cannot be found in standardized traditional diagnostic tests but at the cost of "specific psychometric limitations." A test like the PP can also provide more detailed information about the nature of functionally good and poor communication acts that is not easily obtained on some of the other functional communication instruments (e.g., multifaceted look at turn-taking behaviors).

9

Comprehensive Examinations

Comprehensive examinations of the aphasic patient's language ability have a basic goal. Within an organized set of tasks, they seek to obtain a diverse sampling of performance at different levels of task difficulty along all language dimensions that the test author deems relevant to language disability. Examples of dimensions common to most of these tests include naming, spontaneous speech, oral expression, auditory comprehension, repetition, reading, and writing. Other dimensions may or may not be present, according to the theoretical orientation of the authors.

Schuell (1973) provided perhaps the clearest explanation for the use of comprehensive batteries: "If it is a long time before the complex problems of aphasia are clearly understood, we can at least be confident that careful differential diagnosis is the sine qua non of all responsible clinical procedures in dealing with brain damaged patients" (p. 104).

There is some commonality to this family of diversely organized test instruments. The shared areas of elicited language behaviors noted previously—even though obtained in different ways—are a unifying feature of aphasia assessment and bridge the past with contemporary practices. Also, most of these comprehensive instruments are divided into subtests so that (unlike a screening test) any single aspect of language function is usually examined by a reasonably broad sampling of items.

Comprehensive examinations are different from one another, though, and they do vary in their purpose, structure, utility, and adequacy. Some tests, for example, are constructed to examine presumed clinical–anatomic localization and to provide prognostic information regarding a defined set of standard anatomically based aphasic syn-

117

dromes. Proponents of such tests see the data generated from their work as forming the diagnostic anchors for brain-behavior knowledge. Others are concerned with eliciting behavior that will provide more descriptive information without subscribing to a specific taxonomic system.

For practical purposes, we limit the current review to instruments designed for or primarily used in English. Tests developed and available mainly in another language (e.g., Aachen Aphasia Test, Willmes et al., 1983; Willmes and Ratajczak, 1962; Global Aphasic Neuropsychological Battery, Van Mourik et al., 1992) are excluded. However, we note that the AAT has now been standardized in English in a sample of aphasic and nonaphasic individuals from Scotland, Northern Ireland, and England (Miller et al., 2000) and a commercially available version of this English AAT (EAAT) is forthcoming (N. Miller et al., in press). Psychometric properties of the EAAT are detailed in N. Miller et al. (2000). We also omit some older and infrequently used instruments (e.g., Appraisal of Language Disturbance; Emerick, 1971). Tests available in translation or designed as multilingual instruments are mentioned in a section on bilingualism later in this book.

A common denominator of the instruments we review is the need for adequate training and practice before the examination can be effectively employed. The choice of an assessment instrument is a serious decision that not only involves personal preferences but also takes into account the clinical setting, the type of referrals that the clinician can expect, the stated intentions of the test instrument, as well as the adequacy of the examination as an at least minimally reliable, valid, and useful test.

Aphasia Diagnostic Profiles

The Aphasia Diagnostic Profiles (ADP) (Helm-Estabrooks, 1992; Applied Symbolix, $179) offers a relatively refined and tightly structured aphasia battery allowing for the systematic typing of nonfluent, fluent, and borderline fluent aphasias and—within those categories—global, Wernicke's, Broca's, conduction, transcortical motor, transcortical sensory, anomic, and mixed aphasia subtypes. This "Classification Profile" is one of five profiles provided by the test. Additionally, the ADP offers Aphasia Severity, Error, Alternative Communication (writing, reading, singing, gestural), and Behavioral Profiles.

The ADP comprises a series of nine relatively brief subtests. Subtests include Personal Information, Writing, Reading, Fluency (conversationally elicited and in response to a grocery-store drawing), Naming, Auditory Language Comprehension (following command, single-word comprehension, and understanding of a story), Repetition, Elicited Command Following Gestures, and Singing. The author reports that the test can be completed in 40 to 50 minutes and need not be completed in a single session. Administration is designed to emphasize conversational interactions with the patient being examined. The portable test material includes a Patient Information Sheet and stimulus cards; a letterboard also is provided for use when testing intubated or other nonverbal patients. The test's manual and response forms clearly delineate administration and scoring rules. Standardization of the test was based predominantly on adults with CVAs.

Responses for most tasks are scored on a five-point scale (no response, fully incorrect, some correct, mostly correct immediately or fully correct with prolonged delay or self-corrected, and fully immediately correct). Some subtests (Auditory Language Comprehension and Singing) have a different scoring system. Other subtests (e.g., Naming and Repetition) require use of a standardized error system. The Fluency subtest also allows for the determination of an Index of Wordiness, which is based upon the relation between total words produced and number of "correct informational units."

The ADP represents a new addition to comprehensive aphasia assessment. It includes features not commonly found in other batteries, but at this time lacks the psychometric foundation of other batteries. Its portability and well-written instructions are strong assets. The ADP clearly appeals to clinicians seeking assessment-based information while planning intervention strategies. It has not been part of contemporary research studies. The Behavioral Profile is not a substitute for psychological and neuropsychological assessment findings and would seem to have only modest descriptive value. In reviewing the ADP, van Gorp (1998) pointed toward the test's Index of Wordiness as a potentially useful measure in investigations of language changes in Alzheimer's disease and other neurological processes. The emphasis on alternative communication, such as gestures and singing, clearly dovetails with specific intervention planning and execution of treatments, such as Melodic Intonation Therapy.

Boston Assessment of Severe Aphasia

The purposes of the Boston Assessment of Severe Aphasia (BASA) (Helm-Estabrooks et al., 1989; Pro-Ed, $269) are to provide a full assessment of language and other communicative functions in severely aphasic patients and to "quickly identify and quantify" those preserved abilities that might form the initial steps of directed rehabilitation.

The BASA consists of 61 items organized into 15 subtests: *(1)* Social Greetings and Simple Conversation. Responding appropriately to greeting ("good afternoon," "How are you feeling today?"), name, statement of purpose of visit, etc. *(2)* Personally Relevant Yes/No Questions ("Is this [wrong name] hospital?"]. The patient responds verbally or by using a knob that can be turned one way to indicate "Yes" and the other way to indicate "No." *(3)* Orientation to Time and Place. The patient responds verbally or by pointing to a calendar (for month, part of month), or map ("Where do you live?"). *(4)* Bucco-Facial Praxis. The patient is requested to make mouth movements on command. *(5)* Sustained "Ah" and Singing. *(6)* Repetition. Single words and short sentences ("I love you") are repeated. *(7)* Limb Praxis. Patient is asked to show how to salute, shake a finger at a naughty child. *(8)* Comprehension of Number Symbols. Point to the appropriate number on a four-choice card, or indicate the number of fingers shown by the examiner. *(9)* Object Naming. Patient is asked to name, describe the use, or demonstrate the use of objects (e.g., toy gun). *(10)* Action Picture Items. Patient is asked to choose a picture of an activity demonstrated or verbalized by the examiner (e.g., sleeping), and name the activity. *(11)* Comprehension of Coin Names. Patient indicates the correct coin or coins named by the examiner. *(12)* Famous Faces. Name, describe, or otherwise indicate identity of Hitler, W.C. Fields, and Marilyn Monroe. *(13)* Emotional Words, Phrases, and Symbols. Reading or otherwise indicating comprehension of words (e.g., "pain"). *(14)* Visuospatial Items. Freehand drawing of a man, visual matching, and visual memory for a drawing or stick design. *(15)* Signature. Patient is asked to sign a form; leaves the session with an appropriate farewell.

Several items can be administered in a relatively informal manner or as part of a conversation. The test takes approximately 30 to 40 minutes. Stimulus material included in the test set include a map and photographs. Test users need to provide a felt-tip pen and pennies, nickels, dimes, and quarters.

Items are scored at several levels of performance, depending on task demands: no verbal or gestural response, gestural refusal, noncommunicative gestural response, partially communicative gestural response, fully communicative gestural response, gestural response with affective quality, perseverative gestural response, verbal refusal, noncommunicative verbal response, partially communicative verbal response, fully communicative verbal response, verbal response with affective quality, and perseverative verbal response. For each subtest, exact scoring criteria are provided. Correct responses (verbal response 2 points) are summed across five-item clusters (i.e., auditory comprehension, praxis, oral-gestural expression, reading comprehension, gesture recognition; and across writing and visuospatial tasks). The grand total of correct responses forms the BASA total score. The total of other responses can also be summed across clusters and for the total test.

Norms are based upon the performance of 111 patients with severe aphasia who provided 186 test performances. The age range was 30 to 79 years, with most subjects older than 50 years of age. Aphasia subtypes included 47 patients with global aphasia, 16 with Wernicke's aphasia, 10 with Broca's aphasia, and one anomic aphasic. Of the sample of 111 patients, 25 could not be classified into an aphasic subtype. Most patients had sustained a CVA. Three patients were head-injured; it is not clear into what category some patients in the sample could be placed. As a reflection of the severity of the aphasic disturbance for the bulk of the sample, 80% had BDAE Aphasia Severity Rating Scale scores of 0 or 1 of 5. Norms are divided into those from the full sample and those with a diagnosis of global aphasia.

To use the norms, raw scores for the five areas are converted into standard scores, which in turn can be used to assign a percentile rank within this aphasic population. Norms for normal healthy speakers are not provided because they would presumably achieve a perfect score. Effects of age, gender, or education are not reported.

Internal consistency for the BASA is high: correlations range between .72 and .89 for the five areas and .94 for the total score, slightly lower in global aphasics. Test-retest reliability for 39 severe aphasics after an average interval of 3.7 months ranged from .52 to .73 for the area scores, and was .74 for the total score. Reliability was similar for 23 global aphasics. Interrater reliability ranged from 80% to 100% in two patients.

Concurrent validity with the BDAE is modest to adequate. This is probably to be expected because of the low ceiling of the BASA subtests and the wide range of the BDAE. The correlation for 43 patients between BASA total score and BDAE aphasia severity rating was .67.

Cluster-total score correlations ranged from .44 to .76, suggesting some independence of each area score. A factor analysis showed three factors: an expressive language, a visuospatial, and a comprehensive language factor.

The BASA samples a wide range of low-level communicative functions and easily lends itself to bedside examination of severely language impaired patients. The authors state that a number of items were inappropriate or ineffective when testing (presumably nonaphasic) closed head injury patients. The test has many qualities that make it comparable to the CADL, but is shorter and not suitable for the wider range of aphasia severity covered by the CADL. The BASA has, however, documented significant improvement in 31 global, 5 severe Wernicke's, and 5 other severe aphasics over a 2-year period (M. Nicholas et al., 1993); the authors noted that initial test scores were less accurate than 6-months postonset cluster scores for the prediction of the total BASA score after 24 months. The greatest amount of recovery was found in the first 6 months.

The scoring of affect, perseveration, and of partial verbal and gestural responses can provide useful information for the examiner and others, but so far these have not been further investigated. Towne (1995b) stated that the inclusion of gestural communication is a unique feature of the BASA, but that this also makes extra demands on the examiner's attention during testing.

The BASA is a useful addition to the other comprehensive batteries in that it provides the fullest opportunity for a broad communication assessment in severely aphasic patients by extending the range of items in the lowest range of performance. So far, research with this relatively new instrument has been limited.

Boston Diagnostic Aphasia Examination, 3rd Edition

The original Boston Diagnostic Aphasia Examination (BDAE) (sometimes referred to simply as the Boston) was published by Goodglass and Kaplan in 1972. It became one of the most popular examinations for use in aphasia settings. Beyond traditional aphasia settings, it was among the top five language tests reportedly used by speech-language pathologists who provided services to patients with traumatic head injuries (Frank and Barrineau, 1996). It has been revised twice: the BDAE-R (Goodglass et al., 1983) and the current version of the test, the BDAE-3 (Goodglass et al., 2000). The primary focus of the BDAE is the diagnosis of classic anatomically based aphasic syndromes. This diagnostic goal is attained by comprehensive sampling of language components that have previously proven themselves valuable in the identification of aphasic syndromes.

Goodglass and Kaplan stated in the past that the design of their instrument was based on the observation that various components of language function may be selectively damaged by central nervous system

(CNS) lesions; this selectivity is an indication of the anatomical neural organization of language, the localization of the lesion causing the observed deficit, and the functional interactions of various parts of the language system. A number of studies have validated this stated purpose (e.g., Meffer and Jeffrey, 1984; Naeser and Hayward, 1978; Naeser et al., 1981; 1987).

The BDAE-3 has three formats: standard, short, and extended. This choice of format is a major structural difference from earlier versions of the test. The standard format is the one most closely related to earlier versions of the Boston and, indeed, itself "extended" in terms of numbers of subtests and length of time required to administer relative to other commonly used aphasia batteries, such as the WAB and the MAE. The authors report that the new short form of the test requires only 40 to 60 minutes to complete and refer to it as "a brief, no frills assessment; " the extended version offers clinicians a fuller neurolinguistic assessment instrument. Other structural changes in the current version of the Boston are a new index (Language Competence Index), the formal inclusion of the Boston Naming Test into the battery format, and the elimination of animal naming (fluency), which had been a popular subtest. The current version comes with a very helpful instructional video for novice users, which is more than 2 hours in length and shows the administration of the battery to three different individuals with aphasia.

Like earlier versions, the standard BDAE-3 is divided into five language-related sections: *(a)* Conversational and Expository Speech; *(b)* Auditory Comprehension; *(c)* Oral Expression; *(d)* Reading; and *(e)* Writing. The extended version of the BDAE-3 includes a sixth section: praxis. Each BDAE-3 section contains a variety of subtests. Each subtest attempts to measure the specific function in as purely isolated a fashion as possible.

The detailed manner of examining conversational and expository speech has always been an important and relatively unique aspect of the BDAE; the BDAE-3 offers an even more extensive procedure for this assessment than earlier versions of the test. A Speech Characteristics Profile is derived from samples of free-conversational speech, narrative description of the Cookie-Theft card, and (in the extended-testing format) a new section examining narrative discourse based upon stories from *Aesop's Fables*. The profile indexes verbal prosody (melodic line), fluency, articulation, grammatical level, paraphasias, and word-finding difficulties. Repetition and auditory comprehension are also rated, but ratings are derived from subtest performances. Finally, an overall Aphasia Severity Rating Scale can be determined from these conversational speech samples, ranging from "no usable speech or auditory comprehension" (a score of 0) to "minimal discernible speech handicaps" (a score of 5). The reliability of the Speech Characteristics Profile was first examined for the original BDAE, employing three judges who rated the tape-recorded speech samples of 99 patients. The lowest interjudge correlations were .78 and .79 for word-finding difficulties and paraphasias, respectively; the other dimensions had coefficients of at least .85. Other interrater agreement studies have also shown satisfactory results (Davis, 1993).

In the standard format, Auditory Comprehension tests for Basic Word Discrimination (pointing to objects, body parts, numbers, letters, and colors on cards); Word Comprehension by Categories (tools, foods, and animals on cards); Commands (including 1 to 5 informational units, e.g., "make a fist"); and Complex Ideational Material (yes or no responses to questions like "Will a stone sink in water?" and questions indicating that the patient has comprehended four different paragraphs). For the extended format, a number of other tasks are included in the assessment, including map locations, semantic probing, syntactic processing, reversible possessives, and embedded sentences.

Oral Expression includes Oral Agility (mouth movements and rapid repetition of words); Automated Sequences (e.g., recite days of the week); Recitation, Melody, and Rhythm (e.g., reciting nursery rhyme, singing familiar song, repeating a rhythm tapped on the table); and Repetition (single words and sentences). Oral expression also includes Naming, including responsive naming (e.g., "What do we tell time with?"), the Boston Naming Test,[5] and naming of letters, numbers, and colors.

Reading includes basic symbol recognition (letters and numbers), word recognition (picture-word matching and lexical decisions), phonics (basic homophone matching and advanced phonic analysis), derivational and grammatical morphology, oral reading (basic words, sentence reading and comprehension, and paragraph reading and comprehension). Comprehension responses are based on a multiple-choice format. Extended testing in this section includes fuller assessments of phonics and of oral reading.

Writing includes a rating of the Mechanics of Writing in three areas (i.e., well-formedness of letters, correct letter choice, motor facility), dictation (letters, numbers, and real and nonsense words), spelling to dictation, written naming of objects, actions, and animals, and narrative writing (using the Cookie-Theft card).

---

[5] See Chapter 7.

Praxis examines natural and conventional gestures, use of pretended objects, and bucco-facial and respiratory movements.

Supplementary nonlanguage tests (once called the Boston Parietal Lobe Battery, but now referred to as a Spatial Quantitative Battery) were included as a separate adjunct in earlier versions of the Boston and remain an option for the BDAE-3. These include constructional apraxia (drawing to command—including clock drawing, stick construction copying, stick construction from memory, three-dimensional block design), finger agnosia, right–left orientation, and acalculia and ideational apraxia.

Internal consistency for the BDAE-R ranged from .98 for visual confrontation naming to .68 for body-part identification. Test-retest reliability was not reported for that version.

The BDAE-3 standardization sample is notably smaller than those that defined both the BDAE and the BDAE-R. The sample for the BDAE-3 comprises only 85 aphasic subjects (predominantly CVA) and 15 normal, community-dwelling elderly. In contrast, the original BDAE was standardized on a sample of 207 aphasic patients with relatively distinct CVAs and isolated, well-defined symptoms, and the revised BDAE was standardized on a new sample of 242 patients.

The original BDAE was also standardized on 147 healthy normal adult subjects (Borod et al., 1980) to provide cutoff scores at 2 SD below the mean, and include age and education corrections. These means, ranges, and suggested cutoff scores were included in the original manual. Means, standard deviations, and ranges for the subtests, based on between 147 to 193 aphasic patients in the 1972 sample, and on between 97 to 232 patients in the 1983 sample are presented to provide an index of severity of aphasia in the various areas tested in the manual for the test's first revision.

Emery (1986) found only minimal, insignificant decline of scores on all subtests when comparing 20 healthy adults aged 30 to 42 years with a similar group aged 75 to 93 years. Whitworth and Larson (1989) found no significant effects for gender and education in their sample. Heaton et al. (1991) present norms for the comprehension of complex material of the BDAE-R in scaled scores, corrected for gender, education, and age, that are based on 553 normal subjects. However, these norms should be used with caution because the number of subjects in some of the cells is quite small. Norms based on 180 normal Spanish speakers from Colombia, broken down by educational level and three age ranges (16 to 30, 31 to 50, 51 to 65 years) were presented by Rosselli et al. (1990). These data show a significant effect of educational level for most tasks, and an age effect for some of the tasks, that is, word discrimination, confrontation and animal naming, oral sentence reading, high- and low-probability repetition, symbol discrimination, oral spelling, word-picture matching, sentence-paragraph comprehension, and serial, primer-level dictation, written confrontation naming, and spelling to dictation, all showed a significant drop in the oldest age group. More recent norms and an examination of the role of demographic variables in task performance on the Spanish BDAE by 156 normal adults living in Medellin, Colombia were reported by Pineda et al. (2000), who also found that education had a significant impact on performance on most subtests. Pineda and colleagues provide means and standard deviations on each subtest, broken down by age and education, in an appendix to their paper. Norms for the parietal lobe battery in older subjects (age 40 to 89) were presented by Farver and Farver (1982).

Borod et al. (1984) applied the parietal lobe battery to 163 right-handed aphasics, and found four factors: construction, visual schemata, verbal components of the Gerstmann syndrome, and visual finger recognition. Impairment was strongest in patients with lesions in both left parietal and frontal areas. The spatial-quantitative tests (the parietal lobe battery) together with the WAIS were applied to right- and left-handed aphasics: Left-handed aphasics were significantly poorer on both, especially on tasks involving visuospatial construction, suggesting that in left-handers, the left hemisphere is typically dominant for tasks usually considered as right-hemisphere specific (Borod et al., 1985).

Construct validity has been examined by reviewing the intercorrelation matrix of the 43 language and 23 nonlanguage measures of the BDAE and by factor analysis. In an earlier analysis (Goodglass and Kaplan, 1972), a strong general language factor emerged, as expected, with other factors covering the spatial-quantitative-somatognostic, the articulation-grammatical fluency, the auditory-comprehension, and the paraphasia domains. A second factor analysis (Goodglass and Kaplan, 1983), omitting ratings and nonlanguage tests, resulted in five factors (comprehension/reading/naming, recitation/repetition, writing, oral agility/singing/rhythm, auditory comprehension). When rating scales were included, three additional factors (fluency, reading, paraphasia) were found. The addition of the spatial-quantitative tests resulted in a 10-factor solution including a strong spatial-quantitative factor, a finger identification factor, and a factor labeled "freedom from paraphasia." Discriminant validity between cases of Broca's, Wernicke's, conduction, and anomic aphasia was optimal when the following tests were entered into the equation: body part identification, repetition of high probability sentences, paraphasia rating, word-finding rating, phrase-length rating, and verbal paraphasias.

Divenyi and Robinson (1989) reported correlations of .86 and .93 of the auditory comprehension measured in the BDAE with the Token Test and with the respective part of the PICA. The BDAE and the oral apraxia task specifically were found to be related to other articulation tasks (Sussman et al., 1986).

The BDAE auditory comprehension subtest was not an adequate predictor of auditory paragraph comprehension in independent standardized material (R. Brookshire and Nicholas, 1984); a second study (L. Nicholas et al., 1986) showed that both aphasic and healthy subjects were able to answer a similar number of questions about a paragraph without having actually read the passage, suggesting a high passage dependency of this test. This dependency applied not only to the BDAE but also to similar tasks in the MTDDA and the WAB. Dyadic interaction measures also did not correlate well with the BDAE (Behrmann and Penn, 1984). Decision rules for the diagnosis of the individual subtypes are not always clearly defined, although Reinvang and Graves (1975) attempted such clarification. Crary et al. (1992) tried to isolate subtypes of aphasia empirically by means of a Q-type factor analysis for the BDAE and the closely related WAB; the resulting seven patient clusters (labeled Broca's, anomic, global, Wernicke's, conduction, and two unclassified clusters) agreed only poorly (in 38% of 47 patients) with the classification obtained using the classification rules of the test itself; the results were even worse for the WAB. The study, aside from its limited subject population for factor analytic studies and the use of a somewhat dated cluster-analysis technique, suggests that BDAE classification rules are based on clinical rather than construct validity. Similarly, Naeser and Hayward (1978) and Reinvang (1985) pointed out that scale profiles can aid in the classification, but do not firmly classify patients into subtypes of aphasia. The test authors acknowledge that 30% to 80% of aphasic patients are not classifiable; this finding is also consistent with clinical experience that a majority of aphasic patients show mixed rather than pure symptomatology.

Li and Williams (1990) found that in the Repeating Phrases and Sentences subtest, conduction aphasics showed a greater number of phonemic attempts, word revisions, and word and phrase repetitions; Broca's aphasics showed more phonemic errors and omissions; and Wernicke's aphasics produced more unrelated words and jargon. The BDAE predicted progress in therapy (Davidoff and Katz, 1985; Helm-Estabrooks and Ramsberger, 1986). In aphasics, word reading (Selnes et al., 1984) and confrontation naming (Knopman et al., 1984) showed striking improvement after 6 months had elapsed since time of insult. Specifically, R. Marshall and Neuberger (1994) found that measured pre-treatment effort in self-correction (but not success of self-correction) and good auditory comprehension were related to improvement during treatment as measured by the BDAE and the PICA. Narrative response to the Cookie-Theft card has been examined as a method of gleaning additional information about patients' self-monitoring and self-correction of errors. Nonaphasic and nondemented healthy elderly were noted to self-correct 72% to 92% of their errors in the description of this card (McNamara et al., 1992).

In Alzheimer's disease, Kirshner (1982) found language to be fluent with normal prosody, syntax, and phrase length; few paraphasias were found, but word-finding problems and poor repetition of low-probability phrases were present. Sentence comprehension, but not letter and word reading were found to be related to severity of AD patients (Cummings et al., 1986). Whitworth and Larson (1989) compared 25 AD patients, 25 patients with other dementias, and 58 age-matched controls. They found significant differences compared to controls on all but four of 38 BDAE scores (paraphasia, articulation, primer dictation, word reading). Discriminant function analysis produced correct classification for 95% of the three groups. Nineteen test scores contributed to the discrimination of four levels ("stages") of severity of dementia, resulting in correct classification of 100% of 22 dementia patients. Gorelick et al. (1993) found also that scores on the BDAE Commands and Responsive Naming subtests were lower in 66 patients with multi-infarct dementia as compared to a group of 86 patients with infarcts without dementia. In a comparison of multi-infarct dementia, AD, and normal control subjects, Mendez and Ashla-Mendez (1991) found that the unstructured Cookie-Theft card description discriminated better than structured tests between groups: The multi-infarct group produced fewer words per minute and fewer constructional assemblages.

Two hundred eighteen patients with closed head injury showed significantly poorer word fluency skills than normals; although their strategies were similar to those used by normals, some qualitative differences in semantic associations were found that were related to severity of cognitive disruption (Gruen et al., 1990).

All versions of the test are lengthy (90 to 120 minutes) and probably more useful for assessments in the context of detailed studies of aphasia and aphasia rehabilitation than as a routine language test. The BDAE-

3 now includes a short form, which reduces administration time. The extended format, in turn, provides an even more extensive examination than the standard administration. In addition, the Boston has always included useful directions for observing and recording many specific types of errors (e.g., paraphasias) found in aphasia, reflecting an approach to assessment that has come to be known as the Boston Process Approach (Kaplan, 1988). However, even if the short format of the test is not used, a number of isolated subtests can be useful additions to clinical assessment depending on the presenting symptoms of the patient. In particular, the BNT has frequently been used as a stand-alone test, for example, to evaluate recognition-cued word-retrieval skills in the elderly (LaBarge et al., 1986).

Knowledge of the "Boston school" approach to aphasia classification is necessary to interpret the BDAE (e.g., Benson, 1979a). This is true for both the Speech Characteristics Profile and the Aphasia Severity Rating Scale, which are central to diagnostic decision making with the BDAE—especially its fluency–nonfluency dimension. More detailed diagnoses may incorporate corroborative information from the profile sheet delineating subtest performances. The test manual provides profiles for classic and rarer aphasic subtypes.

Spanish (Goodglass and Kaplan, 1986), French (Mazaux and Orgogozo, 1985), Hindu (Kacker et al., 1991), and Finnish (Laine et al., 1993) versions are available, though they do not employ the newest BDAE-3 format. Computerized scoring and interpretation software is also available (Code et al. 1990).

Multilingual Aphasia Examination

The benefits of having equivalent versions of a single aphasia examination for several language communities has been well stated by Benton (1967; 1969). The Multilingual Aphasia Examination (MAE) has been developed through the efforts of Benton and his collaborators to meet the requirements of such an examination (Benton et al., 1978). The third edition of the MAE is available (Benton et al., 1994; PAR, $299), as is a Spanish version (MAE-S, Rey and Benton, 1991; Rey et al., 1999; 2001; PAR, $239). Chinese, French, German, Italian, and Portuguese versions of this test are being prepared. The different language versions of the MAE are functionally equivalent in content rather than being simple translations. For example, COWA uses letters that have corresponding levels of difficulty in each language rather than employing identical letters. Hence, performance of the task in each language is functionally equivalent.

The MAE, a shortened and highly modified relative of the NCCEA, consists of seven subtests: Visual Naming, Sentence Repetition, COWA, Spelling (oral, written, and using block letters), a version of the Token Test, Aural Comprehension of Words and Phrases, and Reading Comprehension of Words and Phrases. Two MAE rating scales are included. The first is Speech Articulation, based upon verbal performance throughout the test session. Ratings range from 0 ("speechless or usually unintelligible speech") to 8 ("normal speech"). The second is Writing Praxis, scored when possible by performance on tasks of writing to dictation (from the MAE Spelling subtest); scores range from 0 ("illegible scrawl") to 8 ("good penmanship").

A practical and distinctive feature of the MAE is that alternate versions of Sentence Repetition, COWA, Spelling, and Token Test are available for repeat assessment of the patient. In addition to the clinical utility of this feature, it has made the MAE a useful measure to assess language function in protocols that require repeat testing prior to an intervention like neurosurgery and posttesting afterwards. Hermann and Wyler (1988) and Hermann et al. (1995) provide specific examples of the utility of this feature prior to and after temporal lobectomy in patients with medically intractable seizure disorders.

Visual Naming requires naming of line drawings (whole objects and object details), which is more difficult than naming of actual objects. COWA presents three letters progressively increasing in their associative difficulty (see Chapter 7 for a detailed discussion of this subtest). The Spelling subtest is actually a "mini-battery" that employs any combination of three modalities: oral spelling, writing to dictation, or block-letter spelling. The TT comprises 22 commands at two levels of complexity, and items are scored in pass–fail fashion. Aural and Reading Comprehension are administered in a multiple-choice format. Scoring adjustments for age and educational level are provided in the test manual.

The MAE manual provides standardized test instructions, normative information (in the form of percentiles) from a sample of 360 normal Iowa adults (aged 16 to 69 years) without a history or evidence of neurological disability. A second validation sample of 50 aphasic patients is included, which may be used to discern aphasic subtypes. Normative information for 229 children from 6 to 12 years, based on a study by Schum et al. (1989), is included in the manual. The MAE-S manual includes normative information from a sample of 234 normal Spanish-speaking Texas and Puerto Rico adults (aged 18 to 70 years) without history or evidence of neurological or psychiatric disability. Two MAE subtests (COWA and Token Test) have been incorporated into the Mayo Older Americans Normative Studies (MOANS; Ivnik et al., 1996); the authors reported results with a large sample of normal adults between 55 and 97 years of age. Because the Naming subtest may be especially sensitive to cultural experience, separate normative data have been obtained for urban inner-city African American residents (R. Roberts and Hamsher, 1984). COWA was included in a cognitive battery normed on healthy elderly adults between 65 and 84 years of age; there was no suggestion of significant performance decrement over this age span (Benton et al., 1981). The latest edition of the manual reports data by Schum and Sivan (1997) about the MAE performance of a new sample of 61 healthy control subjects, aged 70 to 90 years. Stable performances were noted for subjects in their 70s, but performance decrements were found for those in their 80s, particularly on the Sentence Repetition and Token Test subtests. These studies were conducted with well-educated adults who lived in the community; the authors speculate that subjects with less education may show a steeper decline with age. This was confirmed by Elias et al. (1997) who used a sample of 1893 community residents, stratified by age and education level: the oldest participants with the fewest years of education had the lowest performance, with lower levels of performance for men than women. Rather than looking for poor performance in depressed elderly, La Rue et al. (1995) emphasized good COWA performance in elderly adults scoring high on a measure of "zestfulness," suggesting this as an example where COWA performance at better than expected levels might have functional significance.

Validity was examined by the discrimination between 115 normal and 48 aphasic subjects with six of the MAE subtests. The use of the suggested cutoff scores caused between 2.6% and 7.0% of normals and between 14.4% and 64.6% of aphasics to be misclassified by individual subtests. With failure on one subtest as a cutoff, 15% of controls and no aphasics were misclassified; with failure on two or more subtests, the misclassification rates were 3% and 4%, respectively (Jones and Benton, 1995). The Token Test proved to be the best discriminator between the two groups; the two comprehension subtests were least discriminative. Patients with left temporal lobe epilepsy also showed significant impairment on the MAE (and on tests of verbal learning) compared to epileptics with right hemisphere impairment (Hermann and Wyler, 1988; Hermann et al., 1992). Concurrent validity of the Visual Naming subtest, which has 30 items, and the 60-item BNT (.86) was reported by

Axelrod et al. (1994) in a diagnostically mixed sample of 100 adult patients with neurological or psychiatric histories.

Research has shown that failure on the MAE Token Test is a sensitive indicator of the presence of acute confusional states (delirium) in non-aphasic medical inpatients (G. Lee and Hamsher, 1988). F. Goldstein et al. (1996) found a near-significant trend for Visual Naming to discriminate between normal controls, AD patients, and patients with closed head injury, but naming of low-frequency and high-frequency words was similar in all three groups.

Levin and colleagues (Levin et al., 1976; 1981) employed the MAE to examine the linguistic performance of patients with closed head injuries, documenting a high frequency of naming errors, defective associative word finding, and impaired comprehension of nonredundant aural commands (i.e., Token Test), and revealing their correlation with the severity of brain injury. R. Lincoln et al. (1994) used test performances on the MAE to better understand performances on the WAIS-R in a sample of 79 closed head injured patients. WAIS-R Verbal subtests were correlated most strongly with MAE Visual Naming, with the exception of Digit Span and Arithmetic, which were correlated more closely with performance on MAE Sentence Repetition. As might be anticipated, WAIS-R Performance subtests showed lesser degrees of correlation with the MAE but they showed modest correlations with the MAE Token Test and COWA. Crosson et al. (1993), also studying closed head injury, compared MAE performance with performance on a measure of verbal learning and memory (i.e., the California Verbal Learning Test [CVLT]). MAE Visual Naming showed the strongest relation to performance on the CVLT.

A factor analysis of 16 aphasia battery subtests (including subtests of the MAE, NCCEA, and the WAB), given to healthy Taiwanese volunteers (Hua et al., 1997) suggested a major factor of verbal comprehension (including Token Test, Sentence Repetition, Digit Repetition, Visual Naming, Reading, and Aural Comprehension). A second factor was labeled effortful writing. A third factor involved mainly verbal expression and word production. Other research examined the use of both MAE performance and clinical features of aphasics' language (e.g., paraphasias in conversational speech, *conduite d'approche*) in order to provide an MAE differential diagnosis of aphasic subtypes (K. Hamsher, personal communication, 1988).

In sum, it is hoped that the successful deployment of the MAE in a number of language communities will facilitate direct cross-community comparisons of case and sample data. Regardless of this research goal, clinical use of the English-language MAE suggests that it is an effective instrument requiring relatively brief (usually under 45 minutes) administration time. In addition, use in general clinical practice of individual subtests (e.g., Visual Naming, Token Test, COWA) can serve as a good exploratory examination as to the presence of language deficits, to document performance status, and to determine need for further exploration with additional testing.

Minnesota Test for Differential Diagnosis of Aphasia

The Minnesota Test for Differential Diagnosis of Aphasia (MTDDA)[6] (Schuell, 1955, 1973) has been a cornerstone of aphasia assessment for many years. One reviewer cited its "venerable history in psychological testing" (Reed, 1998). It was ranked among the more popular batteries in 1984 (Beele et al., 1984), and using selective subtests from the test remains a popular choice at many speech and language clinic settings, although few studies using the test have been published in recent years. It is a comprehensive examination designed to observe the level at which language performance is impaired in each of the principal language modalities at different levels of task difficulty. To Schuell, the goal of a careful and comprehensive description of impairment in the aphasic patient should be to provide a guide for effective therapeutic intervention.

The current version of the MTDDA is the result of numerous systematic revisions of the original experimental version of the late 1940s. The author employed empirical factor analytic techniques (Schuell et al., 1962) with large databases as well as clinical experience to construct and revise the test. The construction of the MTDDA reflects Schuell's theoretical view of aphasia as a unitary reduction of language that crosses all language modalities, and that may or may not be complicated by perceptual or sensorimotor involvement, by various forms of dysarthria, or by other consequences of brain damage (Schuell, 1974b; Schuell and Jenkins, 1959; Schuell et al., 1964). The MTDDA consists of five sections: Auditory Disturbances (represented by 9 subtests); Visual and Reading Disturbances (9 subtests); Speech and Language Disturbances (15 subtests); Visuomotor and Writing Disturbances (10 subtests); and Numerical Relations and Arithmetic Processes (4 subtests). Within each section, subtest order is generally arranged from the least to the most difficult. Each section may be started at an estimated level of difficulty corresponding to the patient's ability (the "Binet method"), and then

---

[6] Currently out of print.

continued to the point where the patient fails 90% or more of the items. Both the test manual (Schuell, 1965) and the companion monograph (Schuell, 1973) describe supplementary tests that should be considered as well as the factor and intercorrelation structure for the test sections.

The auditory disturbances subtests include examinations of retention span and comprehension for vocabulary, sentences, and paragraphs. The visual and reading subtests include examinations of form and letter matching, matching printed words to pictures, reading comprehension for sentences and paragraphs, and oral reading. The speech and language subtests include 4 subtests that deal with speech movements and articulation and 11 that deal with language, ranging from overlearned serial tasks to retelling of a paragraph. The visual and writing subtests include five dealing with the reproduction and recall of visual forms and five dealing with written language. The four numerical and arithmetic subtests deal with functional arithmetic ability, minimizing the influence of education on performance.

Differential diagnosis using the MTDDA identified five aphasia syndromes: simple aphasia; aphasia with visual involvement; aphasia with sensorimotor involvement; aphasia with scattered findings compatible with generalized brain damage; and an irreversible aphasia syndrome (Schuell, 1974a). Schuell (1966, 1973) also added two additional "minor syndromes": mild aphasia with persistent dysfluency (dysarthria) and aphasia with intermittent auditory imperception. However, as Zubrick and Smith (1979) pointed out, the MTDDA was not designed to deal with broader issues of aphasic differential diagnosis: distinguishing aphasia from nonaphasic disorders that may manifest language disturbances (e.g., memory loss, dementia, severe hearing loss, and confusional state). The test has been successfully used to measure language recovery after stroke and head trauma, and to show that language recovery is relatively independent from intelligence (Bailey et al., 1981; David and Skilbeck, 1984). Armstrong and Walker (1994) tested older adults with an MTDDA short version to examine any gender differences, but did not find any.

The length of the MTDDA presents a problem for the user of the test. Short forms (Schuell, 1957) and "very short" forms (Powell et al., 1980) have been created, reducing the 43 subtests to as few as 4. Schuell herself was not impressed with the usefulness of short examinations in the diagnosis of aphasic disorders. The large number of subtests include many functions that exceed what some authors would consider the assessment of speech and language functions, and range into material that has been a traditional component of many intelligence tests. Schuell's factor analysis may, on closer inspection, seem to reflect a major first "general" factor that is closely related to the "g" obtained in factor analyses of intelligence tests. Schuell and Jenkins (1959), however, considered this factor a general language factor, supporting their assumption about the unitary nature of language.

In sum, the MTDDA is an extensive examination. At the time of initial publication, the test represented a major breakthrough in the development of comprehensive aphasia test instruments that met the requirements of both standardization and objectivity. Great care was taken in its construction, employing both clinical expertise and empirical technique. Potential users of the MTDDA should consider whether its length will be prohibitive in clinical settings. Users should also examine the theoretical bases of the MTDDA relative to their own conception of the nature of aphasic deficits, and balance its breadth against practical needs.

Neurosensory Center Comprehensive Examination for Aphasia

The Neurosensory Center Comprehensive Examination for Aphasia (NCCEA) (Spreen and Benton, 1977; Spreen and Strauss, 1998) was designed to provide a comprehensive assessment of language comprehension, language production, reading, and writing. Other stated goals of the NCCEA are to provide subtests that are sufficiently complex that the clinician can obtain a relatively exact measure of performance level; to standardize and score performances such that necessary corrections for age, sex, and education can be made; to include nonlinguistic subtests to ensure valid interpretation of performance deficits on language tests as either linguistic in nature or due to other dysfunction; and to include specific subtests that could be employed to investigate research questions in aphasiology (Benton, 1967).

The NCCEA comprises 20 subtests that focus on the language functions stated above and 4 "control" subtests of visual and tactile functioning. The test is designed to yield a description of the patient's profile of abilities and disabilities. NCCEA subtests include stimulus presentation in either the visual, auditory, or tactile modality. The subtests measure visual object naming, description of object use, tactile object naming for each hand, sentence repetition, sentence construction, object identification by name, oral reading of names and sentences, oral reading of names and sentences for meaning, writing of object names, writing to dictation, copying sentences, and articulation. The sequential order of subtests provides a meaningful grouping into tests of name finding, immediate verbal memory, verbal production and fluency, receptive (decoding) ability, reading, writing, and articulation. Eight of the 20 language subtests and 3 out of the 4 control subtests require the use of four sets of eight common objects, displayed on trays. The four sets are matched for item difficulty, and are equivalent in mean and distribution of difficulty for aphasic patients (mean percent correct is approximately 63% for all trays) and young children (mean acquisition age of names approximately 5:8 years); they are rotated throughout the battery. Three object substitutions were made in 1987 to replace outdated items. Unlike other aphasia instruments, provisions for collapsing performance on several subtests into category or modality performance summaries are not provided in the test manual.

Several subtests provide a set of items for initial testing, as well as a second set of items to be used only if errors occurred on the first set. This feature tends to shorten test administration in areas in which a patient has no difficulties. The second set of items provides more detailed quantitative information in problem areas. Isolated errors due to poor attention or other irrelevant causes will be reduced in importance if the second set of items is then passed correctly. The complete test takes between 45 and 120 minutes to administer.

The range of item difficulty is limited. In an attempt to avoid highly specialized or low-frequency vocabulary, the authors used only very common objects for their object naming, identification, and similar tasks. As a result, the test has a rather low ceiling on some of the subtests, with the effect that very mild aphasic symptoms in highly educated patients may be missed. Other subtests, however, are "open ceiling" tests for which this limitation does not apply.

Scores on the NCCEA are determined by response correctness. Incorrect responses and mispronounced correct responses are recorded verbatim, as are unusual features of performance, to yield qualitative performance information. An individual's performance on the NCCEA, when corrected for the influence of age and educational level, can be converted into percentile scores to yield relative levels of performance on each subtest and can be entered on three different profile sheets. These profile sheets allow the clinician to compare the patient's performance to that of samples of normal adults (Profile A), aphasic patients (Profile B), and nonaphasic brain damaged patients (Profile C). The aphasic and nonaphasic brain damaged samples consist of consecutive referrals for neuropsychological evaluation in acute-care hospital settings.

Since the development of the NCCEA, a number of studies have investigated its properties and its practical usefulness. Because it was primarily designed for the examination of patients with aphasia or aphasia-type complaints, patients without language problems and normal controls tend to obtain ceiling scores. Therefore, the test cannot be used to measure language ability in normal adults, although the language development in children has been successfully measured with most subtests up to a ceiling age ranging from 8 to 13 years (Gaddes and Crockett, 1975). Because of the low ceiling of the naming tasks, the Visual Naming subtest can be supplemented by use of the BNT.

An empirical study with 353 children, aged 5:5 to 13:5 (Crockett, 1974) found that seven factors described the content of the NCCEA in that population: reading/writing, verbal memory, name finding, auditory comprehension, syntactic fluency, reversal of digits, and repeating digits.

One-year retest reliability in older adults for selected subtests has been reported as satisfactory (Word Fluency .70; Visual Naming .82; Token Test .50; W. Snow and Tierney, 1988).

Construct validity was examined in two studies by Crockett (1976; 1977). The first studied the discrimination of groups of aphasic patients based on ratings of verbal productions, and divided on the basis of the Howes/Geschwind two-type, and the Weisenburg/McBride three-type typologies. Neither of the two models showed significant multivariate differences. The second study showed significant multivariate differences on the NCCEA between four types of aphasia empirically derived from ratings of verbal production by hierarchical grouping analysis. Two of these four types appear to be similar to Howes's two types, a third appears to reflect Schuell's single dimension of language disorder, and a fourth seems to be characterized primarily by memory impairment. Concurrent validity with the WAB was demonstrated by Kertesz (1979). Concurrent validity for changes in language functioning during therapy was reported by Kenin and Swisher (1972) for overall FCP scores.

Predictive validity was established in a study by Lawriw (1976), who also presented a successful cross-validation between patient groups from Iowa City, New York City, and Victoria, B.C. Kenin and Swisher (1972) and Ludlow (1977) investigated patterns of recovery from aphasia; improvement was best reflected in writing from copy and tests of comprehension, whereas expressive performance showed least improvement. Single-word reception or production was more readily recovered than that of longer verbal units. The authors mentioned that reading, writing, and oral production items were not sufficiently difficult for patients at an advanced stage of recovery. In contrast, Ewing-Cobbs et al. (1987)

reported that a high percentage of 23 children and 33 adolescents with closed head injuries exhibited clinically significant language impairment on the NCCEA. Visual Naming, Sentence Repetition, Word Fluency, and Writing to Dictation best discriminated between mild and moderate-to-severe closed head injuries in children and adolescents. Sarno (1984b) described significant differences between aphasic, dysarthric/subclinical, and subclinical aphasic patients on Visual Object Naming, Sentence Repetition, Word Fluency, and the Token Test. Patients with Alzheimer's disease scored significantly lower in the areas of verbal expression, auditory comprehension, repetition, reading, and writing compared with age-matched nonneurological controls (Murdoch et al., 1987). Using only the Token Test and the Word Fluency subtests of the NCCEA, M. Sarno and Buonaguro (1986) reported that females showed signs of more severe aphasia compared to males, although such sex differences did not occur on the FCP, and that the recovery rate was the same for both genders, with an optimal level of recovery reached at 1½ to 2 years after CVA. M. Sarno and Levita (1981) described recovery from global aphasia during the first 3 months after stroke. In a study unrelated to aphasia per se, Spellacy and Brown (1984) found that better scores on the NCCEA and other tests of mental control and academic achievement predict prosocial behavior in young criminal offenders after brief institutionalization.

The 1977 NCCEA normative data for an aphasic reference group are based on 206 unselected referrals to hospital and clinic services in Iowa City, New York City, and Victoria, B.C. Although the concept of "averaging" across aphasic patients, also used in the BDAE, disregards the different types of aphasia, this procedure allows the profiling of individual patients against that reference group; that is, an individual patient's subtype will stand out more clearly. However, when patients from another referral source (e.g., patients in rehabilitation or patients with residual aphasia) are seen, the reference group may no longer be appropriate. Similarly, Profile C is based on a population of patients with brain lesions referred to a neuropsychological service excluding patients with diagnosed aphasia. Use with other patient groups (e.g., those with dementia) may also show poorer comparability.

Normative data for most subtests remain stable through the age span up to age 64. Results of studies with a geriatric population on some of the tests (Montgomery, 1982) showed only a minor decline of 1 or 2 points, which has been incorporated into the age and education correction rules. A study by Tuokko (1985) of elderly subjects in Vancouver, B.C., for example, showed a mean for Visual Naming of 16 (ceiling score) for subjects below 60 years of age to hold up to age 79, and a drop to a mean of 15.44 for subjects 80 years and older. Similarly, Description of Use showed a ceiling score of 16 up to the age of 74; the mean for subjects 75 years and older was 15.78. Tactile Naming (right hand) showed a mean of 15.66 for subjects up to the age of 79, and of 14.89 for subjects 80 years and older. Tactile Naming (left hand) showed a mean of 16 for subjects under 60, and means between 15.14 and 15.57 for subjects between the ages of 60 and 79 years, but a mean of 12.44 for subjects 80 years and older.

Normative data for children between 6 and 13 years are presented. The means were merged from studies by Gaddes and Crockett (1975) and Hamsher (1980), since the differences between the two sources (Victoria and Milwaukee) were minimal. No sex differences were found on 11 of the 20 subtests; on the remaining subtests, sex differences were transient around ages 6 and 7 when girls did slightly better on the writing and reading tasks, except for Word Fluency on which girls were more productive between ages 9 and 13, and Spelling of Written Names on which boys were poorer at ages 7 to 11 years.

The test has also been adapted into Italian, Japanese, and Spanish. Writing from Dictation and Writing from Copy were used in a Chinese study (Hua et al., 1997).

In summary, the NCCEA provides a comprehensive assessment of language functions for aphasic patients without the use of a specific model of language, and without applying a specific approach to delineating diagnostic types of aphasia. Psychometric development of the test has been slow, and few new studies from the last decade are available. The development of three different profile sheets for score evaluation is a distinct asset. On the other hand, the low ceiling of some subtests suggests that some aspects of language functioning in mildly or borderline aphasic patients cannot be adequately measured.

Porch Index of Communicative Ability

The Porch Index of Communicative Ability (PICA) (Porch, 1967; 1973; 1981) is designed to assess verbal, gestural, and graphic responsiveness subsequent to brain damage. Unlike classificatory instruments, the PICA is designed to categorize the nature of the aphasic's ability to respond, modality of response, and quality of response to task demands. Prime uses of the PICA have been assessing performance on multiple occasions postonset to determine the recovery of language ability and aiding in the structure of treatment (Porch, 2001). The PICA has 18 subtests: 4

verbal, 8 gestural, and 6 graphic. A high degree of homogeneity among subtests is established through the repeated use of 10 common, everyday objects of equal difficulty (e.g., a key, a cigarette) for the subtests; this allows examination of fluctuations of performance over time, although this may introduce a practice effect. Subtest order is arranged so as to introduce only minimal information during earlier subtests that would be needed to perform later subtests. Subtests were created to conform to a model of language functioning involving several possible input modalities and outgoing responses, and several possible output modalities. Five modalities are assessed: auditory comprehension, visual comprehension, written expression, verbal expression, and pantomime. The test takes between one-half and 2 hours to administer. Two short versions of the PICA were developed by DiSimoni et al. (1980), reducing the administration time to one-third; the authors found that the short PICA predicted overall PICA scores with an "acceptable confidence level."

Porch has stressed the need to have examiners formally trained by means of workshops in order for the test to have full usefulness. A persistent problem in recording responses to test items involves assessing and quantifying the given response as one of a wide variety of possible responses. As a compromise between two possible extremes (i.e., long-hand notation of response characteristics and simple pass–fail or normal–abnormal dichotomies), the PICA uses a 16-point multidimensional scoring system, an attempt by the author to integrate the strengths of the two approaches while minimizing their weaknesses.

A given response to a PICA test item is evaluated along five dimensions: accuracy, responsiveness, completeness, promptness, and efficiency. A scoring system that considers all possible permutations of these five dimensions is, for all practical purposes, impossible and meaningless. Hence, 16 categories have been identified that represent various relevant combinations of the five dimensions, resulting in a 16-point ranked scale from "no response" (1) to "complex response" (16). For example, any attempt by the patient to perform on the task is scored at least a 6; all accurate responses are scored at least an 8. Additional points are given for a correct response after repeated instructions, for self-corrected responses, responsive ease, completeness, promptness, and efficiency. Porch (1967) reported the viability of the rank ordering of the 16 categories by examining the clinical literature, as well as by pointing out the high agreement between PICA category ordering and ranking of categories by 12 speech pathologists. The individual item scores (180 possible) are transformed into an overall performance score, several modality scores, and individual subtest scores. The overall performance score is considered the best single PICA index of the patient's general communicative ability. Modality scores yield information of the relative capacity of verbal, gestural, and graphic communicative ability. Use of mean values requires that statistical and conceptual assumptions of equal intervals between category levels be met. Whether this assumption is legitimate for the PICA has been the subject of debate (e.g., N. Lincoln and Pickersgill, 1981; A. Martin, 1977; McNeil, 1979). Although single item responses can be categorized on the 16-point scale (i.e., a score of 12 represents an incomplete response), mean values cannot be so categorized. Hence, mean scores cannot categorize the method by which the patient generally communicates, but can only represent a performance level relative to other normative values or the patient's derived scores.

Data indicating that the PICA shows high interrater reliability as well as high test-retest reliability are provided in the manual. The construct validity of the PICA is addressed logically, but not statistically: Both the model of language functioning upon which the PICA is structured and the behaviors categorized in the scoring system have been noted in the aphasiological literature. Holland (1980) reported concurrent validity of the PICA as .93 with the CADL, .86 with the FCP, and .88 with the BDAE. Lendrem and Lincoln (1985) found that the PICA given at 4 weeks postonset successfully predicted spontaneous recovery at 6 months in 32 male stroke victims between 48 and 80 years of age. Age, but not type of aphasia, was related to rate of recovery in 87 stroke victims between the age of 38 and 92 years (Lendrem and McGuirk, 1988). However, N. Lincoln and McGuirk (1986), examining 124 patients between age 38 and 92, 4 weeks and 34 weeks after stroke, noted that groups with and without treatment did not reach the level of recovery predicted by the PICA, and concluded that such predictions are not accurate enough for clinical practice. Avent et al. (1998) used the PICA to document language impairment in the context of pragmatic behaviors.

Percentile data for all principal transformed scores from normative samples of 357 left hemisphere–damaged patients, 96 right hemisphere, and 100 bilaterally damaged patients are presented in the manual (Porch, 1981). In addition to providing relative information for these transformed scores, percentiles are also utilized to determine a given patient's "aphasia recovery curve," employing the overall test percentile, the mean percentile of the nine highest scored subtests, and the mean percentile of the nine lowest scored subtests. Predictions on the scope of recovery can be attempted from this curve; a recovery ceiling is assumed when the three percentiles coincide (Porch et al., 1980). DiSimoni and Keith (1983) found that "tuning in" and "fading out" patterns of the first, middle, or late PICA subtests were related to overall severity of performance on the test. Studying 110 aphasic patients with the PICA, R. Marshall and Tompkins (1983) found that age, health, etiology, and time since onset were good predictors of improvement during the course of treatment. Training patients in functional communication efficacy, on the other hand, did not result in improved performance on the PICA, although improvement was found on the CADL (Aten et al., 1982).

The underlying factor structure of the PICA has been addressed by Clark et al. (1979a,b). Three definable factors emerged from a factor analysis of Porch's original standardization sample (*n* = 150). The first factor was formed by the four verbal subtests, representing a pure dimension of verbal competence. Factor 2 represented five of the six graphic subtests, factor 3 the eight gestural and the other graphic subtests; however, only four of the eight gestural subtests were principally defined by this factor. A second-order factor analysis indicated the presence of a general language factor. PICA subtests showed loadings on this general factor as a function of task difficulty. A factor analysis of a second sample revealed five distinct factors: verbal competence (fluency), verbal-graphic expression, gestural-verbal expression, gestural-nonverbal comprehension, and graphic-geometric comprehension, accounting for 90.6% of the variance. The first four of these factors were highly intercorrelated, again suggesting the presence of a general language factor. These studies also provided empirical evidence for the diversity of subtests subsumed under the gestural modality (A. Martin, 1977). A cluster-analysis of 118 male chronic aphasics (mean age 54.2 years, Hanson and Riege, 1982) found five categories of aphasia, showing primary impairment in specific areas of the PICA: speaking, writing, comprehension, gesturing, and copying. These clusters accounted for 83.9% of the variance with 100% discrimination between clusters.

DiSimoni et al. (1975) found a high degree of redundancy among PICA subtests and concluded that a shortened form of the test may be more useful. DiSimoni et al. (1980) described two short versions of the PICA that require only one-third of the time used for the full-length test. A Portuguese (Brazilian) version is available (Gunther, 1981). Linguistic phenomena in schizophrenia were studied using the PICA (Landre and Taylor, 1995). Reduced attention was the best predictor of language performance, while the content of the thought disorder was not predictive of performance level.

In sum, the PICA is a well-developed and standardized test instrument that has been extensively employed in rehabilitation settings to track recovery and help refine treatment efforts, although we found few research studies with the test in recent years. The multidimensional scoring system has become the most criticized aspect of the test, only partly remedied in the second edition. Two further relative shortcomings of the PICA include the paucity of sampling auditory comprehension and the unfortunate labeling of several subtests as gestural when they entail other specific behaviors. McNeil (1979) suggested that such criticism should not turn clinicians away from the PICA as a test instrument, but rather should make them more cautious interpreters of PICA results. Porch (2001) recently highlighted clinical experiences in using the test during treatment.

Psycholinguistic Assessment of Language Processing in Aphasia

The Psycholinguistic Assessment of Language Processing in Aphasia (PALPA) (Kay et al., 1992; Psychology Press, $325) is a relative newcomer to the comprehensive batteries, one that was hailed as a new psycholinguistic approach to the assessment of aphasia. The test is based upon "the philosophy of considering language assessment as an iterative procedure of hypothesis testing" (Kay et al., 1996, p. 159). The 1996 paper announced that an American version was in preparation, but so far that has not been available. The test has also been used in Australia, Holland, and Spain (Kay et al., 1996, p. 211).

The battery consists of 60 "rigorously controlled tests of components of language structure such as orthography and phonology, word and picture semantics and morphology and syntax" (Kay et al., 1992). The heavy emphasis on reading and writing tasks reveals the fact that the PALPA was originally designed as a reading test. The 60 subtests that make up the PALPA are referred to as distinct "assessments" that one can pick and choose from as needed on an individual basis. Additionally, each task offers guidance as to what additional PALPA tasks a clinician might move on to in order to follow up on a patient's performance on that task. These "assessments" on the PALPA are organized in four sections, each with its own stimulus booklet. The Auditory Processing module comprises 17 tasks including same–different discrimination, repetition, and phonological processing. The Reading and Spelling module comprises 29 tasks, such as letter discrimination (including mirror reversal, upper-to-lower-case matching and vice versa, and specific letters found in word and nonword strings of letters), oral reading, and spelling to dictation. Picture and Word Semantics has eight tasks, relying upon picture matching, picture naming, and synonym judgment. The authors note that the synonym judgment tasks are structured in such a way that half the items are high (e.g., marriage/wedding) and half are low (e.g., advice/counsel) in their "imageability" (i.e., the ability to form a mental image or picture). Finally, Sentence Comprehension is assessed by six tasks that assess comprehension for oral and written material and for locative relations (e.g., an egg under a chicken, a bucket on top of a box). A number of the tasks, such as the assessment of locative relations, have potential value for use in assessment, but many lack or have only minimal normative data available. The authors of the PALPA do not find the paucity of normative information a weakness for the type of use they propose for the test, but the lack of a psychometric approach is very limiting for potential users looking for an empirically well-grounded instrument. The flexible nature of the instrument, however, might find value for the clinician who is seeking to have at hand a series of exercises that might be used to assess progress of therapy or to test the effectiveness of a potential intervention strategy. This type of use would be in keeping with the authors' statement that the "purpose of the PALPA battery is to allow one to derive hypotheses about the nature of the processing disorder" (Kay et al., 1996, p. 22). Such hypotheses can subsequently be ruled in or out by diagnostic testing or by the clinician's intervention with the patient.

At this time, the battery lacks a full standardization and is without psychometrically satisfactory measures of validity and reliability. It is not clear, for example, how many errors would constitute an aphasic deficit (J. Marshall, 1996). The authors stress that the PALPA "is not designed to be given in its entirety to an individual" (Kay et al., 1996, p. 160). It is suggested that the selection of tests for an individual aphasic patient follow the guidelines in the manual to explore in depth the specific problems presented by the individual. In fact, the PALPA is presented as a test still in development (Kay et al., 1996, p. 210). It does not allow diagnostic conclusions, nor does it suggest a specific treatment program. Rather, it provides the material for testing hypotheses about language processing in an aphasic individual based on an elaborate model of both auditory and written language processing (See Figure 9 from Kay et al., 1996, p. 172). Even this model has been criticized as "simplistic" (Ferguson and Armstrong, 1996). Basso (1996) notes that verb retrieval and sentence production are not adequately tested, and Ferguson and Armstrong (1996) note that discourse analysis and processing, which have been a cornerstone of psycholinguistic research, are not represented.

Although Petheram (1998) optimistically lists the PALPA the second most often used test among speech therapists in the United Kingdom, little research with the test has been published since its original publication. Ogden (1996) used the test in four patients to demonstrate how phonological dysgraphia and dyslexia are affected by right and left hemispherectomy in adults; Franklin et al. (1994) used it in a study of "deafness" for abstract word meaning; Grayson et al. (1997) describe the use of the PALPA in therapy with a single case of jargon aphasia.

From a practical point of view, the PALPA is useful only to the practitioner with a strong interest in psycholinguistics who wants to explore specific deficits in detail in an aphasic patient. It is not a substitute for other comprehensive assessment methods.

Western Aphasia Battery

The Western Aphasia Battery (WAB) (Kertesz, 1979; 1982; Pro-Ed, $119) is a close relative of the BDAE and shares with it the diagnostic goal of classifying aphasia subtypes and rating the severity of the aphasic impairment.

The examination, designed for both clinical and research use, comprises four language and three performance domains. Syndrome classification is determined by the pattern of performance on the four language-domain subtests, which assess spontaneous speech, comprehension, repetition, and naming. Weighted responses on these language subtests yields an overall measure of severity of aphasia, the Aphasia Quotient (AQ). Stepwise regression analysis has shown that, of the AQ constituents, the Information Content rating is most highly correlated with the AQ (Crary and Rothi, 1989). The performance-domain areas —reading and writing, praxis, construction, and Raven's Colored Progressive Matrices—yield a second summary measure: the Performance Quotient (PQ). Finally, the AQ and the PQ are summed to form a Cortical Quotient (CQ). Based on the language subtest responses of 375 aphasic patients with various etiologies (mostly CVA) and 162 normal individuals, criteria for the classification of eight aphasic syndromes are described; these syndromes are global, Broca's, Wernicke's, anomic, conduction, isolated, transcortical motor, and transcortical sensory. Classification is forced into one of these syndromes; unclassifiable aphasia subtypes or mixed presentations are not provided for. In this respect, WAB classification is more rigid than in any other diagnostic aphasia battery. This rigidity may have relatively more appeal to researchers than clinicians.

Spontaneous speech is assessed both in response to questioning and in the patient's description of a line drawing, similar to the BDAE. Speech is rated on two 10-point scales: information content and fluency (the fluency scale incorporates both grammatical competence and the presence of paraphasias). Comprehension is assessed by yes/no questions that may be answered in either verbal or nonverbal fashion; by word recognition; and by performance to sequential commands. Repetition has 15 items that are scored as correct, as phonemic error (partial correct), or as an error. Naming comprises object naming (without cuing or, if necessary, with tactile and/or phonemic cuing), word fluency (animals), sentence completion, and responsive speech. Test items were selected to provide a wide enough range of difficulty for assessing all levels of severity.

An uncommon feature of this test's structure is the dissociation from language performance of reading and writing abilities, which, along with nonverbal measures, form part of the PQ. Shewan (1986) reunited the spoken language section (i.e., the AQ tests) with reading and writing as part of a scale called the Language Quotient (LQ), and provided a detailed account of reliability and validity for this addition to the original WAB format. The LQ is weighted so that 60% reflects spoken language performance, and 40% reflects written language performance. Shewan's report emphasized the relation between the LQ measure and the severity of the aphasic disorder. Crary and Rothi (1989) demonstrated internal consistency for the 10 language subtests with protocols of 100 aphasic patients: all subtests correlated highly with the AQ.

WAB standardization information and reliability and validity data were provided by Kertesz and Poole (1974), and then updated by Kertesz (1979) and Shewan and Kertesz (1980). The WAB clearly meets standard rules of test construction, although it ranked last in a review of nine aphasia tests based on criteria reported by Skenes and McCauley (1985). The WAB manifests good internal consistency and high interrater and intrarater reliabilities. High test-retest reliability has been reported for a sample of 38 chronic aphasic patients. Successful criterion validity has been described by the author. Aphasics were differentiated from non-brain-damaged adults in their WAB performance; the AQ distinguished aphasics from non-brain-damaged controls. Construct validity was assessed in a sample of 15 patients who were examined with both the WAB and the NCCEA; there were high intercorrelations between corresponding subtests ranging from .82 for spontaneous speech subtests to .95 for comprehension subtests. The WAB line drawing, used to elicit spontaneous speech, was found to elicit more enumerations, produced at a slower rate than the pictures in the BDAE or the MTDDA

(Correia, et al., 1990). McClenehan et al. (1992) compared the accuracy of estimation of comprehension problems, using the WAB and the FCP, with estimates made by doctors, nurses, and relatives. The comprehension sections of the two tests usually overestimated the patients' ability compared to the judged estimates, but was more accurate for patients with mild problems. Interestingly, length of relationship or educational background did not affect the correctness of judgment, but high or low level of confidence in the judgment by the individual making it did have an influence. One study examined the validity of cutoff scores on the CQ (Fromm and Holland, 1989; Fromm et al., 1986); a cutoff score of 90 points showed good sensitivity and specificity. The authors stated that the language subtests can be administered in approximately 1½ hours, but that the full WAB might require at least two 2-hour sessions to complete. The test manual is far less detailed than Kertesz's book (1979), which remains a good detailed introduction to the WAB.

The WAB has established itself as a useful classificatory research instrument, helped by its inclusive objective classification rules and its summary measures (e.g., AQ, PQ, CQ), which facilitate the interpretation of group data. The main subtypes obtained with the WAB are global, Broca's, Wernicke's, conduction, and anomic aphasia (Shewan and Kertesz, 1980). Studies with the test included novel cluster analytic taxonomies of aphasic syndromes of different etiologies over time (Kertesz and Phipps, 1980) and the evolution of aphasic syndromes during the course of recovery (Kertesz, 1981) and during therapy (Lesser et al., 1986; Shewan and Kertesz, 1984). Crary et al. (1992) used cluster analysis with a small group of 47 patients and found that cluster membership corresponded only poorly (30% of cases) to the classification suggested by the WAB classification rules. Other research investigated the role of activation of the nondominant hemisphere during word repetition (as shown in PET studies, Ohyama et al., 1996), the relation between aphasia and nonverbal intelligence (Kertesz and McCabe, 1975), the relation between language and praxis (Gonzales-Rothi and Heilman, 1984; Kertesz and Hooper, 1982), comparative diagnostic classification between a Portuguese version of the WAB and a Portuguese aphasia examination (Ferro and Kertesz, 1987), and the efficacy of aphasia treatment. A study with 193 Norwegian aphasics found good agreement (85%) between classifications made with the WAB and the Norwegian Basic Aphasia Test, but only after a large number of mixed or otherwise unclassifiable patients were excluded (Sundet and Engvik, 1985); a cluster analysis of this group showed four types of aphasia: global, Wernicke's, Broca's, and anomia, each at a major and a minor impairment level. Butterworth et al. (1984) found that semantic errors were not related to diagnostic grouping, but to severity of aphasia. Semantic errors occurred on both naming and auditory comprehension, suggesting that both have a common underlying deficit.

Studies with Alzheimer's disease patients showed that aphasia was frequently present, and most pronounced on spelling, suggesting a linguistic form of agraphia (Rapcsak et al., 1989); another study (Emery and Breslau, 1988) showed impairment on all tests, but particularly on name finding. Emery and Breslau (1989) compared 20 AD patients with 20 normal controls, and with 20 elderly patients with major depression; they found that the depressed group performed better than the AD group on three WAB subtests; the difference between depressed and normal individuals was significant, suggesting that language problems in depression may mimic aphasia in some cases. Appell et al. (1982) found that 25 AD patients differed from normal controls on all subtests, but the distinction between patients with CVA was confined mainly to higher fluency and lower comprehension scores; AD patients showed more semantic jargon and circumlocutions, but phonemic paraphasias or target approximations were not more frequent. A second study (Karbe et al., 1993) found that spontaneous speech and word fluency were most impaired in cases of primary progressive aphasia. Horner et al. (1992) found that the WAB reading, writing, LQ, and AQ had good discriminant validity between AD and focal stroke patients with aphasia, although discrimination between patients with right hemisphere cerebral infarctions and those with AD was of limited success. Bryan (1988) compared 30 right hemisphere with 30 left hemisphere CVA patients and 30 controls; she found that patients with right hemisphere lesions did not show clear impairment on the WAB, although a discourse analysis indicated some language deficits after right hemisphere damage.

Mega and Alexander (1994) examined subcortical aphasia in 14 patients, and found what they described as a "core aphasia profile" in frontal-caudate lesions (with serious problems in repetition), based on the WAB, the BNT, and the TT. However, Kirk and Kertesz (1994), in a comparison of 32 stroke patients with cortical lesions and 42 age-matched patients with subcortical lesions, found no clear WAB pattern for subcortical aphasia, nor was the lesion volume significantly associated with aphasia severity; instead, aphasias of a broad spectrum of classification occurred in these patients.

The WAB has been employed to examine changes in aphasia during acute recovery and early intervention (e.g., Buoyer McDermott et al., 1996; Horner et al., 1995). Buoyer McDermott and colleagues, for example, examined WAB performance on two occasions in the first few months after left hemisphere CVA for 39 adults (mean age of 65 years and an average of 10 years of education). Significantly increased AQs on the second administration relative to the first were observed and the evolution of aphasia subtype was related to the magnitude of the AQ improvement. The average AQ improvement was in the order of 16 points, with a range from roughly −2 through 49 AQ points. Patients with evolved subtypes showed an average improvement of 20 AQ points, while those who did not evolve showed an average improvement of 8 AQ points.

At least on a research-use basis, versions of the WAB exist in Portuguese (Ferro and Kertesz, 1987), Japanese (Motomura et al., 2000), Arabic (Safi-Stagni, 1991), and Hebrew (Kasher et al., 1999; Zaidel et al., 2000).

Like the BDAE, the WAB offers a measure of spontaneous speech; the WAB, however, appears to be less comprehensive than the BDAE method; for example, fluency, grammatical competence, and the extent of paraphasic errors are combined into a single scale on the WAB, whereas they are assessed independently on the BDAE. Shewan and Donner (1988) also noted that the WAB spontaneous speech subtest does not provide comprehensive information compared with other tests designed to evaluate this aspect of language. The repetition test does not appear to be as encompassing or as well structured as other repetition tasks (e.g., NCCEA or MAE Sentence Repetition).

Auditory-verbal comprehension, as measured on the WAB, is strongly related to outcome (Mark and Thomas, 1992). This study did not find strong relationships between neuroradiological measures and outcome, whereas Metter and colleagues (1990; 1992) found significant relations between outcome and PET scan findings in the left temporoparietal cortex (left angular, supramarginal, and posterior superior temporal gyri). L. Nicholas et al. (1986) found that passage comprehension could be answered correctly better than chance without reading the sentences that the items purported to test, a finding that also applied to the passage comprehension in the BDAE and the MTDDA. Goren et al. (1996) used the test to describe language deficits in 24 medicated schizophrenics, and found that patients who did not respond to medication showed more severe impairment on the WAB and the BDAE Cookie-Theft picture description; the language impairment did not, however, reach low to moderate aphasia levels.

In sum, the primary use of the WAB, like the BDAE, is diagnostic in nature: the classification of aphasic performances into traditional aphasic syndrome subtypes. Explicit decision rules about which classification applies in an individual case are provided, but the test operates on the assumption that all cases can be clearly classified as one of eight basic types. Such clear-cut classification has limited meaning for the "mixed" aphasias that occur much more often in clinical practice than this classification system suggests. Nevertheless, the WAB offers an additional choice for aphasia assessment that is on par with contemporary research in the field, and has found continuing use in research studies. Beyond traditional use in aphasia-specific settings, the WAB (like the BDAE) is among the top five language tests used by speech-language pathologists providing services in treatment settings for traumatic brain injury (Frank and Barrineau, 1996). The inclusion of a "cortical quotient" is new and unusual in an aphasia battery. The concept of a CQ, using a mixture of language and performance measures (including the Raven Progressive Matrices), seems to compete with the traditional concept of IQ (general intellectual functioning) without providing the solid psychometric and theoretical foundations for an intelligence test.

III

TESTS FOR CHILDREN

10

Issues in the Testing of Children

The major obstacle encountered in designing assessment methods for children is that language ability increases with chronological age in the normal child and there is relatively high variability from child to child within a given age level. Full language competency is not reached until 12 to 14 years of age (depending on the definition of competency). After this age, further development takes place in terms of increased vocabulary (G. Miller, 1991), grammatical complexity, awareness of rules of generative grammar, and so on. For these reasons, any assessment method for children requires the establishment of normative data for each year (or half-year) of age. Because of somewhat different rates of growth of language abilities in boys and girls, separate norms for each sex are also required. Obviously, the construction of suitable tests for children requires much more extensive psychometric work, especially for standardization, than does the construction of tests for adults. However, validity and reliability must also be fully established for each age level and cannot be taken for granted on the basis of studies involving children from all age levels.

Aphasia in children may be acquired or developmental. Much of the assessment of children focuses on developmental language retardation, better known in current terminology as *specific language impairment* (SLI) (Leonard, 1997), which only in its severe form may be described as developmental aphasia. The origin of SLI remains unknown; by definition, obvious accompanying conditions such as mental retardation, neurological damage, or hearing impairment are ruled out. Several subtypes (e.g., verbal auditory agnosia, verbal dyspraxia, phonological programming syndrome, phonological-syntactic deficit, lexical syntactic

153

deficit, semantic-pragmatic deficit) have been proposed (Joanisse and Seidenberg, 1998) but have not been clearly established, nor do they have recognizable distinct anatomical foundations; for these reasons subtypes have found little use in clinical practice. Korkman and Haekkinen-Rihu (1994) described three different forms of SLI on the basis of 18 subtests of the Neuropsychological Investigation for Children (NEPSY) with 80 six-to-20-year-old individuals, and described three different forms of SLI: a global, a specific dyspraxia, and a specific comprehension subtype. These subtypes remained distinguishable in 80.5% during a 3-year follow-up. However, *acquired aphasia* due to brain damage at a young age does occur. It is usually recognized by the sudden onset after a relatively normal development of language. Although it has been hypothesized that acquired childhood aphasia is primarily of the nonfluent type, a recent study (Van Dongen et al., 2001) performed a cluster analysis and confirmed that both fluent and nonfluent clusters similar to the adult pattern exist. In contrast to adult aphasia, however, aphasia in children during a hypothetical "critical period" (below the age of 11 years; Lenneberg, 1967) often shows dramatic and frequently complete recovery (Adam, 1998). Nevertheless, Van Dongen et al. (2001) conclude that the "equipotentiality" and "progressive lateralization" of the two hemispheres hypothesis, which was invoked to account for such recovery, should be discarded: "the anatomic substrate for language representation in the child is similar to that in adults" (p. 351).

The available tests are suitable for both forms of childhood aphasia; most frequently, they have been constructed for the measurement of SLI, and few studies of acquired aphasia in children are available for these tests (Aram, 1998). Because autism frequently affects language development severely, tests should also show adequate discrimination between autistic and aphasic disorders.

Most tests are designed for school-age children, although several tests offer extensions into the lower age range from 3 to 6 years. For the earliest development of language in infancy, the Preschool Language Scale-3, the Fluharty Preschool Speech and Language Screening Test - 2 (Fluharty-2, Fluharty, 2000; Riverside Publishing, $161), and the somewhat briefer Preschool Language Assessment Instrument (PLAI) are available. The Early Childhood Research Institute on Measuring Growth and Development also developed "Individual Growth and Development Indicators" (IGDI) for preschool aged children (McConnell, 2000; McConnell et al., 2001), which include well-designed measurements of picture naming, of utterances during semistructured play, and of early literacy such as alliteration, rhyming, and phoneme blending, designed for prediction of school success and recognition of need for

intervention. However, the IGDI is not yet commercially available. Olswang et al. (1987) developed a test for children below 2 years of age
(Assessing Linguistic Behaviors, ALB) aimed at prelinguistic and early
linguistic behavior. It includes Cognitive Antecedents to Word Meaning
(i.e., nomination, agents, and location); Play Scale (mouthing, banging,
visualizing, and manipulating objects, etc.); Communicative Intention
Scale (commenting, requesting, answering); Language Comprehension
Scale (action games, single words, word combinations); and Language
Production Scale (prelinguistic utterances, meaningful speech production). Unfortunately, the lack of standardization and data on reliability
and validity as well as the length of the ALB leads to the conclusion
that this material should be used for informal evaluations rather than
as a formal test (Atlas, 1992; Bliss, 1992). For similar reasons, Bachman
(1995) made the same recommendation for the Receptive-Expressive
Emergent Language Test, 2nd ed., designed for children from birth to 3
years of age (REEL-2, Bzoch and Leage, 1991; Pro-Ed, $79).

Clinicians also often resort to general tests of early infant development that cover a wide range of abilities but include simple assessments
of language (e.g., smiles, orients to sound, visually tracks voice, interacts). However, the predictive validity of such measures below the age
of 3 years is questionable (Harris and Langkamp, 1994). A large number
of such assessment procedures, usually aimed at the general intellectual
development of the child, but including several measures of language
development, are available (e.g., Battelle Developmental Inventory, birth
to age 8:0; Newborg et al., 1984; Riverside Publishing, $325; Bayley
Scales of Infant Development-2; 1 month through 42 months; Bayley,
1993, Harcourt Brace, $1480; Revised Denver Developmental Screening
Test (DDST) also available in Spanish; Franenburg and Dodds, 1990;
Denver Developmental Materials, $40; Kaufman Assessment Battery for
Children, K-ABC, Kaufman and Kaufman, 1995; Western Psychological
Services, $410; Kaufman Survey of Early Academic and Language Skills,
Kaufman and Kaufman, 1993; Western Psychological Services, $196.50;
NEPSY, Neuropsychological Developmental Assessment, age 3 to 12
years, Korkman; Psychological Corporation, $600; Stanford-Binet In-
telligence Test-4th ed., 1 month to 4½ years; Thorndike et al., 1996;
Riverside Publishing, $777). In a sample of 137 low birth weight infants,
the Bayley scales detected language delay mainly through a detailed analysis of specific language items rather than through the Bayley Mental
Development Index (Siegel et al., 1995). Both the K-ABC and the DDST
have been successfully used for large-scale prekindergarten developmental
screening and between birth and 6 years (Allard and Pfohl, 1988; Diamond, 1990; Diamond and le Furgy, 1988), although a meta-analysis of

five validity studies by Greer et al. (1989) noted poor sensitivity in not identifying 80% of children who had poor outcome. Feeney and Bernthal (1996), however, found a 93.5% positive hit rate with the DDST-2. The NEPSY, originally developed in Finland, has found considerable interest since its extensive North American restandardization, and includes body-part naming, phonological processing, comprehension of instructions, verbal fluency, and oromotor sequences as tests of the language domain. Korkman et al. (1999) report high sensitivity of this test for impairment of phonological awareness in a normal sample and in both children with very low birth weight and with asphyxia followed up to the age of 5 to 9 years (Korkman et al., 1996). Another study by the authors (Korkman and Haekkinen-Rihu, 1994) used NEPSY subtests to identify subtypes of impairment in 6-to-10-year-old children with language impairment; the authors identified a global, a specific dyspraxia, and a specific comprehension subtype.

Among the language screening tests for children is the Joliet 3-Minute Preschool Speech and Language Screen (Kinzler, 1993; Psychological Corporation, $115) for 2½-to-4½-year-olds, together with the Joliet 3-Minute Speech and Language Screen-Revised (Kinzler and Johnson, 1993; Psychological Corporation, $115) for kindergarten, grade 2, and grade 5. Both are designed for quick identification of problems in receptive vocabulary, expressive syntax, and phonology with the presentation of eight plates at each age level, and a subjective rating of fluency and voice. The test has been standardized on a stratified sample of 2587 children. Pragmatics and language comprehension are only minimally covered (Fischer, 1998) and discriminant validity remains questionable (McNeil and Campbell, 1998). The Test of Pragmatic Language (TOPL, Phelps-Terasaki and Phelps-Gunn, 1992; Pro-Ed, $124) focuses on listening and speaking skills in a social context (with subcomponents of physical setting, audience, topic, purpose, visual-gestural cues, and abstraction). It takes about 45 minutes, and is designed for the age range from 5:0 to 13:11 years. The Screening Test of Adolescent Language, Revised (STAL, Prather et al., 2000; Western Psychological Services, $55) is designed specifically for teenagers and takes about 7 minutes with subtests for vocabulary, auditory memory span, language processing, and proverbs explanation.

In addition, a number of tests of *phonological discrimination* are available: the British Auditory Discrimination and Attention Test for children between 3½ and 12 years of age (Morgan-Berry, 1988; NFER-Nelson, $150); Comprehensive Test of Phonological Processing (Wagner et al., 1999; Sopris West, $224); Goldman-Fristoe-Woodcock Test of Auditory Discrimination (American Guidance Service, $99.95); Halstead-Reitan Speech Sound Discrimination Test (older children version, Reitan Neuropsychology Laboratory, $55); Khan-Lewis Phonological Analysis (P. Webster and Plante, 1995; American Guidance Service, $78.95); Assessment of Phonological Processes-Revised (APP-R, Hodson, 1986; Pro-Ed, $109); Lindamood Auditory Conceptualization Test (LAC, Lindamood and Lindamood, 1998; Psychological Assessment Resources, $115); the brief (5 minutes) Test of Auditory Analysis Skills (TAAS; age 5 to 8 years; Rosner, 1999; Academic Therapy Publications, $16); the Test of Auditory Perceptual Skills-Revised (age 4 through 11, Gardner, 1998; Academic Therapy Publications, $87); the Test of Phonological Awareness (TOPA, kindergarten and early elementary versions, age 5 to 8:11; Torgesen and Bryant, 1994; Pro-Ed, $168); Wepman's Auditory Discrimination Test, 2nd ed. (age 4:0 to 8:11 years, Wepman and Reynolds, 1998; Western Psychological Services, $89.50) are useful for the examination of children's ability to recognize speech sounds essential for the development of language and of reading at the preschool and school level. Further, a variety of vocabulary tests are available: Comprehensive Receptive and Expressive Vocabulary Test (CREVT, age 4 to 17; Wallace and Hammill, 1994; Psychological Corporation, $200.50), also published with an adult version; the Receptive One-Word Picture Vocabulary Test, 2000 edition (ROWPVT, age 2:0 through 18:11; R. Brownell, 2000a; Wide Range, $125), is very similar in design. Among children's naming tests, the Expressive One-Word Picture Vocabulary Test, 2000 edition (EOWPVT, age 2:0 to 18:11; R. Brownell, 2000b; Academic Therapy Publications $125) is similar to the BNT but has found limited use so far. The BNT as well as tasks of phonemic and semantic fluency have been used with children between 5:11 and 11:4 years; the results show a linear increase with age (Riva et al., 2000).

For the assessment of related problems in *articulation*, the Arizona Articulation Proficiency Scale-3 (AAPS, 18 months to 18 years of age; Barker-Fudala, 1998; Western Psychological Services, $118); the Frenchay (Enderby and Crow, 1996); the Goldman-Fristoe Test of Articulation-2 (2 to 21 years; American Guidance Service, $169.95); the Photo Articulation Test-3 (3:6 to 8:11 years; Lippke et al., 1997; Pro-Ed, $144) are used to assess the articulatory development in children (Alberts et al., 1995) or to differentiate between articulatory and other motor disability (Gentry et al., 1997). Of these, the Goldman-Fristoe, the AAPS, and the Frenchay Tests have found the most attention in test development and research studies (J. Roberts et al., 1990; Sommers et al., 1994). Sturner et al. (1993) also found that the Fluharty Preschool Speech and Language Screening Test showed good sensitivity for articulation problems when compared to the AAPS and the Templin-Darley Test of Articulation. Pollock (1991) compared the Goldman-Fristoe, the AAPS, the Photo Articulation, the Assessment of Phonological Processes-Revised, and the Fisher-Logeman Test of Articulatory Competence and found that the tests differed widely in the vowels sampled in each test, and suggested that the tests all needed additional stimulus words for an appropriate vowel analysis. A supplemental examination for structural and apraxic problems, the Oral Speech Mechanism Screening Examination - 3 (OMSE-3, St. Louis and Ruscello, 2000; Pro-Ed, $89), is designed to screen in 5 to 10 minutes for problems of tongue, lip, jaw, palate, teeth, velopharyngeal mechanisms, breathing, and diadochokinesis with norms for 5-to-78-year-olds. A new instructional videotape allows better standard administration, which had been a problem in previous editions (Martin, 1992). The Screening Test for Developmental Apraxia of Speech - 2 (STDAS-2, Blakeley, 2000; Pro-Ed, $84), designed for 4-to-12-year-olds, takes about 10 minutes, and includes calculating the difference between expressive and receptive language, and screening for prosody, verbal sequencing, and articulation. Reliability and validity data have been added in the new edition.

For the assessment of *prosody*, the Prosody-Voice Screening Profile (PVSP, Shriberg et al., 1990; Communication Skill Builders, now out of print) used an audiotaped conversational speech sample of 12 to 25 or more utterances for coding of phrasing, rate, stress, loudness, pitch, and quality (Shriberg, 1993). It was designed for young children with intelligibility problems, but can be used for all ages. Coding with this instrument may require considerable training or experience, and takes 15 to 30 minutes. Reliability and validity testing of the PVSP has so far been limited.

The most popular *reading tests* are the brief Wide Range Achievement Test-3, which also covers spelling and arithmetic (WRAT-3, G.S. Wilkinson, 1993; Wide Range Publishers, $148), the Wechsler Individual Achievement Test-2nd edition (WIAT-II, Psychological Corporation, 2001, $321), or the abbreviated WIAT-II ($130) used for screening, the Gates-McGinitie Test, and the Woodcock Reading Mastery Test-Revised (American Guidance Service). A detailed (90 minutes) assessment for children is provided by the Test of Written Language-3rd ed. (TOWL-3, Hammill and Larsen, 1996; American Guidance Service, $210).

Another area of potential overlap with aphasia or SLI are the *central auditory processing disorders* (CAPD). CAPD is characterized by normal hearing, but poor listening skills, short auditory attention span, or difficulty in understanding speech in the presence of background noise, presumed to have a neurological cause. The American Speech-Language-Hearing Association (1996) defines CAPD as deficiencies in one or more auditory behaviors: sound localization and lateralization, auditory discrimination, auditory pattern recognition, temporal aspects of audition (resolution, masking, integration, ordering), auditory performance decrements with competing acoustic signals, and decrements with degraded acoustic signals. Slow learners are specifically excluded. The diagnostic label is still somewhat controversial (Cacace and McFarland, 1998), particularly since deficit in just one of the five areas is sufficient to make this diagnosis. It needs to be differentiated from SLI and acquired receptive aphasia, attention deficit/hyperactivity disorder, and learning disability, all of which show similar symptoms. James et al. (1994) suggest that the underlying deficit lies in the semantic system and immediate phonological working memory.

The Test for Auditory Processing Disorders in Children (SCAN-C-Revised) (Keith, 1999; Psychological Corporation, with CD disk $225) for the 5-to-11-year-old age range (also available as SCAN-A for adolescents and adults, 12 to 50 years; Keith, 1994; Psychological Corporation, with audiocassette $185) was designed as a screening test for CAPD. It includes filtered words, auditory figure-ground, competing words, and competing sentences tasks, and can be completed in 20 minutes. Reliability is good (.47 to .69 for subscores, .77 for total test score). Amos and Humes (1998) report that scores increase on retesting after 6–7 weeks, and Emerson et al. (1997) found that it overidentified children not at risk for CAPD; moreover, SCAN-C results were poorer in a "quiet school setting" (as recommended by the manual) compared to results when testing was done in an audiometric booth. Domitz and Schow (2000) also offer the more detailed preliminary Multiple Auditory Processing Assessment (MAPA), designed for 3rd grade children, a selection of tests including the Selective Auditory Attention Test (SAAT, Cherry, 1980), Pitch Patterns (Pinhiero, 1977), Dichotic Digits (Musiek, 1983), and Competing Sentences (Willeford, 1985), which can be administered in 30 minutes, and compared the results with those of the SCAN-C: They found four factors emerging from the MAPA tests (auditory pattern/temporal ordering, binaural integration, binaural separation, monaural separation/closure), while the SCAN measured only the last two of these factors. Examining 81 eight-to-9-year-old children, MAPA identified 17 as CAPD, while the SCAN showed less sensitivity.

11

Tests for Infants and Young Children

Children's Acquired Aphasia Screening Test

The Children's Acquired Aphasia Screening Test (CAAST) (Whurr and Evans, 1998; Whurr Publishers, appr. $200) was designed in Britain for children between 3 and 7 years of age and follows a model similar to that of the Whurr Aphasia Screening Test (Whurr, 1996). The model is a standard input–output and sensory–motor model. The CAAST comprises 25 subtests, including prespeech and prereading tasks as well as nonlinguistic tasks, for example, drawing and gestures. It was standardized on 108 normal children. Whurr and Evans (1998) demonstrate the results of four cases of acquired childhood aphasia. No further research has been published as yet.

Aphasia Screening Test

The Aphasia Screening Test (AST) is part of the Halstead-Reitan Neuropsychological Battery, Older Children's Battery, Young Children's Battery (Reitan Neuropsychology Laboratory, $59.95 for the individual tests, $2230 for the complete battery). The AST can be administered in 10–25 minutes and consists, similar to the adult version, of 22 items requiring the child to write his or her name; copy figures; name objects; read numbers, letters, and a short sentence; print; count fingers; do simple additions; identify body parts; show tongue; and perform other body orientation tasks ("place finger on nose").

Reitan and Wolfson (1992) reported that the AST discriminated well between 26 normal and 26 brain-damaged children between the age of 6 and 8 years. It also correlated strongly (.82) with the Wechsler Intelligence Quotient. The sample apparently did not include children with aphasia. In general, the AST seems to be misnamed, since its purpose seems to be screening for brain damage rather than aphasia per se.

Clinical Evaluation of Language Fundamentals-Preschool

The Clinical Evaluation of Language Fundamentals-Preschool (CELF-Preschool) is a downward extension of the CELF-3 for ages 3 years to 6 years, 11 months (Wiig et al., 1992), available from Psychological Corporation for $249; 25 record forms, $45.

The test requires between 30 and 45 minutes administration time. Like the CELF-3 (see below), it consists of three receptive and three expressive language subtests. Each subtest is introduced with several familiarization trials. Discontinuation rules for each age level serve to avoid unnecessary testing and failure experiences for the child. The Quick Test, as a preliminary screening device, uses only the first subtest of each of the two parts (Linguistic Concepts and Recalling Sentences in Context) to determine whether administration of the full battery is indicated.

The receptive subtests are:

Linguistic Concepts: After initial familiarization trials to test whether the child understands the vocabulary and commands used in the test, the child is asked to point to an animal on multiple-choice cards. Linguistic demands increase from "Point to one of the bears" to "Point to the giraffe after you point to an elephant and a monkey." (20 items)

Basic Concepts: The child has to point to one of three pictures fitting the concept being asked for, for example, "The one that is inside," referring to the picture of a dog inside a doghouse (as opposed to the other two pictures showing the dog in other places). Concepts range from "inside, up," to "different and last." (18 items)

Sentence Structure: Three pictures are shown and the child must point to the one corresponding to a statement, for example, "The boy is sleepy" to "The boy saw a girl who was carrying a hammer." (22 items)

The expressive subtests are:

Recalling Sentences in Context: The child is asked to repeat 18 verbal expressions contained in short stories, for example, "Robert knew that packing for the move would be hard work. He said 'I will help' What did Robert say?"

Formulating Labels: The child is asked a question that can be answered from a picture presented at the same time. This part essentially tests noun and verb vocabulary, ranging from "sailboat" to "thermometer." (20 items)

Word Structure: The child supplies a word for a sentence presented by the examiner describing pictures, for example, "This boy is skating. This boy will skate. This boy is painting. This boy will _____."

Each item is scored as correct, incorrect, or no response with some subtests using a 2-1-0 scoring for transpositions or other partially correct responses. Scoring rules are quite explicit and easy to follow. A special feature is a list of acceptable dialectical variations. The material is presented in booklets/easels resembling children's books for this age group. The record form includes a behavioral observation checklist, a linguistic breakdown of items for four of the subtests, and a summary page for the transformation of raw scores into standard scores (mean of 10), percentile ranks, and an expressive/receptive and total language score (mean of 100, SD = 15), in 6-month intervals based on norms available in the manual. Norms are based on field testing of 550 normal children with distribution of gender, race, and educational level of primary caregiver similar to the 1988 U.S. census. The manual also contains useful items for extension testing as well as suggestions for intervention, using the Wiig Criterion Referenced Inventory of Language (Wiig, 1990).

Internal consistency ranges from .81 to .96, reliability for 57 children retested after 2 to 4 weeks ranged from .60 to .96. Interrater agreement exceeded 90%. Correlation between CELF-Preschool and CELF-R for 80 language-disordered children between 5 and 6 years ranged from .41 to .86. for 5-year-olds and from .31 to .93 for 6-year-olds. Correlation with the Wechsler Preschool and Primary Scale of Intelligence (WPPSI-R) was .70 for receptive language, .60 for expressive language, and .71 for total language score, with the Differential Abilities Scales (DAS) between .62 and .68. Discriminant function analysis between 80 children with and 80 without language disorder resulted in a misclassification rate of 25% with a criterion of 1 SD, and of 28% with a criterion of 1.5 SD.

To our knowledge, no research studies using the CELF-Preschool have been published. However, because of the strong similarity, research findings and critical comments for the CELF-3 would apply to this version as well.

Fluharty Preschool Speech and Language Screening Test-2

The second edition of the Fluharty Preschool Speech and Language Screening Test (Fluharty, 2000; Pro-Ed, $139) contains five subtests: articulation, repeating sentences, responding to directives and answering questions, describing actions, and sequencing events. It is designed for the identification of preschool children for whom a full speech and language evaluation is indicated, and takes about 10 minutes to administer. It has been restandardized on a sample of 705 children in 21 states, representative of the U.S. census in 1998. Scores for each subtest and a composite score can be transformed into standard scores with a mean of 100 and an SD of 15, as well as percentile ranks. The test manual documents good reliability and content and construct validity. The composite score correlates highly with that of the TOLD-P3.

Sturner et al. (1993) tested 700 children between 4:6 and 5:9 years of age with the first edition of the Fluharty, and compared results with those for the Arizona Articulation Proficiency Scale-Revised, the Templin-Darley Test of Articulation, the Test of Language Development-Primary, and the Test for Auditory Comprehension of Language-Revised. Comparing two stratified samples based on speech/language screening results, the authors found a sensitivity of .43 for speech, of .31 for language outcome, a specificity of .82 and .92, respectively, a predictive value of .43 and .54, percent agreement of 72% and 80%, resulting in overreferral of 14% and underreferral of 5%.

Oral and Written Language Scales

The Oral and Written Language Scales (OWLS) (Carrow-Woolfolk, 1996; American Guidance Service, $264.95), designed for testing language development and school readiness, is suitable for the age of 3 through 21 years (for written expression 5 through 21). It actually consists of two tests, the Oral Language Scale (available separately for $189.95) and the Written Language Scale. The Oral Language Scale includes the Listening Comprehension (LC) and the Oral Expression (OE) scales (total administration time: 20–65 minutes). The LC scale consists of 111 items and the OE scale of 96 items. The child looks at four numbered black-and-white drawings and must point to the correct drawing or say the number; reading or verbal responding is not required for the LC scale. The scale includes comprehension of lexical (nouns, verbs, modifiers, personal pronouns, prepositions, idioms, words with multiple meanings, words representing direction, quantity, and spatial relations), syntactic (noun and verb modulators such as number, tense, gender, voice; constructs such as embedded sentences, coordination, subordination, direct/indirect object), and supralinguistic (figurative language and humor, derivation of learning from context, logic, inference) items. In addition, the OE scale includes items for pragmatic language that require appropriate responses in specific situations such as questions, explanations, etc.

The Written Language Scale consists of four overlapping age-appropriate item sets, ranging from copying written words, writing to dictation, to retelling a story or interpreting a statement in written form.

Explicit scoring rules are provided; computer scoring is available (CD-ROM kit $149.95). Transformation into age- or grade-based standard scores, percentiles, stanines, and test-age equivalents are presented in 6-month intervals for age 3 and 4, and yearly for older children. The standardization for the Oral Language Scale was carried out with 1985 subjects between age 3 and 21 appropriate for the U.S. census, and with 1373 subjects for the Written Language Scale. Clinical validity testing resulted in significant differences between control groups and children with language delay, language impairment, reading disability, learning disability, hearing disability, and mental handicap, but not for children with speech impairment. Internal reliability ranged from .84 to .93, test-retest reliability from .73 to .89, interrater reliability was .95 for both scales. The intercorrelation between LC and OE was .70, between the composites of language and written scales .67. Concurrent validity with the TACL-R was .78, with the CELF-R .91, with the PPVT-R .75, with K-ABC Achievement .82, with WISC-III Verbal IQ .77, with Kaufman Brief Intelligence Test vocabulary .76. Correlations with nonverbal and global IQ scores ranged from .59 to .76, with academic achievement tests from .47 to .88.

No published clinical or research studies with these scales other than those reported in the manual are available at this time.

Preschool Language Assessment Instrument

The Preschool Language Assessment Instrument (PLAI) was developed by Blank et al. (1978) and is available from the Psychological Corporation in English and Spanish (test manual $98.50; record forms $48 each). A Cantonese version is also available (Stokes and Wong, 1996). The PLAI is designed to measure language skills required for school success in children from age 2.9 to 5.8 years, and evaluate integration of knowledge of vocabulary, concepts, and language in following directions, reflecting on information, and solving problems, and to structure appropriate teaching. Each item is evaluated with a 0 to 3 scoring system, judging adequacy, relevance, and completeness of the response. It relies on teacher–child conversational exchanges on a specific topic at four different levels of abstraction.

1. Find one like this (matching object); show me what you heard (object identification by sound); what did you hear (naming object heard); what did you touch (naming object touched); what is this (visual naming); say this (repeating simple sentences); what did you see (remembering pictured object and incidental information).

2. Find one that can . . . (scanning for an object defined by its function); what is happening (describing a scene); what things did I say (recalling items named); what, who, where (recalling specific information); finish this sentence (sentence completion); tell me its . . . (naming characteristics and function); how are these different? (identifying differences); find one that is . . . and . . . (attending to two characteristics); name something that is . . . (citing an example within a category).

3. Find one to use with this (integrating verbal and visual information in object finding); what will happen next (events subsequent to a scene); what would he say (assuming role of another person); do this . . . , then this (set of directions); make these into . . . (arranging picture sequence); tell me how . . . (formulating set of directions); what happened to all of these (generalization about a set of events); tell this story (formulating statement to combine sequence of pictures); how are these the same (identifying similarities); find the things that are not . . . (selecting by exclusion); what is a . . . (definition).

4. Where will . . . (predicting changes in position); what will happen if . . . (predicting changes in structure; why will . . . (justifying a prediction); what made it happen (identifying causes of event); what could you do (formulating a solution); what could she do (formulating a solution from another perspective); what could we use (selecting means to a goal); how can we tell (explaining an inference); why can't we . . . (explaining an obstacle to an action).

The manual shows findings that confirm that the four levels are achieved in a progressive order. It also reports differences based upon family economic status: 83% of middle-class 5-year-olds had achieved "mastery," defined as an average score of 1.5, whereas only 33% of lower-class children obtained this score.

Fagundes et al. (1998) developed a thematic interaction instruction (PLAI-T) in which exactly the same questions were asked, but questions were interwoven with stories telling an arts and crafts activity, and a snack activity. This modification resulted in scores for African American children that were not significantly different from those of Caucasian children, except for the highest level of abstraction where Caucasian children scored higher. The Caucasian children did not show an improvement of their scores when the PLAI and PLAI-T were compared. The study also confirmed the progression of abstraction level with age. Skarakis-Doyle et al. (1998) complained about the small standardization sample, since the test is often used to measure delayed language development. They produced new normative data for 152 three- to 5-year-olds in Ontario, Canada. They found scores for age groups similar but more stable in their sample compared to the standardization group, due to sample size, thus confirming the originally published norms. Santiago (1995) used the test to evaluate factors of home-language environment affecting the performance in Spanish-English bilingual preschoolers. Schetz (1994) found that the use of computer software in tandem with extensive instructor interaction improved the results on the PLAI in low-functioning preschoolers. The test correlates strongly with the Reynell Developmental Language Scales (Stokes and Wong, 1996).

Van Kleek et al. (1997) found that parents' discussion of book reading with their youngsters correlated significantly with the children's gain in abstract language development. Culatta and Young (1992) found that children with spina bifida hydrocephalus performed comparably to controls on concrete tasks of the PLAI but produced more irrelevant and "no-responses" than controls.

Readers familiar with other assessment procedures will recognize that many of the questions overlap with the verbal part of several intelligence tests. However, in early language testing such an overlap cannot be avoided. The test appears to be a promising addition to preschool language testing.

Preschool Language Scale-3

The Preschool Language Scale-3 (PLS-3) (Zimmerman et al., 1992a) examines language comprehension and production, and is available from the Psychological Corporation for $185 for the complete kit. It is designed for infants and children from the age of 2 weeks to 6 years, 11 months. A Spanish edition is available (Zimmerman et al., 1992b).

The test includes direct testing and supplementary testing with an Articulation Screener, a Language Sample Checklist, and a Parent Questionnaire. For children under 12 months, the PLS-3 focuses on language precursors including attention, vocal development, and social communication, although one reviewer (Walker, 1994) found the item gradient quite steep for infants, and the ceiling too low for older children; she recommends the PLS mainly for the age range from 3 to 5 years. For older children the receptive composite score includes tests of attention, semantics (context), vocabulary and concepts (including quality, spatial, and time sequence), structure (form), morphology and syntax, and integrative thinking skills (classification, word definition). The expressive composite score includes the areas of vocal development, social communication, semantics (content), vocabulary and concepts, structure (form), morphology and syntax, and integrative thinking skills. In addition, a total language composite is calculated. Raw scores are transcribed into standard scores and percentile rank equivalents. Administration time ranges from 20 to 50 minutes.

The PLS-3 has been standardized on a sample of 1200 children representative of the age range and the U.S. census for region, race, parental education, and gender. This may remedy the overestimation of large rural and suburban samples reported by Hilton and Mumma (1991) for the earlier (revised) edition of this test. For the current edition, Allen et al. (1990) also reported that test results were more closely related to socioeconomic status than medical risk in children with congenital anomalies. As discussed in an earlier section about the range of item difficulty (Chapter 4), Norris (1998) notes that the standardization excluded children with less than average language ability, evidence of language disorder, or who were at risk for such a disorder; this exclusion leads to misjudgments, that is, a score 2 SDs below the mean is still in the average language ability range, and may lead to overidentification of children as language disordered, a problem not unique to this test. However, the authors found 66%, 70%, and 80% correct classifications when these norms were used for the discrimination between language-disordered and non-language-disordered children at the age of 3, 4, and 5, respectively, using a cutoff of 1.5 SD. Norris considers this a problematic finding, perhaps due to the exclusion of items appropriate for language-disordered children. The large SEM also makes it difficult to distinguish between minimal, mild, and more severe language disorders.

Reliability (internal consistency [.47 to .94, total test .92 to .94], test-retest coefficients [.81 to .94], interrater reliability [89%]) is satisfactory. Concurrent validity with other standardized instruments as reported in the manual ranged from .66 to .88.

Nor surprisingly, the PLS correlates between .47 and .69 with the Stanford-Binet Intelligence Scale-IV in 120 referred preschool children with a mean age of 47 months (Tedeschi, 1995). It correlates reasonably well with the Denver Developmental Screening Test-II (Franenburg and

Dodds, 1990), and the receptive, expressive and total language composite correlates .66, .86, and .88 with the respective parts of the CELF-R, suggesting that the two tests measure very similar concepts. Correlation with total communication measures, including word meaning fluency, phoneme segmentation fluency, naturalistic observation of infant-toddler communication, communication-evoking situations, caregiver communications measure, semistructured play, picture naming, story telling) was reported as .86. Auditory comprehension and verbal ability were significantly related to locomotor skills as measured with the Test of Gross Motor Development in 4-year-olds (Merriman et al., 1995). It was also sensitive to deficits on the Pediatric Language Acquisition Screening Tool for Early Referral (PLASTER-R, Shulman and Sherman, 1996; Sherman and Shulman, 1999). Modifications of the test for severely physically handicapped children were described by Moran (1989).

The test has been used to evaluate outcome of prenatal cocaine and polydrug exposure at the age of 3 to 6 years (El-Khatib, 1997; Phelps and Cottone, 1999; Phelps et al., 1997) and of perinatal HIV exposure (Mcneilly, 1999) at the age of 1:3 to 3 years. It has also been shown to be sensitive to socioeconomic and family variables as well as medical risk factors in low birth weight children at the age of 3 years (Hershberger, 1996). The PLS also indicated progress in autistic 4-year-olds under treatment (Handleman et al., 1991; Harris et al., 1991). No studies of aphasic children are available.

In sum, the PLS-3 is a well-developed instrument that has shown its sensitivity to a number of disorders in research studies. Clinicians should be aware of the standardization problem in the low range of ability and in the item range for infants and 6-year-olds, which may require considerable judgment in identifying and classifying degree of impairment. Fourth editions of the English and Spanish versions are forthcoming in 2003.

Reynell Developmental Language Scales-III

The Reynell Developmental Language Scales-III (RDLS-III) were designed for children from age 1 to 6 years (Reynell and Gruber, 1990; Western Psychological Services, $499; Reynell and Huntley, 1971). The 134-item battery can be administered in 30 minutes, and was also adapted into Dutch (Zink and Schaerlaekens, 2000) and Finnish (used with a sample of infants between 8 months and 29 months of age; Lyytinen et al., 1994). Edwards et al. (1999) presented a revised British edition that extends to age 7. The test consists of the verbal comprehension scale (including a parallel version normed for children who can respond only by pointing) and the expressive language scale, which includes items for testing structure, vocabulary, and content. The RDLS-III, originally published in 1977, appears to be the most popular and best-established comprehensive children's test, although it does not assess the pragmatics of communication (Lees, 1999). Lees et al. (1998) also published an RDLS study of children with acquired epileptic aphasia (Landau-Kleffner syndrome).

Norms are based on a sample of 600 children selected to be representative of the U.S. population.

Ball (1999) criticized the reliance on elicited speech samples rather than the use of spontaneous speech samples, although this method lacks the standardized scoring of the RDLS. Rome-Flanders and Cronk (1998) investigated the age at which measurement of infant linguistic abilities begins to be reliable. They found a parent-report instrument to be reliable from the age of 9 months, whereas the RDLS showed significant correlations from age 1:3.

Marinac and Ozanne (1999) presented a refinement of scoring for 3:0-to-4:5-year-olds by subdividing comprehension scale answers into "random answering," "probable reasoning," and "semantic probability." This hierarchy of comprehension strategy prior to full language comprehension was documented and found to be replicable. Hagtvet and Hagtvet (1990) examined the construct and discriminant validity of the RDLS by comparing the test to constructs of the ITPA; they found a high degree of concurrence. Lyytinen et al. (1997) found no general correlation between symbolic play and RDLS language score, but the RDLS scores related to symbolic play scores in 110 late talkers at age 1:6.

Cornish and Munir (1998) used the RDLS to investigate the language skills of children with cri-du-chat syndrome, and found that in these children language skills still increase beyond age 10. Children with Down syndrome showed a range of pragmatic skills and communicative intentions when compared to controls matched for mental age (F. Johnson and Stansfield, 1997). Petrie (1975) found that progress in 5- and 6-year old children in a residential school with difficulties in listening skills and language acquisition could be measured with the RDLS, although progress was small, and the differentiation between deafness and receptive language disorder was difficult in this group.

Test of Early Language Development, 3rd Edition

The Test of Early Language Development, 3rd ed. (TELD-3)(Hresko et al., 1999) is a version of the Test of Language Development (TELD-P3) and of the TOLD-I3, both designed for older children. It is available from Pro-Ed for $264. The TELD-3 is designed for children from age 2:0 to 7:11 years and takes about 20 minutes to administer. It has two subtests, receptive and expressive language, and also yields an overall language score, which can be expressed in standard scores, percentile ranks, and age equivalents. The authors claim that the test shows little or no bias toward gender, disability, racial, socioeconomic, or ethnic groups.

The normative sample for the TELD-3 consisted of 2217 children, representative of U.S. population statistics for 1997. It has been used for the assessment of the effect of environmental factors on language development in toddlers (Gray, 1996), the effect of early intervention programs (Cole et al., 1993), and the relationship between language development and phonological awareness in preschool children (Webster and Plante, 1995). Another study investigated the relation between theory-of-mind development and language in a longitudinal study of 3-year-olds (Astington and Jenkins, 1999).

12

Tests for School-Age Children

Several tests of normal language development in children are available. Unfortunately, the popular Illinois Test of Psycholinguistic Abilities (ITPA, Kirk et al., 1968) was out of print for several years. However, a revised and updated version—the ITPA-3—has recently become available (Hammill et al., 2002; Western Psychological Services; $179.50). The ITPA-3 includes a new standardization sample. The original ITPA had been used to analyze the deficit of 237 children with severe oral language disorders (Luick et al., 1982). The authors found that auditory associations and grammatical closure showed the most severe impairment, consistent with a deficit in the central organization process, that is, central aphasia or inner language. It has been successfully used to measure progress in an ITPA-structured teaching program for children with language disorders (Evesham, 1977). The McCarthy Scales of Children's Abilities, though designed for an overall evaluation of child development from age 2:6 to 8:0 years, includes a strong language factor (Forns-Santacana and Gomez-Benito, 1990), and has been used to evaluate children with speech/language disorders (Morgan et al., 1992). It correlates well with the Goldman-Fristoe Test of Articulation in 4-to-5-year-old children, and shows little difference between ethnic groups (Alberts et al., 1995). A Comprehensive Assessment of Spoken Language (CASL, Carrow-Woolfolk, 1990; American Guidance Service, $299.95; Macintosh/Windows computer disk $149.95), designed for individuals age 3 to 21, takes about 30 to 45 minutes, provides a detailed assessment of comprehension and expression, but is primarily aimed at use with children who have learning disabilities. The 15 subtests measure comprehension, expression, and retrieval in lexical-semantic, syntactic, supralinguistic, and pragmatic areas and require only verbal or pointing responses, not reading or writing. The Speech and Language Evaluation Scale (SLES, Fressola et al., 1990; Hawthorne Educational Services, $112) is designed for the hand of the teacher, and uses 68 three-point ratings in a "pre-referral checklist," covering articulation, voice, fluency, and form (speech), content and pragmatics (language). It comes with a PC or Apple computerized quick-score program and speech and language intervention manual. The SLES was designed for children between 4:6 and 18 years of age, takes about 15 to 20 minutes, and provides separate norms for boys and girls. However, not all items are appropriate for the entire age range, and the recommendations for intervention are questionable (Hall, 1995). Few tests have been constructed or restandardized for children for the specific purpose of aphasia assessment (see review by Eisenson, 1972; Sattler, 1988). The Pediatric Evaluation of Disability Inventory (PEDI, Haley et al., 1992) provides a first functional profile of ratings designed for children. It includes ratings based on observation or parent report for self-care, mobility, and social function; the social function domain includes detailed ratings of comprehension of word meaning, comprehension of sentence complexity, functional use of expressive communication, and complexity of expressive communication.

Among the number of brief or specific-purpose assessment methods, adaptations are common. Several adaptations of the sentence repetition method, described fully in Chapter 7, have been attempted. The CELF-R contains a similar subtest with 26 items, designed for children and adolescents, age 5 to 18 years. The CELF-Preschool offers an 18-item version for children aged 3 to 6 years. A specific test suitable for children and adults is a part of the Woodcock-Johnson-III Cognitive Abilities battery (Memory for Sentences) (Isaki and Plante, 1997; Riverside Publishing). Special sentence repetition tests for prekindergarten children are the Sentence Repetition Screening Test (Sturner et al., 1993; Sturner et al., 1996) and the Carrow Elicited Language Inventory (CELI; age 3:0 to 7:11; Carrow-Woolfolk, 1996).

One experimental technique that used 24 sentences that vary according to grammatical complexity was used in a population of congenitally aphasic children (Bliss and Peterson, 1975). Adaptations of the COWA (see Chapter 7) rely less on words starting with a given letter than on animal names or similar categories or words beginning with a specific sound ("*sh*-words") for children who cannot be expected to have a sufficient knowledge of spelling.

The Token Test (TT) has been employed as a measure of language development. DiSimoni (1978) published an adaptation of the Token

Test for Children (Riverside, $116), standardized with 1304 children from preschool (age 3) to grade 6 (age 12:6), drawn from a mixed suburban population. The test manual also reviews several other studies investigating the scoring criteria as well as aspects of concurrent validity with other tests of auditory comprehension, including the ITPA and the PPVT. Hall and Jordan (1985) created a TT standardization sample for children in kindergarten through ninth grade. The TT has also been investigated as a discriminator between aphasic and other brain-damaged children, in relation to socioeconomic status of the home, an important aspect of language development in children (Gutbrod and Michel, 1986), and in relation to speech training in language-delayed children (D. Alexander and Frost, 1982). Syntactic comprehension in children was also examined with the TT and the BDAE Auditory Comprehension subtest, and compared with adult forms of aphasia (Naeser et al., 1987). Other tests of auditory comprehension not specifically designed for the assessment of aphasia but potentially useful are the Assessment of Children's Language Comprehension (ACLC, 2nd revision, Foster et al., 1983; Consulting Psychologists Press, $22.50) and Carrow's (1972; 1973) Test for Auditory Comprehension of Language (Tallal et al., 1985).

A frequently used test of receptive vocabulary, the PPVT-III (see Chapter 7) is appropriate for children from age 2:6. For example, it has been used, together with the ITPA, to study the effects of recurrent otitis media during infancy on the auditory comprehension of 9-year-old children (Luotonen et al., 1996). An Australian naming test, the Hundred Pictures Naming Test (J. Fisher and Glenister, 1992; Jordan and Ashton, 1996; Jordan et al., 1997), has seen limited use.

Comprehensive examinations designed for children include the already mentioned ITPA (which has been used for the assessment of aphasia and severe oral language disorders in some studies, e.g., Luick et al., 1982; Paul and Cohen, 1984), the Northwestern Syntax Screening Test (Arndt, 1977; Lee, 1970), the Porch Index of Communicative Ability in Children (PICAC, Porch, 1981; Riverside, $210), and the Utah Test of Language Development-3 (Mecham et al., 1967).

Adaptations of comprehensive examinations for aphasia for use with children have been presented for the NCCEA, the MAE (Schum et al., 1989), and the children's revision of the AST (Tramontana and Boyd, 1986). The NCCEA adaptation (Gaddes and Crockett, 1975) merely provides norms for children between ages 6 and 13 for each of the NCCEA subtests but has not been used in research studies with aphasic children. The presented norms show an acceptable gradual increase with age for some subtests, whereas other subtests show a rapid increase within a limited age span, after which the test scores remain at ceiling level.

The Porch Index of Communicative Ability in Children (PICAC, Porch, 1981) contains a "basic battery" for 3-to-6-year-olds, and an "advanced battery" for 6-to-12-year-olds. With the exception of some floor effects, score progression with age is satisfactory. Reliability data are provided, but so far no validity studies with aphasic children have been reported. As with the PICA, the multidimensional scoring system can pose difficulties and requires extensive training.

Clinical Evaluation of Language Fundamentals-3

The aim of the Clinical Evaluation of Language Fundamentals-3 (CELF-3) is to provide a comprehensive assessment of language development in school-age children. The test kit includes an examiner's manual, a technical manual, two stimulus manuals, and record forms (Psychological Corporation, $348). A parallel Spanish edition is available for $348. The technical manual provides full details of the revision of the test and information regarding reliability and validity. The stimulus material is presented in two stimulus manuals that fold up into easel form. The CELF-3 Screening Test uses a shortened selection of items from each of the subtests (10–15 minutes) and is available separately for $172. In addition, a CELF-3 Observation Rating for teachers, parents, and students, and a summary form are available for $55. A CELF-3 Clinical Assistant or computer scoring and report writing is available on four PC diskettes for $129.

The test battery (Semel et al., 1987; 1995) consists of three receptive and three expressive language subtests, which differ by age group (6 to 8 years, 11 months; 9 to 21 years, 11 months). In addition, the test includes two supplementary subtests. Approximately 30 to 45 minutes are required for the complete CELF-3. Administration for all subtests is described in detail in the manual, but essential instructions are also provided on the record form. Age-appropriate entry points and discontinuation rules allow considerable time-saving. The subtests are as follows:

Ages 6 to 8—Receptive:

Sentence Structure: The child has to point to one of four line drawings that corresponds to the statement read by the examiner (e.g., "The man comes home from work"). This subtest measures comprehension of negative, passive, infinitive, and other phrase structures. (20 items)

Concepts and Oral Directions: The child has to follow instructions by pointing to white or black circles, triangles, or squares, increasing in length and complexity of modifiers, similar to the Token Test (e.g., "Point to the last large black triangle to the left of the small black circle." (30 items)

Age 6 to 8—Expressive:

Word Classes: The child must identify two words that "go together best" out of three or four read by the examiner (e.g., chair, table, plant, dog). Relationships include semantic, opposite, spatial, and temporal. (34 items)

Word Structure: The child has to complete sentences requiring regular and irregular plurals, pronominalization, and other derivational forms. (32 items)

Recalling Sentences: The child must repeat phrases similar to the Sentence Repetition Test, but increasing not only in length but also in syntactic complexity. (26 items)

Formulated Sentences: The child has to create a sentence containing a given word, either describing a stimulus card or making up a sentence of his or her own. Words range from "car" to "unless." (22 items)

Age 5 to 7—Supplementary. These tests may be substituted for the calculation of expressive or receptive language score.

Listening to Paragraphs: The child listens to two stories read by the examiner, and then answers four questions about the content of each story.

Word Associations: The task requires generating as many words from a given category (animals, ways to get from one place to another, work people do) as possible in 60 seconds. The task is one of category-based fluency. (3 trials)

For ages 9 to 21 years, 11 months, the following subtests are given:

Receptive: Concepts and Directions, Word Classes, Semantic Relationships.

Expressive: Formulated Sentences, Recalling Sentences, Sentence Assembly.

Supplementary: Listening to Paragraphs, Word Associations.

Optional: Rapid automatic naming. The individual must name as rapidly as possible colors, then shapes, then colors and shapes ("green triangle"). (36 items each)

The record form provides scoring not only for each answer and each subtest's raw score but also for major types of errors, depending on the stimulus material (e.g., Concepts and Directions for time, inclusion/exclusion). Raw scores are translated into standard scores by referring to tables in the examiner's manual in 1-year age intervals up to the age of 16 years, 11 months. The final age interval (17 years to 21 years, 11 months) shows no further gain for most subtests. The standard scores are summed to provide a receptive, expressive, and total standard language score with a mean of 100 and an SD of 15, as well as an age equivalent. For each subtest, points above or below the mean, a confidence interval, percentile range (with its own confidence interval) are also entered on the record form; the form also provides for calculation of receptive/expressive differences with a notation of the prevalence of such differences.

A study of Native American 6-to-11-year-olds found scores significantly below the norms on the CELF-R, especially in the expressive domain (Atkinson, 1995). A study of 20 twelve-year-old Scottish children (Young and Gibbon, 1998) showed means well below that of the U.S. standardization sample, suggesting that the test norms may not be suitable for the United Kingdom.

Internal consistency ranged from .54 to .91 for subtests, and from .83 to .95 for expressive/receptive/total language scores, depending on age. Retest reliability after 4 to 8 weeks for a subsample of 116 children ranged from .50 (for word associations at age 6) to .90 (for recalling sentences at age 6), and from .77 (for receptive language score in 13-year-olds) to .93 (for total language score in 7-year-olds).

Criterion-related validity was based on the comparison of 136 students with language-based learning disability and 136 matched normal learning age peers at 7, 9, 11, 15, and 16 years. Correct classification was 71.3% for the total language score. Concurrent validity of the CELF-R had previously been reported as .68 against the PPVT-R (n = 53), .52 (receptive .44, expressive .46); against an intelligence test (WISC-R, n = 48), .42 (receptive .32, expressive .37). The CELF-3 correlated .75 with the WISC-III Full Scale IQ (n = 203; receptive language score .71, expressive language score .71). T. Powell and Germani (1993) reported moderate correlations between the CELF-R and the Vineland Adaptive Behavior Scale (Sparrow et al., 1984) and the Test of Nonverbal Intelligence (L. Brown et al., 1998). Children with central auditory processing disorders tend to show expressive language difficulties (Howard and Hulit, 1992; L. Martin and Bench, 1997), and even children with unilateral hearing impairment showed difficulties on receptive and expressive morphosyntactic and semantic tasks tapped by the CELF-R (Byrd, 1997). However, stutterers are not necessarily impaired in their language development (Nippold et al., 1991).

The test has been used to examine the language abilities of juveniles in a correctional facility (Sanger et al., 2000) and children with specific reading disability (Gillon and Dodd, 1994). A study by Miniutti (1991) showed that children with behavior disorders and children with learning disabilities both showed significant differences when compared with normally achieving children. Similar results were found for school-refusing adolescents (Naylor et al., 1994).

A study of 11 adolescents with brain injury (Turkstra, 1999) confirmed previously diagnosed language impairment, but did not identify individuals with verbal processing impairment. The author concluded that the test did not allow identification of strengths and weaknesses. A study of 5-to-10-year-old children with HIV infections compared to their uninfected siblings showed impairment of both expressive and receptive language functions that were proportionate to CNS defects shown on CT scans (Wolters et al., 1995). No studies of specific aphasiological interest have been presented so far. However, the test provides downward extensions or modifications of at least three tests that have been extensively used with aphasic populations: Word Associations (category-based word fluency), Recalling Sentences (sentence repetition), and Concepts and Oral Directions (Token Test). When testing children, the examiner may wish to use these as welcome substitutes with a good normative database. The full-length CELF-3 is suitable for the exploration of both developmental and acquired language deficits in children. While it may not satisfy everybody's model of language functions, it covers the major areas of syntax and semantics in both the receptive and expressive mode. It does not cover phonological (articulatory) problems.

A factor analysis for the CELF-R extracted two major factors, a "general language" and a "metalinguistic activity" factor. The authors stress, however, that the CELF-R is basically a one-factor test.

The test has been well standardized in 2450 children representative of the United States in terms of region, age, sex, and ethnicity. White–African-American and male–female differences are reported and discussed in the technical manual but are not used in the standard-score transformations. However, the manual provides rules on the interpretation of dialectical variants for Word Formation (morphology) and Sentence Structure (syntax) are provided in the manual. The authors stress the need for local norms to be developed by the test user, since they can differ considerably from the norms presented in the manual. One particular strength of the manual is the provision of sources for additional testing and instructional resources throughout the examiner's manual for each subtest. The constant reminders of confidence intervals for each test and for differences between tests on the summary page are also a welcome addition to this test.

Test for Auditory Comprehension of Language-3

The Test for Auditory Comprehension of Language (TACL-3) (Carrow, 1973; Carrow-Woolfolk, 1998) is designed for children between 3:0 and 9:11 years of age, and consists of an examiner's manual and a spiral-bound picture book as well as 25 profile/examiner record booklets, available from Academic Therapy Publications for $254. The test is un-timed and requires approximately 20 minutes.

The test consists of three subtests with a total of 142 items: vocabulary, grammatical morphemes, and syntax. The current edition has been thoroughly revised by elimination of nonfunctional items and the addition of 31 items to the first 111-item version. All items are written in English and Spanish.

The TACL-3 is a measure of oral language comprehension in children between 3:0 and 9:11 years. The examiner reads the name, descriptor, function, or sentence, and the child points to the correct answer on a multiple-choice card for each item (e.g., cat; two that are alike; look at the third picture, then point to the baby of this animal). Items are arranged in order of increasing difficulty. The test form allows a breakdown into vocabulary, grammatical morphemes, and syntax scores as well as specific categories (e.g., verbs, noun-phrase with two adjective modifiers, etc.).

Norms are based on 1102 children, which allows raw scores to be transferred into percentile ranks on age-appropriate tables. Consistency between English and Spanish versions has been demonstrated. Retest reliability is reported as .94 for English, .93 for Spanish.

Statistically significant differences have been shown between deaf children and those with articulatory deficit, between aphasic children and those without linguistic deficit, and between children with and without articulation disorders.

The test allows testing of language comprehension in a fashion similar to the Token Test with items more appropriate for this age group. The linguistic breakdown of item scoring is useful although not fully systematic.

Using the second edition of the TACL, Ruhl et al. (1992) assessed the language skills of 30 public school students with mild to moderate emotional behavior disorders, aged 9:4 to 16:2, and found that these students fell a minimum of 1 SD below the normative means, except for the Word Classes and Relations subtest. This finding was confirmed in the PPVT-R and the Expressive One-Word Picture Vocabulary Test. The authors suggested that students with behavior disorders tend to have problems with both expressive and receptive language. Chapman et al. (1991) found differences between PPVT and TACL scores in Down syndrome, but not in normal children, suggesting that development of syntax was more impaired than vocabulary in this group.

Test of Adolescent and Adult Language-3

The Test of Adolescent and Adult Language (TOAL-3), now available from Stoelting ($145) in its third edition (Hammill et al., 1994), is a collection of eight subtests designed to assess adolescent and adult competence in expressive and receptive language: Listening/Vocabulary, Listening/Grammar, Speaking/Vocabulary, Speaking/Grammar, Reading/Vocabulary, Reading/Grammar, Writing/Vocabulary, Writing/Grammar. From these, 8 composite scores (listening, speaking, reading, writing, spoken language, written language, vocabulary, grammar) and 2 summary scores for receptive and expressive language, as well as a general language quotient, can be calculated. Phonetics, morphology, and pragmatics are not tested. The test takes between 1 and 3 hours to complete.

Normative data are based on over 3000 subjects, but most of them already served for the earlier two editions of the test, so that changes in norms are not readily evident. Also, regional, gender, or racial differences are not explored. C. Johnson et al. (1999) found the normative data inadequate and provide local norms for the area of Ottawa, Canada. Internal consistency is good, and reliability acceptable (.80 to .96 for retesting after 2 weeks); interrater agreement ranges from .70 to .99, based on a limited rescoring of only 15 records. Factor analysis yielded only a single factor.

The test is designed mainly for the identification of school children in need of special assistance, not for aphasia. The adult norms are available only for age 18 to 25. A review by Richards (1998) finds the administration lengthy and complicated, and the norms inappropriate for students in urban school systems. Because of its design, lack of discriminant validity studies in the aphasia area, and its length, the test is not recommended relative to its peers.

Test of Language Competence—Expanded Edition

The Test of Language Competence—Expanded Edition (TLC-EE) is a measure of higher-level language functioning and strategy (Wiig and Secord, 1989; Psychological Corporation; $405). The test has two age-based levels: Level I for children aged 5 through 9 years and Level II for children, adolescents, and teen-agers ages 10 through 18 years. Administration of the full TLC-EE takes about an hour, but the test format allows for a shorter screening format should the clinician be unsure as whether a full administration would be warranted.

The TLC-EE is composed of five subtests: Ambiguous Sentences, Listening Comprehension, Inference Making, Recreating Speech Acts, and Figurative Language. Ambiguous Sentences requires the child to recognize and interpret different distinct meanings for the same sentence. Inference Making requires that the person make an inference given two causally related events. Recreating Speech Acts requires the person to formulate sentences using several key words and a specific context. Figurative Language requires metaphor interpretation as a function of the context of the figurative verbal information.

The test has been used by Barnes and Dennis in several studies of TBI (Dennis and Barnes, 1990; Barnes and Dennis, 2001) and hydrocephalus (Barnes and Dennis, 1998). It has also been employed in studies of severe TBI by Jordan (Jordan and Ashton, 1996; Jordan and Murdoch, 1994). Significant impairment on the measure by head-injured children is a common finding; three-quarters of one of the Barnes and Dennis samples performed defectively on at least one subtest. As might be anticipated, TLC-EE performance is more highly correlated with Verbal IQ than Performance IQ (Dennis and Barnes, 1990), but individual subtests show different correlational patterns with intelligence-test subtests.

Test of Language Development—Primary, 3rd Edition and Intermediate, 3rd Edition

The Test of Language Development—Primary is designed for 4-to-8:11 year olds (TOLD-P3, Newcomer and Hammill, 1999a; Academic Therapy Publications, $278.50) with nine subtests (picture vocabulary, relational vocabulary, oral vocabulary for expressive functions; grammatical understanding, sentence imitation, grammatical completion for different aspects of grammar; word articulation, phonemic analysis, word discrimination for receptive functions). The Test of Language Development—Intermediate is for 8:6-to-12:11 year olds (TOLD-I3, Newcomer and Hammill, 1999b; Academic Therapy Publications, $174) with six subtests including picture vocabulary, malapropisms, sentence combining, word ordering, and grammatical comprehension. Both tests are extended versions of the TELD-3.

IV

CONTEMPORARY CLINICAL PRACTICE

13

Issues in General Clinical Practice

This section presents some general considerations regarding the assessment of aphasia in clinical practice. In particular, we discuss the decision-making process before, during, and after the clinical assessment for questions of diagnosis, treatment planning, and prediction of recovery. Such decisions cannot be made by an assessment procedure, no matter how well constructed or "comprehensive" it may be; they remain the responsibility of the clinician in cooperation with related professionals involved with the individual patient.

Decisions about the Presence or Absence of Aphasia

In clinical practice, some patients are referred with an obvious presentation of aphasia. In a fair number of patients with mild or questionable language disorder, however, a decision that rules out aphasia should be made before proceeding to other questions. On the surface, it would seem that well-validated tests of a more comprehensive nature, or even of a screening type, would be sufficient to determine whether aphasia is present. It should be remembered, however, that no test has a discrimination accuracy of 100%, and that the gray areas of false positive and false negative decisions encountered with any given test lie necessarily in the borderline area between mild (or residual) aphasic features and normal language. Relying solely on a test's cutoff score in patients with borderline impairment would, in effect, not be much better than guessing.

Additionally, disordered language need not indicate the presence of aphasia. Significant nonaphasic language changes or deficits can be observed in other neuropsychological syndromes, such as an emerging dementia or an episode of acute confusion, and even in psychosis. Because the traditional aphasia subtypes are best seen when the etiology is a nonhemorrhagic CVA, language deficits may display different features when there are different etiologies, such as diffuse and severe traumatic brain injury. Experience in acute medical and rehabilitation settings suggests to us that the terms "aphasia," "expressive aphasia," or "receptive aphasia" tend to be overused as descriptions of language behavior, and that a review of the medical history and a formal evaluation would reveal language problems of other origin, such as acute confusion or psychopathology in some patients.

The clinician must use informed judgment to arrive at her or his own diagnosis that significant language changes are present, and that they actually represent an aphasic disorder as discussed in Chapter 15. Nondefective language changes may be observed in the population of normal, healthy elderly (e.g., Obler et al., 1985). Language disorders are frequently seen in dementing diseases and may be described by many linguistic parameters, although not necessarily as aphasic disorders (e.g., Bayles, 1984; Bayles et al., 1989a; Bayles and Tomoeda, 1983; Fromm and Holland, 1989). Language and communication deficits are also common after traumatic head injury, again in the absence of frank aphasia (e.g., Hagen, 1981; Levin et al., 1976; Marquardt et al., 1988; M. Sarno et al., 1986).

Premorbid Language Function and Intelligence

One major consideration in making an informed diagnosis is the determination or estimation of a given patient's language ability and intelligence before the onset of illness. Because premorbid test results are rarely available, a careful consideration of the patient's educational history, occupational record, language background, and reading and writing habits must be made. Relatives may be consulted with regard to this information, and their judgment may be invited as to whether any language impairment is noticeable to them. The judicious clinician often can arrive at a reasonable estimate of the premorbid level of intellectual functioning by obtaining demographic information, such as years of education, age, sex, and race, and using it in specifically developed formulas for calculating premorbid IQ scores (Barona et al., 1984; Krull et al., 1995). Such estimates of premorbid functioning are, however, of limited value in the presence of premorbid illiteracy (Lecours et al., 1987).

Additional information may be provided by concurrent administration of tests of general intelligence. Gross discrepancies between intelligence tests and aphasia tests usually suggest selective language impairment. However, it must be remembered that many intelligence tests rely heavily on subtests involving verbal functions; only the so-called nonverbal component of intelligence tests is useful in this regard. Caution in the interpretation of such "nonverbal" measures must be exercised, because the instructions of many seemingly nonverbal tasks (e.g., coding digits into symbols, arranging cartoon pictures in a meaningful sequence) are given verbally, and task performance itself may benefit from verbal mediation. Specific nonverbal intelligence tests have also been developed to facilitate these decisions (TONI-3, L. Brown et al., 1998; C-TONI, Hammill et al., 1996; Raven Progressive Matrices, Raven, 1938). Once this information has been collected, an expected level of language functioning may be determined. Some tests allow a score correction based on the premorbid educational level to be added before interpretation; many other tests leave this consideration open.

A related, but more difficult consideration concerns the sociocultural habits of the home and job environment of the patient. The need for verbal expression varies greatly from one setting to another, and cultural influences may tend to affect such factors as verbal fluency, general fund of information, vocabulary, articulation (and intelligibility), and prosody.

The Nature of the Speech and Language Deficit

After a diagnosis of aphasia has been made, the description of the exact nature of the deficit becomes of paramount importance. Does the presentation conform to a known clinical–anatomic subtype? What exactly is it that the patient cannot do? What degree of impairment is present in each of the areas under examination? How much will the impairment interfere with day-to-day communication? A description of areas of strength is as important as the description of areas of deficit, since any reasonable approach to treatment will rely on both types of information.

Information about the nature of the deficit continually influences the process of assessment. As we find out about specific areas of weakness over the testing session(s), a more detailed description of those areas and related deficits will be required. Specialized tests may be added to gather this information. Occasionally, it is necessary to continue the examination in this manner after the initial assessment results have been obtained.

Diagnostic subtyping of aphasia has led many test authors to develop a test pattern for each type, either empirically or descriptively. As was pointed out earlier, the range of types of aphasia described varies from test to test, depending on the theoretical orientation of the authors. It is perhaps obvious from the preceding text that fitting a patient into a particular type on the basis of test results is of only preliminary value. Types of aphasia have been related to location of lesion or psycholinguistic models as well as to rate and stage of recovery, but, as with the borderline between aphasic and normal language functioning, the gray area between types presents serious problems. Perfect fit for individual patients into such types is rare, and general or mixed impairment defying any typology is the norm. However, even if a subtype diagnosis is elusive or untenable, the attempt may still benefit the patient and family, as Benton (1994) suggests, by focusing professional decision making and sometimes identifying unsuspected or nascent syndromes. For all these reasons, the description of the nature of the language deficit must proceed beyond a typology and produce an individual profile for each patient.

Affective and Adjustment Considerations

Depressed mood is frequently observed during the phase of neurological stabilization from aphasia-producing CVAs, when a number of patients begin to realize the extent of their acquired problems. Though other patients emerge from this period with persisting deficits in self-awareness, those who do realize why they have been hospitalized may be confronted by problems that they are ill-prepared to understand, let alone adapt to. Depressed mood, poor adjustment, and the stress of excessive frustration may persist beyond the acute recovery period for a proportion of patients, especially those with Broca's aphasia. J. Sarno and Gainotti (1998) describe the classical stages of denial, frustration, depression, and acceptance after the onset of language disorders, all of which can affect test-taking behavior and increase the impact of observed language deficits. These affective and adjustment problems are important not only for appreciating their impact on both testing and test results, but also because they are essential areas for the clinician to consider as part of the overall assessment and treatment process.

Obviously, it is not common in traditional language assessment for a full evaluation of mood and adjustment to be included, alongside aphasia tests, to determine whether problems in these areas need addressing in psychotherapeutic fashion during treatment and, at a more severe level, whether they require medical attention and subsequent psychopharmacological intervention. When language testing forms part of a neuropsychological examination, these features may indeed be part of the assessment. Short of that, though, there are tests that might be of value for the speech clinician to learn about.

Given the importance of knowing the patient's emotional and adjustment status as well as the context of excessive demands on the clinician's time, the clinician in general practice should be aware of some of the rating scales, subjective questionnaires, and other relatively brief screening devices that are available. These measures may help track the emotional status of a patient during treatment and allow the clinician to maintain a sense of when specialist consultation for identifying and treating mental disorders might be warranted (e.g., S. Williams, 1996).

Some of these measures derive from general mental health practice. Others were created to gauge the mental health of elderly patients; a common need for these geriatric instruments is the differential diagnosis of depression and dementia (Kunik et al., 1994; Theml et al., 2001). A smaller number of tasks were designed specifically for patients after experiencing a CVA and, within this set, designed for aphasic patients.

The most common of the general short or screening measures for symptoms of depression is the Beck Depression Inventory–II (BDI-II) (Beck et al., 1996; Psychological Corporation, $66). Another instrument is the Hamilton Rating Scale for Depression (M. Hamilton, 1960). The Geriatric Depression Scale (GDS) (Brink et al., 1982) was developed as a basic screening measure of depression for use with elderly individuals. Sutcliffe and Lincoln (1998) described their Stroke Aphasic Depression Scale, a short 10-item scale.

Two instruments that have been examined in some detail in post-stroke samples are the Code-Muller Scale of Psychosocial Adjustment (Hermann and Wallesch, 1989; Müller and Code, 1983) and the Visual Analog Mood Scales (Arruda et al., 1999). The Code-Müller scale is designed specifically for patients dealing with aphasia. The task items ask the person to consider and then rate ten different situations (e.g., ability to work, ability to speak with strangers, ability to cope with the embarrassment of having speech problems). Ratings are on a scale that ranges from the experience becoming much worse than it is presently to it becoming much improved. This can provide a sense as to the degree of optimism, realism, or pessimism a person might be experiencing at a given point in time. Equivalent versions are available for caregivers and therapists for comparison purposes and, by extension, supportive counseling and guidance.

Assessment of mood and adjustment is not just an issue for the clinician to be concerned about regarding the aphasic patient per se. There has been an increase in interest over the past 20 years in including caregivers in treatment planning, as well as being mindful of the emotional and other adjustment problems of caregivers (Le Dorze et al., 1999; Servaes et al., 1999; Tompkins et al., 1999). This, of course, reflects good overall clinical care—identifying problems that might benefit from intervention and promoting the best use of language and communication in the aphasic patient's everyday life. This level of care is mindful that communication is a social task and that either side of the communicative dyad of aphasic and loved one may be a hindrance to successful and sustained communication. The psychological value of sustained good socially-based communication is a foundation of models of long-term aphasia management (e.g., Fink and Schwartz, 2000).

Attentional and Motivational Considerations

Language is not an isolated cognitive function. Attentional factors may seriously affect the results of testing, especially in children. Specific testing for attention with nonlinguistic stimuli may be a useful adjunct procedure (e.g., Test of Everyday Attention, TEA, Thames Valley Test Company). Some of these tests are available in a computerized version.

Some patients deny their deficits or are unaware of them and are unwilling to submit to testing procedures. These emotional reactions are not limited to patients with aphasia or with left hemisphere lesions (e.g., Gass and Russell, 1986). Patients with accompanying acute confusion, another frequent manifestation after the onset of neurological disease, may be too disoriented or agitated to yield valid performances (e.g., Lipowski, 1980). Confused patients typically show impaired levels of verbal comprehension, regardless of whether or not they are aphasic, complicating evaluations for aphasia. For these reasons, it is quite common that willingness or ability to communicate is drastically reduced, and test performances are defective due to lack of motivational and attentional defects or changes in consciousness. Interpretation of test findings will call on the judgment of the clinician rather than blind reliance on test results.

A special case of lack of cooperation is presented by patients who are unintentionally or deliberately exaggerating their impairment. "Faking bad" can be encountered in depressed patients who feel that they are so severely handicapped that they will not even attempt simple tasks. A deliberate attempt at feigning or exaggerating deficits is occasionally encountered in patients undergoing evaluation for the purpose of determining compensation claims, legal responsibility, or mental competence. In such cases, suspicious behavior should be noted for fuller evaluation to rule out malingering.

When a clinician encounters such behavior, a first response will be to explain to the patient why an assessment should be conducted. Both adults and children will often respond with greater effort when the importance of the assessment for future treatment is explained to them; unintentional lack of will may improve and deliberate exaggeration may cease when the patient learns that the examiner is aware of such tactics. It may be necessary to discontinue testing with a face-saving suggestion that a new date can be arranged when the patient is in a better condition to concentrate.

The practicing clinician will occasionally encounter patients who for a variety of reasons do not make an optimal effort during assessment. They may find the procedure tiresome, silly, or unnecessary; they may follow instructions only superficially, giving simplistic or inappropriate answers, and trying to finish tasks as quickly as possible. In cases where litigation is pending (for financial compensation, or forensic aspects of culpability, e.g., competency to stand trial, etc.), there may be motivation for the patient to exaggerate the inability to cooperate or to simply fake defective performance. Other patients are unresponsive because of depression. In children, rebelliousness, distraction, poor concentration, or test anxiety may lead to refusal or the production of responses that reflect poor effort. Obviously, the results of assessments in such cases may be invalid, and should be interpreted with great caution.

Test results from patients who exaggerate or simulate their symptoms or who give poor effort can be recognized by inconsistencies in performance that seem grossly out of the expected range when compared to other results. For example, when performance on several tests is in the normal range, other test results may be 2 or even 3 standard deviations below the norm. Few dissimulating patients can estimate the scores expected at their age and education level, and consistently score at a lower level. In scanning the test results, it should be remembered, however, that some forms of aphasia may produce unexpected failure in a specific response modality, for example, naming of visually presented objects versus objects presented as sounds (Sound Recognition Test). In such cases, the clinician must explore the deficit by using additional material to verify whether such a specific deficit is the cause of failure or whether poor effort was responsible.

The task of detecting poor effort can also be accomplished by comparing the results of tests or test items that appear at face-value more difficult than those that appear to be easy. Examiners who wish to explore this further are referred to Chapter 17 in Spreen and Strauss (1998), which describes specific tests designed to assess symptom validity.

Neuropsychologists and forensic psychologists with interest in the consequences of exaggeration and malingering have developed a number of "symptom validity tests," which include simple tasks that may appear difficult to the patient. These tests include the Rey 15-Item Test, Victoria Symptom Validity Test, and the Portland Test; see Lezak, 1995). Another approach to this problem is to compare a patient's performance on simple items with performance on the more difficult items of a test. This latter approach can be used during speech/language testing.

Children may pose a special challenge to the clinician: While to older children the testing situation may be similar to that encountered daily in school, younger children need to be gently coaxed into cooperation by establishing a supportive contact and, if necessary, interactive play before the examination can proceed. Occasionally, we encounter a defiant child who simply refuses to cooperate. It should be noted that children's language behavior may be of significance itself: pervasive or primarily receptive language disorders at age 5 have been related to aggressive and hyperactive behavior and social incompetence when tested 7 years later (Beitchman et al., 1996).

14

Brain Injury and Right Hemisphere Populations

One of the notable advances in language assessment over the past 20 years has been the increased interest of speech clinicians in language functions of neurological patients for whom the incidence of aphasia is significantly lower than in the traditional population of dominant hemisphere stroke. In many respects, the state of testing in this area is just emerging. There is an admixture of isolated tests (many of which have only limited psychometric support), ad hoc tasks that vary from setting to setting, a number of scoring systems, and various clinical approaches, but without any organized, broadly accepted, and well-standardized comprehensive instruments. At the same time, however, this realm is an active "proving ground" for operationalizing and applying functional and psycholinguistic concepts and laboratory techniques into daily clinical practice. One might look toward this realm over the next few years to see what may coalesce into standardized and more broadly accepted instruments. Curiously, several instruments frequently cited are measures with a history of only modest or limited psychometric research effort: the Discourse Comprehension Test, the Pragmatic Protocol, and the CETI (all discussed earlier in this book). Ideally, interest in their use with nonaphasic patients might well generate more empirical interest in improving their psychometric foundation than has their more limited use among aphasic patients.

Two specific neurological populations of patients—those with traumatic brain injury (TBI) and those patients with lesions of the nondominant (typically right) hemisphere—have captured both testing and

191

treatment interest among speech clinicians. It is now common for con-temporary texts in speech and language pathology, such as those by R. Brookshire (1997) and Chapey (2001), to include chapters devoted to these populations, and the past few years have also seen an increase in full-book coverage of each topic (e.g., Halper et al., 1991; Myers, 1999; Tompkins, 1995).

The compelling feature of examinations in this area is that while the incidence of aphasia is low, the incidence of acquired difficulties in com-munication can be notable. Even though they do not show severe losses in basic language abilities, these individuals may be far less able to use and coordinate their core language skills in terms of everyday activities and in terms of communication with others. Additionally, the relatively young age of patients in the TBI population adds diversity to the daily communicative environments (i.e., academic and vocational) that need to be considered. Although defining these difficulties varies from source to source, these acquired problems relate most fully to impairments in pragmatics and discourse skills (e.g., Cherney and Halper, 2000) and in the cognitive processing of communication in a social environment.

These difficulties include, but are not limited to, problems in partic-ipating in conversations with others, both in terms of being a listener and understanding the different threads of discourse and of being a con-versant, producing material in ongoing conversation. The efficiency and specificity of conversational discourse may be reduced relative to pre-morbid levels of function. Depending upon premorbid levels of dis-course, the patient's productions may be found to be quite shallow and off-track. Though superficial interactions may appear to be at levels of expectation, a drop-off of performance quality may be notable at more complex levels. The processing speed and level of ability in appreciating what knowledge may coexist between conversants (i.e., "shared knowl-edge") and what is unique to the patient may be noticeably hindered (e.g., Myers, 1999). The affective tone surrounding conversation and ambiguous or abstract meanings in informal conversation may be sig-nificantly more difficult to comprehend.

It has become common to speak of "cognitive-communication," "cognitive-communicative," and "cognitive-linguistic" problems when referring to these nonaphasic problems in communication, especially af-ter a major professional society offered the "cognitive-communicative" label in the late 1980s (i.e., American Speech-Language-Hearing Asso-ciation, 1996). As such, there is overlap in assessment goals between speech-language pathologists and neuropsychological examiners and, to some degree, occupational therapists. This overlap will—in reasonable settings—contribute to multidisciplinary cooperation, while in other settings it can create conflict and so-called turf issues. Our focus in this chapter is on some of the more unique aspects of speech and language testing of these populations in multidisciplinary settings.

Assessment of these so-called cognitive-communicative problems in many respects has centered upon the functional and pragmatic aspects of communication covered earlier in this book. Whereas in the setting of aphasia, problems with basic language skills created by aphasia are clearly the object of professional and family attention, a nonaphasic patient with cognitive-communication problems can use these retained basic language skills, but their application is impaired, counterproductive, or ineffective (e.g., Tompkins, 1995). Functional assessment instruments have already been addressed earlier in Chapter 8; therefore, our coverage in this chapter is relatively brief.

When examining the applications of pragmatics and discourse in these two populations, one can see some consistencies across individual research efforts and clinical approaches, especially for discourse assessment. For example, in examining the state of discourse assessment in TBI, P. Snow and Douglas (2000) offer a useful quadrant model for identifying four basic approaches to what and how to test. The quadrant distinguishes two axes: the range of behavior-sampling methods available to the clinician and the type of analysis that the clinician could employ. At one end of the sampling axis are structured tests and, at the other, naturalistic observations. Analysis ranges on its axis from the purely "microlinguistic" (i.e., the utterance-by-utterance dissection of verbatim transcripts of communication), to the "macrolinguistic," such as clinical rating scales that rely upon listener judgment. However, for the most part, generally agreed-upon task areas and psychometrically sound ways to assess performance are contemporary goals, rather than established findings.

Traumatic Brain Injury

Damage to the brain by mechanical force as a result of motor-vehicle accident, fall, violence, sports-related accidents, etc., can result in a variety of primary and secondary neuropathological changes. These changes and the cognitive consequences of their occurrence depend, in large extent, on the severity of the traumatic brain injury (TBI). Damage on the more severe end of the spectrum usually is multifocal and diffuse in nature, involving multiple brain regions. Acquired communication problems are typically accompanied by alterations in self-awareness, problem solving, and by subjective perceptions of one's abilities and social skills that are often at odds with both objective findings and the perceptions of significant others; these problems form important targets for comprehensive neuropsychological rehabilitation efforts (Prigatano, 1999).

Aphasia is not a common consequence of TBI, though isolated basic language deficits and functional impairments in the use of language may be present. It is useful to keep in mind, however, that assessment of language functioning is important even when aphasic disturbance is not present, but when the nature of the brain condition is such that non-aphasic changes in language and the ability to employ language need to be examined. Identification and attempts to remediate what Sohlberg and Mateer (2001) have called the "socially punishing" communication problems of the TBI have emerged as key facets of contemporary cognitive treatment and were included in an evidence-based exploration of suggested treatment guidelines and recommendations for cognitive rehabilitation (Cicerone et al., 2000).

There is a full literature exploring aphasia and specific aphasic features in TBI, perhaps best represented by the work of Levin and colleagues (e.g., Levin et al., 1976), who employed subtests from the MAE and the NCCEA in their work and have also included a significant amount of exploration of child and adolescent TBI. Additional work can be found by M. Sarno and colleagues (Sarno, 1984b; Sarno et al., 1987), employing subtests of the NCCEA. This type of work has evolved and expanded to include broader explorations of communication (e.g., Chapman et al., 1998). More recently, Hinchliffe and colleagues (1998), for example, employed a language battery that included subtests of the WAB, BDAE, NCCEA, the Test of Language Competence, and a right hemisphere battery to be discussed later (i.e., Right Hemisphere Language Battery).

There have not been many specific tests created and standardized for specific assessment of language in TBI patients. Several measures that have been offered and are discussed briefly are the Dice Game (McDonald and Pearce, 1995), the Brief Test of Head Injury (Helm-Estabrooks and Hotz, 1990), and the La Trobe Communication Questionnaire (Douglas et al., 2000; P. Snow et al., 1998).

There have been detailed examinations of communication problems in patients who have sustained serious head injuries. P. Snow and Douglas (2000) offered a conceptual and methodological review of assessment issues directly related to the topic. Recently, Ylvisaker et al. (2001) provided an integrated assessment-treatment approach to explore three factors for communication assessment in TBI: impairment-oriented assessment (e.g., standardized test instruments), disability (activity)-oriented assessment (e.g., customized functional tasks and functional scales like the ASHA-FACS), and handicap (participation)-oriented assessment (e.g., observational scales, quality-of-life inventories, interviews) for treatment planning.

Much attention has centered on the communicative impact of pediatric TBI. Jordan and colleagues put together a research battery of language tests that included traditional aphasia tests as well as measures of communication and examined children with TBI and also adults who had sustained TBIs during childhood in a series of examinations (Jordan and Ashton, 1996; Jordan et al., 1996; Jordan et al., 1988; Jordan and Murdoch, 1990; 1994). The authors also examined a more specific facet of communication (i.e., comprehension of linguistic humor) in TBI adolescents (Docking et al., 1999; 2000). Research by Dennis and colleagues employing the Test of Language Competence was discussed briefly in Chapter 12. More recently, Dennis and colleagues have explored additional pragmatic aspects of communication after pediatric TBI, such as irony and deceptive messages (Dennis et al., 2001). While even mild TBI had an impact on comprehension, deficits were related to level of severity in their sample of 42 six-to-15-year-old children. Finally, Turkstra et al. (1995) examined the use of a battery of measures considered to reflect pragmatic communication skills in a small sample of adolescents with TBI.

The Pragmatic Protocol (PP) (see Chapter 8) has been used in this population and held in good standing by those concerned with the role of testing in TBI rehabilitation (e.g., Sohlberg and Mateer, 2001). Milton et al. (1984) provided an early examination of the PP in TBI, albeit using a small sample of only 10 subjects: five TBI and five intact adults matched for age, sex, and educational level. On the PP, 76% of behaviors in the TBI group were rated as being appropriate, contrasted with 99% in the normal group. The specific number of inappropriate behaviors in the TBI group ranged from 6 to 10, while three of the five intact subjects showed no inappropriate behaviors and the remaining two showed one each. Common inappropriate behaviors by the TBI group included prosody, affect, topic selection and maintenance, and facets of conversational turn-taking. The PP was subsequently employed by Penn and Cleary (1988) in another sample of six head-injured adults who were between the ages of 22 and 29 years. In addition to the PP, the subjects were assessed on selective tasks from the oral language subtests of the WAB and the CADL. The authors reported that inappropriate performances on the PP were consistent with those reported earlier by Milton et al. (1984). As a group, subjects performed at a better level of functioning on the CADL than they did on the PP; the authors interpreted this as perhaps indicating lowered sensitivity of the CADL to the interactive aspects of communicative adequacy, especially in this type of (nonaphasic) population. Putting the findings in the context of potentially useful treatment planning, Penn and Cleary also examined conversational samples in terms of spontaneous compensatory strategies, from a taxonomy of strategies reported earlier by Penn (1988). The most common compensations (regardless of whether they were effective) were repetitions, simplifications, and circumlocutions. So-called sociolinguistic strategies appeared difficult and ineffective for the sample. Turn-taking in conversation was particularly noted as a problem for TBI patients.

Psycholinguistically influenced scoring systems of conversational discourse have been employed in research exploring acquired communicative problems in TBI. Friedland and Miller (1998), for example, examined Conversation Analysis (CA) in the context of additional cognitive testing in a detailed examination of a single adult TBI patient. The authors conceded that the CA approach was time-consuming (a typical limitation in examining the pragmatics of language), but suggested that the results of the assessment allowed a fuller sense of the patient's conversational difficulties than that provided by measures of naming and verbal fluency. Other conversational scoring methods have been applied to the discourse of TBI patients. For example, Clinical Discourse Analysis (Damico, 1985) was applied to a sample of 26 TBI patients and two control groups (orthopedic patients and healthy university students; 26 members in each group) in a detailed initial examination with 2-year follow-up testing by Snow and colleagues (Snow et al., 1997; 1998).

The Dice Game

The Dice Game, which is not commercially available but offered for use in publications by McDonald (1993; McDonald and Pearce, 1995), is derived from a test exploring children's role taking by Flavell (1987). In a format somewhat like the Reporter's Test (see Chapter 7), the patient is required to offer the description of a game to an imagined listener who cannot see the stimuli and is naïve to the rules. The game is a race between two players, one using a red toy car and the other using a green one on a "race track" of spaces, with movement dictated by the toss of the dice. The format varies in the amount of time that needs to be committed by the examiner, as the examiner must begin playing the game with the patient without offering explicit rules; only once the clinician believes that the patient is appreciating the rules is the patient instructed to provide a description of the game to an imagined third person. Details of the scoring system and analysis of performances by normal and TBI adults are provided in McDonald and Pearce (1995). Use in pediatric samples is reported by Turkstra et al. (1995).

McDonald and Pearce's sample consisted of 43 neurologically intact and 20 TBI adults. Interrater reliability was assessed by the use of six speech pathologists and neuropsychologists. Some variability was noted in identifying individual propositions in transcribing subject responses. However, consistency was present in classifying propositions once they were identified. The publication includes scoring suggestions in an appendix.

Performance with intact adult controls found that age and educational level exerted some influence on test performance, with older and more-educated individuals offering modestly more essential features of the game in their descriptions. Gender had no impact on performance. In a comparison of brain-damaged patients and intact controls, both produced an equivalent quantity of information, but the groups differed in that the TBI group offered fewer essential features and made more irrelevant comments in their descriptions.

The Brief Test of Head Injury

The Brief Test of Head Injury (BTHI) (Helm-Estabrooks and Hotz, 1990) is a "cognitive-communication assessment designed to identify and measure a variety of deficits in patients with traumatic brain injury" (p. 1), with an emphasis on linguistic tasks. The authors note that the test used the BASA as its model. Designed to be completed in 30 minutes or less, the test provides items that examine orientation/attention, ability to follow commands, linguistic organization, reading comprehension, naming, memory, and visuospatial skills. Patients can respond using speech, gestures, or both. The communication quality of each response on the test is assessed on a five-point scale. Field testing of 50 patients provided initial reliability and validity data. Internal consistency was reported as being .96. Interrater reliability was only reported on an anecdotal basis. A subset of 19 patients were subjected to a test-retest assessment after an average 57-day interval. Test-retest reliability for the overall BTHI score was .85. Concurrent validity was assessed by comparing BTHI scores with initial Glasgow Coma Scale scores: a correlation of .52 was reported. A factor analysis of the BTHI was performed, with a two-factor solution reported. The first factor was interpreted as being a "cognitive-linguistic" one and the second as a "visual-spatial" one. At the time of its 1990 publication, the test manual indicated that publication of the test's normative data would be made available the following year. As the test has apparently not been revised or republished in the time since its original publication, potential users might need to contact the author directly for this additional information.

La Trobe Communication Questionnaire

The La Trobe Communication Questionnaire (LCQ) is an instrument "designed to measure perceived communicative ability" as noted by a brain-damaged person and by significant others (Douglas et al., 2000). The authors note that the measure has its foundations in two specific psycholinguistic sources: Grice's (1975) theory concerning conversational discourse and a subsequent operationalization of that theory by Damico (1985): Clinical Discourse Analysis.

The LCQ comprises 30 items that the individual responds to on a four-item scale. The instrument has one form for patients and an equivalent one for significant others. Items are phrased in terms of "When talking to others do you (or: does _____) . . ." and examples include ". . . leave out important details?" ". . . keep track of the main details of conversation?" and ". . . know when to talk and when to listen?" All 30 items are available in O'Flaherty and Douglas (1997).

The test was piloted and standardized on Australian samples of normal individuals and those with traumatic brain injuries. The standardization study of normal performance on the measure involved a sample of 147 primary subjects and 109 significant others. Studies of patients have looked at performance within the first year of recovery and another examination of patients at least 2½ years after their injuries.

Psychometrically, reliability as assessed by Cronbach's alpha was .85 for primary subjects and .86 for others. Split-half reliability was .78 for primary subjects and .83 for others. Test-retest correlations (with a testing interval of 8 weeks) was .76 for a subsample of 24 primary subjects, but only .48 for others. The authors concluded that a methodological weakness of not having a way to assure that the same significant other completed the LCQ on both occasions may have caused the poor test-retest reliability for significant other. LCQ performance was not associated with age (which ranged from 16 to 40 years) nor with educational level. A factor analysis was performed, which yielded a six-factor solution.

O'Flaherty and Douglas (1997) performed a detailed qualitative examination of LCQ performance by five TBI–other dyads, in the context of additional detailed interviews with the dyads. Ten items in particular were noted to be reported by both patients and their significant others as occurring at a frequency greater than "sometimes"—though on an individual item basis, some of the 10 items were noted as being more significant by patients and other items by the significant others. A cautionary finding reported by the authors as a result of their interviewing was that no patient or other cited "communication" as being a significant problem, even when LCQ results indicated otherwise. They noted that these problems may be underreported because of differences between what clinicians may mean by the term and how the general public interprets it: noting that their sample interpreted communication as "being able to speak and sound okay" rather than having a language-related basis. Additional data on LCQ performance in adult TBI can be found in McNeill-Brown and Douglas (1997).

Currently, data on the LCQ have been obtained in a broader adult age span (through the age of 85 years) and in patients with right hemisphere lesions (J. Douglas personal communication, 2001).

Right Hemisphere Lesions

Clinicians examining language functioning in patients with right hemisphere damage deal with patients who are not significantly different in the underlying etiology that caused their difficulties or in basic demographic attributes (e.g., age) than patients with left hemisphere lesions. A primary difference is the lower expectation for presence of aphasia and the correspondingly lower need to rule out aphasic language deficits. A speech clinician still needs to remain vigilant in terms of aphasia in this population: though a traditional diagnosis of aphasia would be uncommon, it does occur in patients with atypical language lateralization or in a minority of left-handed individuals who are right hemisphere language dominant. Thorough reviews of assessing and treating aphasic and nonaphasic language deficits in these patients have been offered by Tompkins (1995) and Myers (1999).

Until the recent increased interest in examining language in patients with lesions of the right hemisphere, it might have been relatively simple to overlook language problems in these individuals because obvious aphasic features would not typically be expected, and thorough language examinations might have been reserved for the rarer cases of patients with language dominance in the right hemisphere.

In addition to considering more traditional aphasic word-retrieval difficulties and auditory language comprehension problems, Tompkins's approach, for example, places emphasis on examining the "pragmatics domain" (including prosody, emotional processing, intention in speech acts, sensitivity to listener's needs, humor, and inference) and "discourse and conversation" (including discourse production, discourse comprehension, and conversational behavior).

Providers of language services for these patients often look, at least initially, at packaged "batteries" of right hemisphere functioning. In the present discussion, we are less concerned with these batteries, because they are often centered on those facets of cognitive function that relate to visuocognitive (i.e., visuoperception, visuospatial, and visuoconstructional) functioning for which some good standardized neuropsychological instruments exist. A number of thorough conceptual reviews of visuocognition and overviews to relevant test instruments exist (e.g., Benton, 1979; Lezak, 1995). Our attention focuses on the subtests of those packaged tests that are specific to language and other specialized language instruments that have seen use in this population. However, many clinicians seem to prefer an individualized clinical or descriptive approach. Two emerging clinical approaches (Myers, 1979; Tompkins, 1995) to assessment in this population may serve as examples. Both have some elements of psychometrics but have yet to coalesce into well-standardized and normed individual tests or a set of subtests within a comprehensive battery.

Rehabilitation Institute of Chicago Clinical Management of Right Hemisphere Dysfunction, 2nd Edition

The Clinical Management of Right Hemisphere Dysfunction (Burns et al., 1985) was one of the first compilations of tasks that could be used to explore language functioning in this population. The second edition by Halper et al. (1996) includes a pragmatic rating scale, a behavioral profile employing observation, conversation, and clinical interview, and proverb/idiom interpretation (e.g., "Save it for a rainy day."). Observational ratings rely upon direct interviewing as well as observing the patient as he or she interacts with family and with hospital/rehabilitation staff. The pragmatic scale assesses both verbal and nonverbal areas, as well as narrative discourse (employing a subtest from the Bayles and Tomoeda [1990] Arizona Battery for Communication Disorders). Normative information from small samples of intact and right brain–damaged patients is presented.

Right Hemisphere Language Battery, 2nd Edition

The Right Hemisphere Language Battery (RHLB) (K. Bryan, 1995) is a revision of the original battery (K. Bryan, 1989). The test consists of seven subtests that examine awareness of metaphors, comprehension of inferences, humor appreciation, and discourse production. As such, it is a first attempt to offer a standardized stand-alone set of subtests looking at the pragmatics of communication in this specific population.

The instrument was standardized on relatively small samples of healthy controls, patients with right hemisphere damage, and those with aphasia-producing left hemisphere damage. Tompkins (1995) concluded that data related to the test's psychometric properties as reported in the original edition of the test were "sparse."

K. Bryan and Hale (2001) explored RHLB performance alongside the WAB in samples of adult patients who had sustained a unilateral left-sided (n = 30) or right-sided (n = 30) CVA or who were neurologically intact (n = 30). The groups were matched for age, gender, educational level, and socioeconomic status. The clinical groups were examined within 6 weeks of their CVAs. Discriminant-function analysis indicated that both clinical groups experienced communication difficulties, but with expected differences related to hemispheric lateralization and as indexed by the use of the two different assessment instruments, with 95% accuracy. The WAB aphasia battery differentiated defective left hemisphere patients from both right-sided patients and controls (who performed equivalently). The RHLB distinguished the low performance level of the right-sided patients from the other groups and, also, distinguished the intermediate performance level of the left-sided group from the better performance of the intact group.

The Rusk Rehabilitation Institute of NYU, like the Rehabilitation Institute of Chicago, also published detailed information about the tests it used in the assessment and treatment of patients with right hemisphere lesions, some of which relate to language and verbal reasoning (Gordon et al., 1984). Other published tests include the Mini Inventory of Right Brain Injury (MIRBI; Pimental and Kingsbury, 1989b), portions of the Burns Brief Inventory of Communication and Cognition (Burns, 1997), and the Ross Information Processing Assessment (D. Ross, 1986). The MIRBI is simply a 27-item screening test. There is not much to report about this test, other than that several of its items include affective communication. The test has been examined by Tompkins (1995), who criticized the test's limited consideration of validity.

Clinical Approaches

We consider now two of the more fully formulated clinical approaches for examination of language and communication in patients with right-hemisphere lesions.

Tompkins's approach

In the functional-communication realm, standardized tests are not available to deal with specific issues faced by patients with right hemisphere lesions. Tompkins's (1995) presentation includes considerations of how to apply any of a number of other standardized functional measures in this population. One part of her approach employed standardized instruments and included consideration of the Pragmatic Protocol, the Profile of Communicative Appropriateness (Penn, 1988), the CETI, and the CADL, as well as specific measures of nonverbal communication (e.g., Profile of Nonverbal Sensitivity by Rosenthal et al., 1979), sensitivity to listener (e.g., the Adult Social Communication rating scale by Hough and Pierce, 1994) and Sherratt and Penn's (1990) right hemisphere discourse analysis format.

In practice, assessment of pragmatics and discourse span the use of preexisting tests, ad hoc tasks, and interpretation of samples of the patient's communication. Tompkins also examines testing pragmatics and discourse in a broader assessment of cognitive functioning, including the use of traditional aphasia measures, such as the Token Test and the Boston Naming Test.

Pragmatics. Pragmatics testing can proceed with a selection from existing tests (e.g., the PP) and case-by-case individualized tasks in what Tompkins terms "referential communication." These referential tasks place the patient and the clinician on opposite sides of the communicator (sender) and listener dyad and explore how well the patient can communicate a message about a stimulus hidden from view of the listener. The clinician assesses not only accuracy but also how well the patient appears to infer whether the message is inadequate and what adaptive steps he or she takes to modify the message. This can be performed even if the message is accurate, as the clinician may take on the role of a listener who misunderstands and needs further clarity. Alternating roles allows the clinician to see how the patient comprehends as a listener. The structure of the approach can be mined further based upon initial findings at the discretion of the clinician. Tompkins recognizes the need to have a very good appreciation for the patient's premorbid levels of functioning in order to fully employ such an unnormed approach. As an ad hoc approach, however, it may be easily integrated into ongoing intervention as a way to assess what is and is not working.

Discourse. Discourse is examined in different approaches, using two basic facets: text-based discourse and conversational discourse. Production, processing, and comprehension can be explored separately for each facet. On the text-based side, Tompkins reports using the Discourse Comprehension Test, as well as ad hoc tasks. Such tasks can be subjected to a variety of scoring systems; Tompkins mentions systems by Joanette and Goulet (1990) and Sherratt and Penn (1990) as methods employed in her approach. Tompkins (1995) offers several pages of guidance for creating sample testing tasks (pp. 125–127). Further, she notes a hybrid approach by J. Webster and colleagues (1992): these clinicians employed the Logical Memory subtests of the Wechsler Memory Scale, scoring performance not by the standard method of information recall, but by scoring performance of propositional elements that were labeled as being either essential or nonessential to the story's plot. There is risk of invalidating a test also used for diagnostic purposes if the patient has been preexposed to the stimulus material for that test; therefore, the use of such "borrowed" material should be undertaken only with consultation of clinicians who may rely on that material for primary testing.

On the conversation-based side, Tompkins discusses how to create and record a conversational sample and how to then examine three areas of discourse she considers to be of key value: topic control, turn-taking, and conversational repair. Tompkins places testing of these phenomena in the context of formulating hypotheses based upon earlier interactions with the patient and the need to consider premorbid functioning for any areas of apparent deficit by querying family members and significant others. Testing here also may require some further modifications of interactions as the examination proceeds in order to gain a clearer sense about the nature and impact of any apparent problems.

Assessment of conversational discourse is a specific area where a diagnostician may look to see what type of standardized instruments might emerge from these varied scoring systems and ad hoc testing tasks with more and more experience in this population (and the TBI population) over the next few years. The three areas of conversational discourse discussed by Tompkins are important to consider in the acquired communication deficits of nonaphasic adults and can easily be influenced by neurobehavioral deficits in other domains, such as executive functioning. All three conversational areas require the ability to identify, process, and act upon social cues, self-awareness of performance, taking account of the perspective of others, and the like. The amount of time currently needed to record and transcribe 15 to 30 minutes of loosely structured conversation and subject the result to exceedingly detailed and idiosyncratic scoring systems may make this an area too time-consuming and cumbersome for regular assessment deployment but might lend itself to development and standardization of a shortened and more accessible evaluation instrument.

Myers's approach

The approach developed by Myers has been reported in a number of publications (e.g., Myers, 1978; 1979; 1997; 2001), though presented most fully in her 1999 book. Her approach includes assessing and treating visual neglect and attentional problems, but in this context we note only those features that relate directly to language and communication. The basic goal of assessment for facets of cognition is to discern whether someone with known or suspected lesions of the right hemisphere has difficulty communicating consistently and to be able to outline the communicative strengths and weaknesses as they may affect planned intervention and functional outcome. Myers's approach to assessment in this realm is a "pick and choose" assessment technique based upon the clinician's experience base and the individualized needs of the person being evaluated.

Myers's approach to communication problems in patients with right hemisphere damage includes an initial screening with emphasis on a clinical interview and "scene interpretation" (i.e., performance on the BDAE Cookie-Theft card or an equivalent scene). Her goal of completing this testing in 20 minutes or less appears overly ambitious but provides an ideal to aim for. Based upon the results on this screening, she then provides descriptions of a set of subsequent "formal and informal tests" in the areas of discourse deficits, prosody, and affective communication.

Interview. The clinical interview detailed in Myers's book is not much different from other reasonable approaches. Though her presentation appears to assume that the clinician has already ruled out the presence of aphasia prior to any evaluation, this type of screening interview can give a gross sense of both aphasic and communicative deficits.

Scene interpretation. Myers provides a detailed elaboration on how to interpret performance on scene-interpretation tasks as being relevant to understanding the types of communication problems of concern to a patient with nonaphasic communication deficits. Rather than following the traditional use of the BDAE Cookie-Theft card, she examines responsiveness to it in terms of how well the individual is able to distinguish between relevant and irrelevant details, can integrate information across the story as it emerges, and can draw inferences about the events depicted on the card (e.g., does the patient appreciate that the depicted female adult is most probably a "mother"?). She provides a scoring system to delineate literal and interpretative concepts on the Cookie-Theft card based upon an earlier paper (i.e., Myers, 1979), as well as using an approach developed by L. Nicholas and Brookshire (1995) for scoring each of seven concepts (e.g., the stool is tipping, the woman is not paying attention) from the card for the presence, accuracy, and completeness of each concept.

In addition to borrowing the Cookie-Theft picture from the BDAE, Myers relies upon the batteries of so-called right brain damage for her set of formal tests, such as the RHLB (Bryan, 1989) and the Rehabilitation Institute of Chicago battery tests (Halper et al., 1991). However, she also details how one can integrate tests more specialized than these batteries and additional informal tasks into the assessment process.

Discourse. Myers's approach assesses discourse in a manner to include both comprehension and production and indicates that comprehension testing can include both narrative and nonnarrative material. Like Tompkins, she points to the use of the Discourse Comprehension Test for assessing narrative discourse, a test that was normed using only a small sample of right hemisphere patients. Editorials and opinion columns (rather than fact-laden news stories) from newspapers and other stimuli can be employed in an ad hoc fashion. She notes that the goal of this part of testing is to determine the degree to which the patient develops and maintains control over the main events and specific details and the degree to which the patient comprehends nonexplicit material relative to explicit information.

Discourse production tasks and scoring methods need to be carefully considered, especially if other cognitive deficits might impair performance. Three types of tasks can be considered: story repetition, interpretation of pictured scenes (as done during screening), and open-ended questions. This small spectrum can be seen to vary in terms of clinician control over the range of responsiveness. Three types of scoring methods can be employed dealing with the correctness of information, in content of information (e.g., Cherney and Canter, 1993), and the concepts employed (i.e., so-called macrostructure and supporting inferences). Myers (1999) presents the main features of her own conceptual scoring system. She cautions that employing these tasks can be difficult to interpret in the absence of norms and standardization.

Pragmatics. Myers recommends obtaining some type of conversational analysis of the person being assessed. This can be obtained by recording the initial interview with the patient or observing a conversational interaction between the patient and a family member or friend. Examining performance to see if the patient has difficulties in topic maintenance, turn-taking, and recognizing that shared knowledge has its limits (e.g., that a new listener might not have the same recognition of information as a family member). Although they are not integrated into her approach, Myers does indicate that measures like the Pragmatic Protocol and the Discourse Abilities Profile (Terrell and Ripich, 1989) can serve as useful guides for the clinician.

Prosody. Myers points to the absence of standardized measures of prosodic comprehension and recommends that the clinician develop his or her own assessment stimuli and tasks. She suggests that the following elements be examined: identifying emotional tone at the sentence level, identifying emphatic stress, and distinguishing between declarative and interrogative sentences. Prosodic production is noted by Myers to be assessable via published test instruments; but she suggests that individualized schemes may still need to be created to cover the same areas noted above for comprehension. She provides a number of tasks that might be used by a clinician (1999, p. 201/202).

Affective communication. Myers indicates that it is useful to explore both verbal and nonverbal emotional expression and comprehension of the emotional expressions of others in an overall assessment of communication problems in patients with right hemisphere lesions. Nonverbal expressions, such as facial changes, contribute to the overall conversational milieu in the everyday environment.

Like Tompkins, Myers clearly places assessment roles as leading directly toward developing and implementing treatment and does not thoroughly examine any fuller diagnostic or consultative roles. As preface to intervention, a substantial portion of her description of her approach deals directly with treatment planning and execution.

In sum, this look at two nonaphasic neurological populations suggests the increasing diversity beyond aphasia assessment and treatment that has been added to the practice of speech clinicians over the past few years. Tompkins (1995) suggests that caseload demands have exceeded educational training in some of these applications for speech pathologists, but that the discrepancy is dissipating. Services for patients in nonaphasic, communicatively impaired populations may well provide the germination of a new generation of standardized test instruments—examination instruments guided not only by treatment expectations but also by a relatively rich literature in the pragmatics of language in everyday, psychosocial communication environments. Turn-taking in conversation, for example, is a problem noted in patients with either traumatic brain injury or vascular right hemisphere lesions. Though a standardized test (or subtest in a larger battery) of this behavior is not yet available, it would seem relatively straightforward to develop such a test, employing the results from available research findings and continued ad hoc testing and observations. One might further anticipate that short versions of whatever instruments might be developed could also be useful in the original and traditional population of interest—aphasic patients —who, in spite of far more basic language impairments, still seek to improve their use of language to communicate in everyday psychosocial environments. However, successful developments in this realm face the same difficulties that clinical researchers faced in earlier times when developing aphasia batteries, with the additional restriction that many testing formats here require some type of conversational recording and transcription followed by scoring systems that, thus far, are often impractical because of length and time demands.

15

Assessment of Language in the Healthy Elderly and in Dementia

For several of the tests described in previous chapters we have referred to the availability of separate norms for healthy elderly subjects. Other tests, for example, the BNT, have been used extensively for research in patients with dementia. This chapter describes briefly the age-related changes found in the assessment of language and the use of assessment instruments for aphasia in subjects with dementia (see also Huntley and Helfer, 1995; Luzzatti, 1999; Lichtenberg, 1999).

Elderly Subjects

Elderly individuals frequently report difficulties in word finding. Such failures in lexical retrieval have been demonstrated in both cross-sectional and longitudinal studies (e.g., Au et al., 1995) and include not only the finding of referents to a definition but also of verbs and proper names, beginning as early as the late 50s and increasing as the individual reaches the 70s. Elderly healthy subjects in their 80s declined by more than 2.5 SD relative to individuals in their 30s in verb retrieval (M. Nicholas et al., 1998). Goulet et al. (1994), in a review of 25 studies, noted, however, that decline with age in the ability to name pictures was an inconsistent finding, due to many uncontrolled factors (e.g., gender, health status, medication, education, etc.).

Analyses of procedural discourse (i.e., verbal instructions that tell how a task is accomplished) also show an age-related decline, evident in the use of simpler, less memory-demanding syntactic constructions, although mean length of utterance, number of sentence fragments, and filler words did not change with age (Kynette and Kemper, 1986). Le Dorze and Bedard (1998) found speech production during the description of the picture of a bank robbery to be less productive in healthy subjects with lower levels of education, while older subjects tended to produce repetitions and some word-finding difficulties, making them less effective in lexicosemantic transmission. McNamara et al. (1992) compared the speech production of healthy elderly subjects, patients with Alzheimer's disease, and patients with Parkinson's disease (PD) and their ability to detect and correct errors. They found that healthy elderly relied on lemma repairs, while Alzheimer's patients used mostly reformulation repairs, and PD patients used both types of repairs.

Another study (Ulatowska et al., 1992) also found preservation of strategies of reduction, generalization, and interpretation of narratives. In contrast, patients with Alzheimer's disease produced fewer statements and longer utterances; they also showed sharp decline over time, more questions, and fewer optional steps (Ripich et al., 1997).

In addition, language comprehension shows a considerable decline with advancing age. Older subjects do not benefit from phonemic cues as much as younger ones (Au et al., 1995) and often complain about difficulty in everyday remembering (where they put things, why they went into a room, etc.). Extralinguistic factors such as decreasing working memory ("benign forgetfulness"), cognitive slowing, and decreasing inhibition of irrelevant information (Engle et al., 1995) as well as poorer functioning of the auditory system all may be involved in this decline. Comprehension in elderly individuals appears particularly sensitive to "linguistic stress," such as not being able to watch the face of the person speaking or the presence of concurrent background noise (Obler et al., 1995). Juncos-Rabadan (1994) and Juncos-Rabadan and Iglesias (1994) state that "all linguistic levels (phonology, morphology, lexicon, and semantics) deteriorate in the elderly although some linguistic skills (comprehension, repetition, lexical access and propositionizing) are impaired"; the authors also claim that this finding can be confirmed for 14 languages considered in their study. A study of 628 elderly (65+ years) subjects in the acute ward of a department of medicine by Sweeney et al. (1993) found that 73% of them had speech or language problems (based on the Frenchay Aphasia Screening Test), 11% had visual deficits, 36% had hearing problems, and 56% had a cognitive deficit on admission.

The immediate neurological correlates of these changes in the elderly are not well known: age related changes in brain anatomy include gyral atrophy, decreased brain weight, ventricular dilation, and loss of myelin. Other changes include loss of dopamine receptor density affecting attentional activity and executive system function. M. Nicholas et al. (1996) argue that such neurological changes relate to the loss of connectivity of the semantic and lexical networks rather than of content. This is partly confirmed by Swaab et al. (1998) who presented 12 Broca's aphasics and 12 healthy elderly subjects with ambiguous words in concordant context, in a context that biased the meaning of the ambiguous word, and in a discordant condition (i.e., incompatible with the target word). They used the electrophysiological index known as N400, which was initially reported in 1980 by Kutas and Hillyard as reflecting the brain's processing of semantically anomalous or inappropriate words. It appears that changes in the amplitude of this evoked response potential can reflect, for example, whether a word is expected or unexpected in a specific context or other decisions that need to be made about verbal information. Swaab and colleagues showed that elderly subjects were able to access the appropriate meaning of the ambiguity; in contrast, Broca's aphasics were not able to find the meaning at short interstimulus intervals (ISI), while at long ISI even the aphasics completed the selection process successfully.

In the elderly, aphasia tends to be more often of the fluent rather than the nonfluent type: on average, fluent aphasics tend to be a full decade older than nonfluent aphasics. This phenomenon was examined further by Annoni et al. (1993), who found more cases of Wernicke's aphasia in an older group (age 70–91 years) of 117 elderly patients as compared to the younger group (age 50–69 years). Ceccaldi et al. (1996) explored this finding in nonaphasic elderly: comparing 32 normal subjects from a younger (45–55 years) and an older age group (70 years and older), they found that elderly subjects used many more morphemes in their discourse than younger subjects. The authors speculate that both biological and sociological age-related characteristics may be responsible.

From a psychometric point of view, the age-related changes described here may easily lead to low scores on aphasia tests of discourse, comprehension, and word finding, and to making a misdiagnosis of aphasia in healthy elderly adults, unless age-appropriate corrections are made. The Framingham Heart Study (Elias et al., 1997) with 1893 participants between the age of 55 and 88 years clearly showed the effects of age as well as gender and education: the lowest level of performance was found for older men in the least educated cohort.

Speed of cognitive processes may be impaired in elderly patients, patients with Alzheimer's disease, or head injury with or without aphasia. Baddeley et al. (1995) published the Speed and Capacity of Language-Processing Test (SCOLP, Western Psychological Services, $175), which consists of the "speed of comprehension" test, which requires the patient to indicate which of a pair of simple statements is true; and to complete as many items as possible in 2 minutes, and the "spot the word" test, which requires the patient to indicate which of a pair of words is a real word, without time limits. The discrepancy between the two scores (speed minus vocabulary) is used as a measure of cognitive slowing in patients without evidence of aphasia. The test has norms for the age range from 16 to 60 years.

As suggested here, the speech clinician must be mindful of language-related changes in otherwise healthy elderly that may account for a number of subjective complaints, yet be very careful not to conclude an aphasia is present when such a diagnosis is unwarranted.

Dementia

Dementia is defined as an acquired impairment of intellectual capacity that includes abnormality in several of the following functions: (*1*) language; (*2*) memory; (*3*) visual-spatial ability; (*4*) cognitive ability; (*5*) personality. It is ascribed to widespread structural and biochemical damage to cortical and subcortical structures. Though Alzheimer's disease (AD) is most frequently investigated, many different disorders can cause dementia, which in turn can also produce aphasia. The most common aphasia in AD is frequently limited to anomia but is almost always present. Leikin and Aharon-Peretz (1998) report that single-word comprehension is preserved in patients with mild and severe AD, but sentence comprehension and especially the ability to grasp grammatical meaning were affected.

The underlying neuropathological correlates have been described as neuritic plaques, paired helical filaments, and granulovacuolar bodies, primarily in the parietal-tertiary areas, the inferior temporal cortex, and the limbic cortex. In addition, reduction in neurotransmitter substances has been noted. Since these changes can be verified only at autopsy, the careful examination of language and other accompanying cognitive deficits becomes crucial in the diagnosis of probable AD. In addition, the presence of aphasia in dementing patients has been associated with poor survival rates (Boersma et al., 1999). A widely used mental status examination for dementia was presented by Mattis in 1976 and has since been revised (Mattis et al., 2001).

Other forms of dementia include multi-infarct pathology, that is, a number of separate cerebrovascular accidents that produce both aphasia and dementia as well as other neurobehavioral sequelae. Aphasia and dementia may also accompany intracranial tumors (with widespread mental changes due to increased intracranial pressure, obstruction of outflow of cerebrospinal fluid, compression of arterial blood vessels, and necrosis of the tumor), intracranial trauma, intracranial infection, subarachnoid hemorrhage, etc.

Preclinical stages of dementia are characterized by memory impairment, changes in abstract reasoning, and confrontation naming ability at the early stages (Jacobs et al., 1995). Because anomia is the most obvious language defect in dementia, testing with word lists (semantic word fluency, e.g., animal naming) is particularly useful, especially if the patient does poorly on word fluency but well on confrontation naming (Benson, 1979b). Many psycholinguistic analyses of AD patients have been published. An interesting description of discourse in four conversations with AD patients (Garcia and Joanette, 1994) may serve as an example: the use of semantic or syntactic cohesion devices (e.g., repetition) was found to be a poor indicator of language deterioration in AD, but the authors describe topic shifting (a macrolinguistic feature) via topic shading: to get to a more familiar topic, failure to continue (with an unfinished topic), anecdotal shift (desire to get to a tangential topic they would like to talk about) by the interviewer as occurring more rapidly because the AD patients ran out of things to say.

LaBarge et al. (1992) found that agraphia, defined as in the inability to write a complete sentence on demand, was not correlated with three different indices of aphasia.

Testing Elderly and Dementing Patients

To establish a diagnosis of dementia, the presence of other defects, for example, constructional problems, memory disorders, or personality alterations must be considered. Testing patients with severe dementia may be impractical because such patients may be unlikely to cooperate meaningfully with further language or cognitive assessment: Pearsall et al. (1995) suggest that the Mini-Mental State Examination be given first; patients scoring eight or less on this test were untestable. Rates of decline are similar in women as in men, although one study found that naming and word recognition skills were generally poorer in women than in men (Ripich et al., 1997).

It should be obvious that in testing elderly patients and patients suspected of dementia the availability of age-appropriate norms is crucial. We have included appropriate references in the discussion of individual tests in the preceding chapters. However, two instruments may serve here as examples: the BNT, because of the large amount of research conducted with the test, and the Arizona Battery for Communication Disorders of Dementia (ABCD) as a first comprehensive language test designed specifically for patients with dementia. A third relevant test area—word fluency measures—was presented in Chapter 7.

Boston Naming Test in elderly and dementing patients

Age stability is a common finding on the BNT in healthy elderly subjects up to the age of 70 (see Chapter 7). Mitrushina and Satz (1995) reported that scores were essentially stable during three yearly administrations of the test in 122 normal adults, aged 57 to 85 years. Ganguli et al. (1996) reported no significant changes between baseline and 2-year follow-up examination with 1017 elderly adults. Lansing et al. (1999) examined various short forms with a population of 717 controls and 237 AD subjects in the age range of 50 to 98 years. They found significant correlations with age and education as well as gender effects for all forms, including the original full-length version. Correct classification rates varied from 58% to 69% for AD patients, and from 77% to 87% for normal controls. Based on a discriminant function analysis, the authors developed a new empirical 15-item version balanced for gender. Hawkins et al. (1993) also found correlations between .74 and .87 between the Gates-McGinitie Reading Vocabulary Test and the BNT across normal and clinical adult populations; they demonstrated that norms for the test may lead to many false-positive errors for naming deficit, and that corrections should be applied, especially for subjects with lower than average reading level. Concurrent validity with the MAE Visual Naming subtest (Benton et al., 1994a) was described by Axelrod et al. (1994).

Jacobs et al. (1995) noted that lower BNT baseline scores were significantly associated with subsequent AD at follow-up, controlling for the effects of age, education, sex, and language of test administration. Poor naming has been singled out as a poor prognostic sign in AD with a more rapidly progressive course (Knesevich et al. 1986). Once AD is diagnosed, the BNT showed the most rapid decline in a sample of 51 AD patients examined at 6-month intervals during a 2-year period (Rebok et al., 1990). Kazniak et al. (1988) found that elderly subjects make one error on average, whereas patients with AD with a mild degree of impairment obtain a mean of 5.5 errors, and those with moderate impairment make about 7.5 errors. Eighty percent of AD patients showed anomia with 11 or more errors on the BNT (Freedman et al., 1995). LaBarge et al. (1992b), Petrick et al. (1992), and Zec et al. (1992) found the test highly sensitive to very mild AD; it also discriminated well between AD and vascular dementia (Barr et al., 1992). Cahn et al. (1995) found that the test discriminated well among 238 normal elderly, 77 at-risk for AD, and 45 AD patients. Poor performance of patients with AD can exceed the impairment shown in patients with anomia (Margolin et al., 1990); the authors explain this on the basis of the amount of semantic processing required for the BNT, as compared to phonological processing in COWA. Lindman (1996) came to similar conclusions in a comparison of BNT and animal fluency data of 68 AD and 80 control subjects, and, in addition, found that female AD patients performed significantly worse than males. Loewenstein et al. (1992) compared the performance of 33 AD patients on the BNT and seven other tests with eight functional tasks (reading a clock, telephone skills, preparing a letter for mailing, counting currency, writing a check, balancing a checkbook, shopping with a written list); the BNT correlated (.40) with only the ability to shop with a written list and did not contribute to a stepwise regression analysis of the eight tests in predicting functional competence. All tests combined accounted for less than 50% of the explained variance. However, C. Baum et al. (1996) conducted a canonical analysis of a variety of measures of activities of daily living and a set of neuropsychological tests in AD patients. The BNT had a loading of .88 on the first canonical variate, indicating good ecological validity in this population.

Arizona Battery for Communication Disorders of Dementia

The purpose of the Arizona Battery for Communication Disorders of Dementia (ABCD) is to provide a comprehensive assessment of language and other communicative functions in patients with dementia. As such, it is not a traditional aphasia assessment instrument in the manner of the other batteries discussed earlier (Chapter 9). The test (Bayles and Tomoeda, 1990; Canyonlands Publishing, $200) includes four screening tasks: Speech Discrimination, Visual Perception and Literacy (reading sentences), Visual Field (circling all As on a page of randomly scattered letters), and Visual Agnosia (naming or describing pictured objects) are designed to alert the examiner to other disorders that may interfere with communicative functioning. The main test consists of 14 subtests. A number of these subtests reflect traditional items found in most aphasia batteries, such as confrontation naming, category (animal) fluency, comprehension (at the yes/no level), and repetition. The battery also includes assessment of mental status (i.e., orientation), free-speech description of three pictured objects, a subtest similar to the Wechsler Intelligence Scale Vocabulary subtest, figure copying, and object drawing. Importantly, the ABCD differs from more typical aphasia batteries by measuring immediate and delayed recall of a story (containing 17 pieces of information).

The response record provides relatively clear scoring guidelines, allowing one point for each item or part of an item. The authors suggest converting raw scores into "summary scores" between 1 and 5 in order to make subtest scores comparable to each other. The summary scores are based on the performance of 50 healthy elderly subjects (mean = 71 years) with a mean premorbid IQ of 105, and a mean education of 13 years. A summary score of 5 was achieved by most normal subjects, a score of 3 to 5 by patients with mild, and a score of 2 to 5 by patients with moderate dementia. A construct summary score can be obtained by averaging summary scores across subtests contributing to each of five major areas (Mental Status, Episodic Memory, Linguistic Expression, Linguistic Comprehension, Verbal Visuospatial Construction). An overall performance score can be calculated by averaging across all subtests.

The ABCD has been used in only a few published studies. The manual reports 1-week retest reliability for 20 patients with AD as ranging from .01 (Reading Comprehension, Words) to .86 (Figure Copying) and concordance rates from .65 to .87. Internal consistency is high for all subtests (.63 to .98). The test has been successfully used in the United Kingdom without a change of items (Armstrong et al., 1996).

Criterion validity has been explored by correct classification rates between 50 normal and 50 AD subjects. Chi-squares for all except three subtests were highly significant. Correlational validity of individual subtests with measures of the severity of dementia in 50 AD patients ranged from .63 to .82 with the Global Deterioration Scale (Reisberg et al., 1982), from .62 to .85 with Folstein's Mini-Mental State Examination (MMSE), and from .59 to .75 with the WAIS-R Block Design subtest. Concordances with the ABCD total summary scores were .78, .84, and .75, respectively. The test has also been used in a study of patients with multiple sclerosis (Wallace and Holmes, 1993) and in a comparison of semantic and phonemic word fluency by Bayles et al. (1989b).

Multidimensional scaling and cluster analysis with a woefully inadequate sample of 50 AD subjects resulted in 17 clusters, and suggested that five of the linguistic expression subtests (Object Description, Generative Naming, Confrontation Naming, Concept Definition, Picture Description) form a closely correlated cluster, while linguistic comprehension subtests are only loosely related. Principal component factor analysis suggested a general and an episodic memory factor.

It is not clear whether the ABCD is subject to age, education, or gender effects, or whether a profile of subtest scores may contribute to differential diagnoses. The test can be viewed as being still in a preliminary or research stage, since derivation of summary scores and studies of discriminant and construct validity based on a sample of 50 AD and 50 normal elderly subjects requires further work and independent confirmation. The test provides a wide range of measures of language and other communicative functions similar to the WAB or the NCCEA. However, it also includes a general measure of mental status, several measures of memory, and diverse screening measures for visual perception, visual fields and/or neglect, auditory discrimination, and visual agnosia. These additional features are suitable and useful for a quick, superficial assessment of the status of mental functions of dementing patients in the context of considering treatment choices. However, diagnosticians may wish to use more detailed and better validated tests for these areas. In fact, one could use the MMSE, the BNT, the F-A-S test or the MAE COWA, and a list-learning task in half the time, and obtain information similar to that tested in the ABCD. The transformation into summary scores is probably premature; it is useful to provide comparability of subtests, but summary scores hide a wide range of raw scores that may be useful for further test exploration. Although designed for elderly patients with dementia, the ABCD may be suitable for a larger age range of patients. It is hoped that additional research with the instrument will help refine its applications and psychometric structure.

16

Aphasia Testing in Non-English Language and Bilingual Patients

Patients whose first language is not English pose a special problem in the assessment of aphasia. For such patients (e.g., Hispanic/Latin Americans, French Canadians, immigrants), it is difficult to judge premorbid English language ability. Moreover, the matter of a differential impairment in the two languages requires investigation. Various theories have proposed that the "older," the "more affectively favored," the "most frequently used" language is less affected by aphasia, and may recover faster (i.e., the notion of differential recovery), whereas other studies point out either that little difference actually exists between languages (Albert and Obler, 1978), or that the language environment during recovery from brain damage is the crucial factor. Another study points out that, at least in a listening task, a second language acquired after the age of 7 years uses other cerebral networks (i.e., is less lateralized and includes the right hemisphere) than the first language (which uses the expected left temporal area) (Dehaene et al., 1997). It is sensible to refrain from such generalizations, focus on the establishment of the premorbid language competence, and assess impairment for both languages. One such study with 16 bilingual aphasics, equally fluent in French and English prior to their illness (P. Roberts and Le Dorze, 1998), found no difference between the two languages on a semantic fluency (animals, food) task both in terms of number of words produced and in semantic organization.

At any rate, it is important that bilingual or multilingual aphasics be tested in all premorbidly spoken languages, because the findings may be of serious cultural and clinical consequences during treatment: the patient may be unaware which of the two languages is more affected, or erroneously believe that one of them is better recovered. On the other hand, specific symptoms may be detectable in only one of the patient's two languages, either because of the particular structural features of that language or because of differential recovery in which the language not tested is the more severely affected.

Frequently, the examination in the second language is carried out by using the same assessment methods with or without the use of an interpreter. Although this provides seemingly close comparability of the assessment in the two languages, such comparability may be tenuous at best and is not acceptable in clinical practice. Frequently, an "instant" translation of this type only poorly approximates the difficulty level of vocabulary and grammar, because of basic differences in the frequency of word use and grammatical structure in the two languages. In addition, cultural differences in the experience of taking tests must be considered. For example, in spite of some modifications, the Category Fluency Test (animals), administered to Nigerian subjects resulted in a mean of 13.8, in Jamaicans of 9.0, whereas means in a U.S. population were 18.7 (Guruje et al., 1995; Unverzagt et al., 1999; Welsh et al., 1994); in the same studies, the 15-item BNT produced means of 8.2 in Nigerians, 9.3 in Jamaicans, and 14.7 in U.S. subjects. Such differences are likely due not only to language differences but also to differences in familiarity with a test situation, with the test material, and differences in test-taking attitudes. Theriault-Wahlen and Beaudichon (1997) express similar reservations regarding the French adaptation of the PPVT. The MAE, described in Chapter 9, attempts to address some of these problems and to provide fully equivalent forms in several languages. For example, the German version uses the letters *B*, *F*, and *L* instead of *F-A-S*. Even this version, though seemingly equivalent in the frequency of letters used in English and German, does not take into account that in German many words start with the prefix "be-," although this is only infrequently used as a strategy by German-speaking individuals (Niemann, 2001, personal communication).

A bilingual test can be used to best effect only when the examiner is fluent in the two languages. More broadly, any translated or interpreted verbal performance on an aphasia evaluation is subject to bias on the part of the translating resource, whether technical (i.e., quality of translation) or understandably interpersonal (i.e., a family member who despite best intentions may "normalize" the aphasic patient's speech).

Table 16-1 Tests available in English and in translation or adaptation

Test	Language
Aachen Aphasia Test	German (Huber et al., 1983), English (N. Miller et al., 2000), Dutch (Graetz et al., 1992), Italian (Luzzatti et al., 1992), Thai (Prachritpukdee et al., 1998)
Aphasia Language Performance Scale	Spanish (Keenan and Brassel, 1975)
Aphasia Screening Test	Punjabi
Assessment of Bilingual Aphasia (BAT)	French (Paradis and Libben, 1993), Spanish
Bilingual Verbal Abilities Test (BVAT)	French
Boston Diagnostic Aphasia Examination	Chinese, Norwegian (Reinvang and Graves, 1975) Finnish (Laine et al., 1993), French (Mazaux and Orgogozo, 1985), Spanish (Garcia-Albea et al., 1986)
Boston Naming Test	Spanish (Taussig et al., 1988; Ponton et al., 1992), Dutch, Finnish (Laine et al., 1993), Korean (Kim and Na, 1999), French
Communication Abilities in Daily Living	Italian (Pizzamiglio et al., 1984), Japanese (Sasanuma, 1991; Watamori et al., 1987)
Controlled Oral Word Association	Spanish (Taussig et al., 1988)
Denver Developmental Screening Test	Spanish (Franenburg and Dodds, 1990)
Multilingual Aphasia Examination	Chinese, French, German, Italian, Portuguese, Spanish (Examen de Afasia Multilingue, Benton and Hamsher, 1994)
NCCEA	French, Italian, Japanese
PALPA	Dutch (Bastiaanse et al., 1995)
Verb and Sentence Test	Dutch (Bastiaanse et al., 1999), English, German*, French*
Western Aphasia Battery	Chinese, Hebrew (Leikin and Sharon-Peretz, 1998), Japanese (Sugishita, 1988), Thai

*Test is in preparation.

Individual tests have been deliberately constructed for the assessment of bilinguals (e.g. Assessment of Bilingual Aphasia; Paradis and Libben, 1987; 1993; $49.95; Multilingual Aphasia Examination; Benton and Hamsher, 1994). Translations or adaptations of other tests are available (e.g., Aachen Aphasia Test, BDAE, CADL, PALPA, WAB, but some are still at an experimental stage or without adequate psychometric studies. A recent language proficiency test (Bilingual Verbal Abilities Test

[BVAT], Munez-Sandoval et al., 1998; Riverside Publishers; suitable for French, Creole, and 15 other languages) was designed for nonaphasic bilingual subjects. Yiu (1992) reports on an adaptation of the WAB into Cantonese. The Language Assessment Scale (DeAvila and Duncan, 1986; Linguametrics Group) was specifically designed in English and Spanish to assess language competency in bilingual school children (B. Goldstein et al., 1993; Secada, 1991).

Unless adequate adaptations are available, it is far more preferable to use tests developed in foreign countries. Examples of well-developed non-English tests are the German Aachen Aphasia Test (AAT; Huber et al., 1983; Willmes and Ratajczak, 1962; De Bleser et al., 1986) and the Japanese Standard Language Test of Aphasia (Kusunoki, 1985; Tamura, et al., 1996).

It should also be remembered that cultural and regional differences must be taken into account when using a test that has been standardized in another country, even though it is presented in the same language. For example, Barker-Collo (2001) found that New Zealand university students made up to 60% more errors compared to U.S. norms on certain items (e.g., pretzel, beaver, globe, funnel, tripod) and native New Zealanders (Maori) performed even worse than those of European origin.

17

Test Choice and Interpretation of Assessment

Choice of Tests

The choice of a test instrument will depend on the purposes of the assessment, as well as on individual preference and theoretical orientation. If quick or routine screening for a possible aphasic deficit is desired, one of the well-established and validated screening instruments described in Chapter 6 will suffice. However, it should be remembered that the hit-rate of any screening instrument is less than perfect, and that false positive (i.e., indicating aphasia even if it is not present) and false negative conclusions can occur, especially in poorly educated, bilingual, or socially disadvantaged clients. To clarify such findings, a follow-up with other tests may be required, especially if other professionals such as teachers, physicians, occupational therapists, and nurses, or relatives have indicated the need for a diagnostic workup.

If a full assessment for diagnostic or therapeutic purposes is required, an optimal description may be gained by using one of the more comprehensive, well-validated instruments and one of the functional communication instruments described in Chapters 9 and 8, respectively. The tests chosen should be supplemented with other test procedures: specific-purpose tests (or parts of another comprehensive battery), tests for associated deficits, a clinical examination of specific problems, and, if possible, specially constructed tasks suitable for retraining.

No formal battery of tests can or should be recommended as sufficiently comprehensive to arrive at an optimal description of the nature of the speech and language deficit for an individual patient. In clinical practice, we, as well as many other clinicians, tend to use a flexible approach for which a comprehensive test battery is only the beginning. Complete reliance on a given test battery tends to introduce an element of rigidity that may result in failure to fully explore the patient's problem.

The approach advocated here requires full knowledge of a very broad range of available instruments as well as clinical skill and judgment. Although parts of the examination are likely to be conducted in many settings by a trained psychometrist, the full involvement of the experienced clinician is necessary to understand and interpret assessment results and their implications.

Although computerized test administration (including touch-screen technology) and scoring are becoming available for many tests and can be time-saving, close supervision of the client during the early testing procedure is necessary to ensure that instructions are fully understood and followed. On the other hand, computer programs for test *interpretation* should be used only with considerable caution, because such programs are suitable only for the translation of test results into existing norms, which may or may not be suitable for a given client; and interpretations generally are worded for general use, not necessarily for the individual taking the test. The need remains for the clinician to review the test scores and interpret the test protocol with suitable adjustments for the individual case.

Other considerations in the choice of assessment methods are (*a*) psychometric adequacy of a test; (*b*) portability of the test material; and (*c*) time requirements. In the first part of this book, psychometric requirements for a well-constructed test were explicitly stated. The closer a test meets the ideals of a psychometrically well-developed test, the more likely it is that valid and reliable results are obtained. Attention should also be paid to research conducted with a given instrument, since this provides additional information about the validity of a test and about making specific decisions concerning diagnosis, treatment, and prognosis. Portability tends to be no major concern in a hospital-based clinic or evaluation service, but does become a problem if bedside examinations are frequently carried out. In this latter case, one would prefer a handy portfolio of pictures rather than a suitcase full of objects, even though any pictured item tends to lose some value on a "reality" dimension. Time is a crucial consideration in many facilities with heavy patient loads; however, time requirements should be carefully weighed against the information that might be gleaned from a given test. Brevity is no virtue if crucial information is not collected. In fact, the approach advocated here suggests that time requirements should be of secondary importance, and that experimental variants and additional exploratory procedures that may be of benefit in the long run should be used in the course of the assessment.

A last point should be mentioned: assessment is not an end in itself but must be considered in relation to its potential value to the patient and the treatment and management of the patient's deficits. As Messick (1980) pointed out, the adequacy of a test is not dictated solely by psychometric soundness. Rather, the concept of construct validity should include the "ethics" of assessment; that is, it must provide a rational foundation for prediction and relevance as well as take into account the implications of test interpretation per se.

Interpretation of Assessment Results

Every clinician has his or her own model of how best to survey a summary sheet of assessment results, with frequent glances at the actual test records and notes on the behavior of the patient during testing. Many of the comprehensive tests provide, of course, their own grouping of the test information and hence a suggested approach to interpretation (e.g., summary scores for dimensions such as auditory comprehension and verbal expression). Other test authors leave the interpretation open to the clinician using the test.

Our own approach (and that of many other clinicians) tends to be *"syndromatic"* in the sense that we tend to focus first on the most seriously abnormal scores in the assessment record and scan the record for related information and corroborative test findings. For example, if the patient's most serious problem is on a test of word finding, we scan all related test results, as well as information about the patient's ability to find words in conversational settings, for higher order performance on verbal and nonverbal memorization/new-learning tests, and so forth. This allows a better description of the deficit, that is, whether the deficit is generalized or specific to the test setting, whether it is related to a specific sensory modality, whether it is a secondary manifestation of a nonaphasic amnestic or attentional disorder, and so forth. Additional assessment procedures may well be necessary to fully evaluate this first "syndrome."

We then proceed to the next syndrome that appears to be reasonably independent of the first, and again search for associated task failures and other corroborative evidence. In this fashion, we can move toward the least deviant score on the assessment record, keeping in mind the estimated premorbid intelligence of the patient. Such syndromes may or may not be related to each other; they may or may not reflect a "classical type" of aphasia with localizing significance. Our primary purpose is to gain a detailed picture of the patient's deficits in order of severity and in the context of other deficits. We then proceed in the opposite direction, searching for the best score in the test record or the best preserved function until the information in the assessment record is exhausted.

Finally, we reexplore the noted syndromes by evaluating the actual behavior of the patient *qualitatively* on individual tests or other assessment procedures, as well as on follow-up tests given after the initial interpretation of test findings. Such a qualitative analysis also includes a review of errors made by the patient and the meaning of such errors; the examiner attempts to understand why a particular error was arrived at. Typically, this step results in a fuller description of the patient's performance. Interpretation of findings in the broader neurobehavioral context of the patient's level of adjustment to his or her current deficits, the patient's awareness of her or his deficits, family cohesiveness and ability to provide support, and appreciation for individualized community reentry needs all are likely to influence the clinician's understanding of the patient. For instance, we would no longer be describing "anomia for visually presented real objects," but can now include details of whether this deficit is part of a fuller diagnostic syndrome, what the associated impairments are, how the deficit affects the patient, his or her job, his or her family, and how remediative treatment might approach the deficit by building on strengths and working on weaknesses.

The approach described here is highly idiosyncratic in a deliberate attempt to avoid preconceived models of language and brain functions. However, until a more generally accepted model of language disorders and generally accepted standards of procedure for generally accepted standard questions are developed—and little progress has yet been made in that direction—this outline of objective procedures for interpretation may provide the fullest utilization of assessment results at the present state of knowledge.

References

Abrahams, S., Leigh, P.N., Harvey, A., Vythelingum, G.N., Grise, D., and Goldstein, L.H. (2000) Verbal fluency and executive dysfunction in amyotrophic lateral sclerosis (ALS). *Neuropsychologia*, 38, 734–747.

Acevedo, A., Lowenstein, D.A., Barker, W.W., Harwood, D.G., et al. (2000) Category Fluency Test: Normative data for English- and Spanish-speaking elderly. *Journal of the International Neuropsychological Society*, 6, 760–769.

Adam, D.M. (1998) Acquired aphasia in children. In: M.T. Sarno (Ed.), *Acquired aphasia*, 3rd ed. San Diego: Academic Press.

Adamovich, B. and Henderson, J. (1992) *Scales of Cognitive Ability for Traumatic Brain Injury (SCATBI)*. Chicago: Riverside Publishing.

Adams, M.L., Reich, A.R., and Flowers, C.R. (1989) Verbal fluency characteristics of normal and aphasic speakers. *Journal of Speech and Hearing Research*, 32, 871–879.

Adolphs, R., Tranel, D., and Damasio, H. (2001) Emotion recognition from faces and prosody following temporal lobectomy. *Neuropsychology*, 15, 396–404.

Albert, M.L., Goodglass, H., Helm, N.A., Rubens, A.B., and Alexander, M.P. (1981) *Clinical aspects of aphasia*. New York: Springer.

Albert, M.L. and Obler, L.K. (1978) *The bilingual brain: Neuropsychological and neurolinguistic aspects of bilingualism*. New York: Academic Press.

Albert, M.S., Heller, H.S., and Milberg, W. (1988) Changes in naming ability with age. *Psychology and Aging*, 3, 173–178.

Alberts, F.M., Davis, B.L., and Prentice, L. (1995) Validity of an observation screening instrument in a multilingual population. *Journal of Early Intervention*, 19, 168–177.

Alexander, D.W. and Frost, B.P. (1982) Decelerating synthesized speech as a means of shaping speed of auditory processing of children with delayed language. *Perceptual and Motor Skills*, 55, 783–792.

Alexander, M.P. (1997) Aphasia: Clinical and anatomic aspects. In: T.E. Feinberg and M.J. Farah (Eds.), *Behavioral neurology and neuropsychology* (pp. 133–150). New York: McGraw-Hill.

Alexander, M.P. and Annett, M. (1996) Crossed aphasia and related anomalies of cerebral organization: Case report and a genetic hypothesis. *Brain and Language*, 55, 213–239.

Al-Khawaja, I., Wade, D.T., and Collins, C.F. (1996) Bedside screening for aphasia: A comparison of two methods. *Journal of Neurology*, 243, 201–204.

Allard, A.M.F. and Pfohl, W. (1988) The Kaufman Asssessment Battery for Children: A validity study with at-risk preschoolers. *Journal of Psychoeducational Assessment*, 6, 215–224.

Allegri, R.F., Mangone, C.A., Villavicencio, A.F., Rymberg, S., Taragano, F., and Baumann, D. (1997) Spanish Boston naming norms. *The Clinical Neuropsychologist*, 11, 416–420.

Allen, R., Wasserman, G.A., and Seidman, S. (1990) Children with congenital anomalies: The preschool period. *Journal of Pediatric Psychology*, 15, 327–345.

Altepeter, T.S. (1989) The PPVT-R as a measure of psycholinguistic functioning: A caution. *Journal of Clinical Psychology*, 45, 935–941.

Altepeter, T.S. and Johnson, K.A. (1989) Use of the PPVT-R for intellectual screening with adults: A caution. *Journal of Psychoeducational Assessment*, 7, 39–45.

American Psychological Association (1985) *Standards for educational and psychological tests*. Washington, D.C.: APA Press.

American Speech-Language-Hearing Association (1990) *Functional communication scales for adults project: Advisory report*. Rockville, MD: ASHA Press.

American Speech-Language-Hearing Association (1996) Central auditory processing: Current status of research and implications for clinical practice. *American Journal of Audiology*, 5, 41–54.

Amos, N.E. and Humes, L. (1998) SCAN test-retest reliability for first and third-grade children. *Journal of Speech, Language, and Hearing Research*, 41, 834–845.

Anastasi, A. and Urbina, F. (1996) *Psychological testing*, 7th ed. New York: Prentice-Hall.

Annoni, J.M., Cot, F., Ryalls, J., and Lecours, A.R. (1993) Profile of aphasic patients in a Montreal geriatric hospital: A 6-year study. *Aphasiology*, 7, 271–284.

Appell, J., Kertesz, A., and Fisman, M. (1982) A study of language functioning in Alzheimer patients. *Brain and Language*, 17, 73–91.

Aram, D.M. (1998) Acquired aphasia in children. In: M.T. Sarno (Ed.), *Acquired aphasia* (pp. 451–480). San Diego, CA: Academic Press.

Armstrong, L., Borthwick, S.E., Bayles, K.E., and Tomoeda, C.K. (1996) Use of the Arizona Battery for Communication Disorders of Dementia in the UK. *European Journal of Disorders of Communication*, 31, 171–180.

Armstrong, L. and Walker, K. (1994) Preliminary evidence on the question of gender differences in language testing of older people. *European Journal of Disorders of Communication*, 29, 371–378.

Arndt, W.B. (1977) A psychometric evaluation of the Northwestern Syntax Screening Test. *Journal of Speech and Hearing Disorders*, 42, 316–319.

Arruda, J.E., Stern, R.A., and Somerville, J.A. (1999) Measurement of mood states in stroke patients: Validation of the Visual Analog Mood Scales. *Archives of Physical Medicine and Rehabilitation*, 80, 676–680.

Arvedson, C.J., McNeil, M.R., and West, T. (1985) Prediction of Revised Token Test overall, subtest, and linguistic unit scores by two shortened versions. *Clinical Aphasiology*, 15, 57–63.

Astington, J.W. and Jenkins, J.M. (1999) A longitudinal study of the relation between language and theory-of-mind development. *Developmental Psychology*, 35, 1311–1320.

Aten, J.L., Caligiure, M.P., and Holland, A. (1982) The efficacy of communication therapy for aphasic patients. *Journal of Speech and Hearing Disorders*, 47, 93–96.

Atkinson, M.H. (1995) Comparison of volunteer and referred children on individual measures of assessment: A Native American sample. *Dissertation Abstracts International*, 56 (1-A), 139.

Atlas, J.A. (1992) Review of Assessing Linguistic Behavior. *11th Mental Measurement Yearbook* (p. 38). Lincoln, NE: University of Nebraska Press.

Au, R., Joung, P., Nicholas, M., Obler, L.K., Kass, R., and Albert, M.L. (1995) Naming ability across the adult lifespan. *Aging and Cognition*, 2, 300–311.

Avent, J.R., Wertz, R.T., and Auther, L.L. (1998) Relationship between language impairment and pragmatic behavior in aphasic adults. *Journal of Neurolinguistics*, 11, 207–221.

Axelrod, B.N., Ricker, J.H., and Cherry, S.A. (1994) Concurrent validity of the MAE Visual Naming test. *Archives of Clinical Neuropsychology*, 9, 317–321.

Azrin, B.L., Mercury, M.G., Millsaps, C. et al. (1996) Cautionary note on the Boston Naming Test: Cultural considerations. *Archives of Clinical Neuropsychology*, 11, 365–366 (abstract).

Bachman, L.F. (1995) Review of Receptive-Expressive Emergent Language Test. In: J.C. Conoley and J.C. Impara (Eds.), *The 12th Mental Measurement Yearbook*. Lincoln, NE: University of Nebraska Press.

Bacon Moore, A., Paulsen, J.S., and Murphy, C. (1999) A test of odor fluency in patients with Alzheimer's and Huntington's disease. *Journal of Clinical and Experimental Neuropsychology*, 21, 341–351.

Baddeley, A., Emslie, H., and Nimmo-Smith, I. (1995) *The Speed and Capacity of Language Processing Test* (SCOLP). Los Angeles: Western Psychological Services.

Bailey, S., Powell, G.E., and Clark, E. (1981) A note on intelligence and recovery from aphasia: The relationship between Raven's Matrices scores and change on the Schuell Aphasia Test. *British Journal of Disorders of Communication*, 16, 193–203.

Baines, K.A., Heeringa, H.M., and Martin, A.W. (1999) *Assessment of language-related functional activities*. Austin, TX: Pro-Ed.

Baker, C.L. (1995) Utilization of the Reitan-Indiana Aphasia Screening Test in identifying learning-disabled and low-achieving children. *Dissertation Abstracts International*, 55(8-B), 3631.

Baldo, J.V., Shimamura, A.P., Delis, D.C., Kramer, J., and Kaplan, E. (2001) Verbal and design fluency in patients with frontal lobe lesions. *Journal of the International Neuropsychological Society*, 7, 586–596.

Ball, M.J. (1999) Reynell Developmental Language Scales III: A quick and easy LARSP? *International Journal of Language and Communication Disorders*, 34, 171–174.

Ball, M.J., Davies, E., Duckworth, M., and Middlehurst, R. (1991) Assessing the assessments: Comparison of two clinical pragmatic profiles. *Journal of Communication Disorders*, 24, 367–379.

Barker-Collo, S.I.. (2001) The 60-item Boston Naming Test: Cultural bias and possible adaptations for New Zealand. *Aphasiology*, 15, 85–92.

Barker-Fudala, J. (1998) *Arizona Articulation Proficiency Scale*, 3rd ed. Los Angeles: Western Psychological Services.

Barnes, M.A. and Dennis, M. (1998) Discourse after early-onset hydrocephalus: Core deficits in children of average intelligence. *Brain and Language*, 61, 309–334.

Barnes, M.A. and Dennis, M. (2001) Knowledge-based inferencing after childhood head injury. *Brain and Language*, 76, 253–265.

Barnsley, G. (1987) Repair strategies used by aphasics and their conversational patterns. B.Sc. dissertation, Department of Speech, Newcastle University.

Barona, A., Reynolds, C.R., and Chastain, R. (1984) A demographically based index of premorbid intelligence for the WAIS-R. *Journal of Consulting and Clinical Psychology*, 52, 885–887.

Barr, A., Benedict, R., Tune, L., and Brandt, J. (1992) Neuropsychological differentiation of Alzheimer's diesase from vascular dementia. *International Journal of Geriatric Psychiatry*, 7, 621–627.

Barth, J.T. (1984) Interrater reliability and prediction of verbal and spatial functioning with a modified scoring system for the Reitan-Indiana Aphasia Screening Examination. *International Journal of Clinical Neuropsychology*, 6, 135–138.

Basso, A. (1996) PALPA: An appreciation and a few criticisms. *Aphasiology*, 10, 190–193.

Basso, A. and Cubelli, R. (1999) Clinical aspects of aphasia. In: G. Denes and L. Pizzamiglio (Eds.), *Handbook of clinical and experimental neuropsychology*. Hove, East Sussex, UK: Psychology Press.

Bastiaanse, R., Bosje, M., and Visch-Brink, E. (1995) *PALPA—Nederlandse Versie*. Hove, UK: Lawrence Erlbaum.

Bastiaanse, R., Maas, E., and Rispens, J. (1999) *Werkwoordenen Zinnen Test* (WEZT). Lisse, Netherlands: Swets & Zeitlinger.

Baum, C., Edwards, D., Yonan, C., and Storandt, M. (1996) The relation of neuropsychological test performance to performance on functional tasks in dementia of the Alzheimer type. *Archives of Clinical Neuropsychology*, 11, 69–75.

Baum, S.R. and Pell, M.D. (1997) Production of affective and linguistic prosody by brain-damaged patients. *Aphasiology*, 11, 177–198.

Baum, S.R. and Pell, M.D. (1999) The neural basis of prosody: Insights from lesion studies and neuroimaging. *Aphasiology*, 13, 581–608.

Bayles, K.A. (1984) Language and dementia. In: A. Holland (Ed.), *Language disorders in adults* (pp. 209–244). San Diego: College-Hill Press.

Bayles, K.A., Boone, D.R., Tomoeda, C.K., Slauson, T.J., and Kaszniak, A.W. (1989a) Differentiating Alzheimer's patients from the normal elderly and stroke patients with aphasia. *Journal of Speech and Hearing Disorders*, 54, 74–87.

Bayles, K.A., Salmon, D.P., Tomoeda, C.K., Jacobs, D., and Caffrey, J.T. (1989b) Semantic and letter category naming in Alzheimer's patients: A predictable difference. *Developmental Neuropsychology*, 5, 335–347.

Bayles, K.A. and Tomoeda, C.K. (1983) Confrontation naming in dementia. *Brain and Language*, 19, 98–114.

Bayles, K.A. and Tomoeda, C.K. (1990) *Arizona Battery for Communication Disorders of Dementia (ABCD)*. Tucson, AZ: Canyonlands Publishing Inc.

Bayley, N. (1993) *Bayley Scales of Infant Development-2*. Chicago: Riverside Publishing.

Beatty, G. and Shovelton, H. (1999) Mapping the range of information contained in the iconic hand gestures that accompany spontaneous speech. *Journal of Language and Social Psychology*, 18, 438–462.

Beatty, W.W. and Monson, N. (1989) Lexical processing in Parkinson's disease and multiple sclerosis. *Journal of Geriatric Psychiatry and Neurology*, 2, 145–152.

Beauregard, M., Chertkow, H., Bub, D., Murtha, S., Dixon, R., and Evans, A. (1997) The neural substrate for concrete, abstract, and emotional word lexica: A positron emission tomography study. *Journal of Cognitive Neuroscience*, 9, 441–461.

Beck, A.T., Steer, R.A., and Brown, G.K. (1996) *Beck Depression Inventory-II: Manual*. San Antonio, TX: Psychological Corporation.

Beckers, N., Netz, J., and Hoemberg, V. (1999) The measurement of outcome in day care neurological rehabilitation: Discrepancies between changes in FIM and Barthel scores and achievement of treatment goals. *Neuropsychological Rehabilitation*, 9, 437–446.

Beele, K.A., Davies, E., and Muller, D.J. (1984) Therapists' views on the clinical usefulness of four aphasia tests. *British Journal of Disorders of Communication*, 19, 169–178.

Behrmann, M. and Penn, C. (1984) Non-verbal communication of aphasic patients. *British Journal of Disorders of Communication*, 19, 155–168.

Beitchman, J.H., Wilson, B., Brownlie, E.B., Walters, H., Inglis, A., and Lance, W. (1996) Long-term consistency in speech/language profiles: II. Behavioral, emotional, and social outcomes. *Journal of the American Academy of Child and Adolescent Psychiatry*, 35, 815–825.

Bell, B.D., Davies, K.G., Hermann, B.P., and Walters, G. (2000) Confrontation naming after anterior temporal lobectomy is related to age of aquisition of the object names. *Neuropsychologia*, 38, 83–92.

Benson, D.F. (1967) Fluency in aphasia: Correlation with radioactive scan localization. *Cortex*, 3, 373–394.

Benson, D.F. (1979a) Aphasia. In: K.M. Heilman and E. Valenstein (Eds.), *Clinical Neuropsychology*. New York: Oxford University Press.

Benson, D.F. (1979b) *Aphasia, alexia and agraphia*. New York: Churchill-Livingstone.

Benson, D.F. and Ardila, A. (1996) *Aphasia. A clinical perspective*. New York: Oxford University Press.

Benson, D.F. and Geschwind, N. (1982) The aphasias and related disorders. In: A.B. Baker and L.H. Baker (Eds.), *Clinical neurology*. Philadelphia: Harper & Row.

Benton, A.L. (1961) The fiction of the "Gerstmann Syndrome." *Journal of Neurology, Neurosurgery, and Psychiatry*, 24, 176–181.

Benton, A.L. (1964) Contributions to aphasia before Broca. *Cortex*, 1, 314–327.

Benton, A.L. (1967) Problems of test construction in the field of aphasia. *Cortex*, 3, 32–53.

Benton, A.L. (1969) Development of a multilingual aphasia battery: Progress and problems. *Journal of the Neurological Sciences*, 9, 39–48.

Benton, A.L. (1979) Visuoperceptive, visuospatial, and visuoconstructive disorders. In: K.M. Heilman and E. Valenstein (Eds.), *Clinical neuropsychology* (pp. 186–232). New York: Oxford University Press.

Benton, A.L. (1982) Significance of nonverbal cognitive abilities in aphasic patients. *Japanese Journal of Stroke*, 4, 153–161.

Benton, A.L. (1994) Neuropsychological assessment. *Annual Review of Psychology*, 45, 1–23.

Benton, A.L. and Anderson, S.W. (1998) Aphasia: Historical perspectives. In: M.T. Sarno (Ed.), *Acquired aphasia*, 3rd ed. San Diego: Academic Press.

Benton, A.L., Eslinger, P.J., and Damasio, A.R. (1981) Normative observations in neuropsychological test performances in old age. *Journal of Clinical Neuropsychology*, 3, 33–42.

Benton, A.L. and Hamsher, K. (1994) *Examen de Afasia Multilingue (MAE-S)*. San Antonio, TX: Psychological Corporation.

Benton, A.L., Hamsher, K., Rey, G.J., and Sivan, A.B. (1994a) *Multilingual aphasia examination*, 3rd ed. San Antonio, TX: Psychological Corporation.

Benton, A.L., Hamsher, K., Varney, N.R., and Spreen, O. (1994b) *Contributions to neuropsychological assessment*, 2nd ed. New York: Oxford University Press.

Berndt, R.S. (1998) Sentence processing in aphasia. In: M.T. Sarno (Ed.), *Acquired aphasia*, 3rd ed. (pp. 229–268). San Diego: Academic Press.

Berndt, R.S., Basili, A., and Caranazzo, A. (1987) Dissociation of functions in a case of transcortical sensory aphasia. *Cognitive Neuropsychology*, 4, 79–107.

Berthier, M.L., Fernandez, A.M., Celdran, E.M., and Kulisevsky, J. (1996) Perceptual and acoustic correlates of affective prosody repetition in transcortical aphasia. *Aphasiology*, 10, 711–721.

Binetti, G., Magni, E., Cappa, S.F., Padovani, A., Bianchetti, A., and Trabucchi, M. (1995) Semantic memory in Alzheimer's disease: An analysis of category fluency. *Journal of Clinical and Experimental Neuropsychology*, 17, 82–89.

Bishop, D.V. and Byng, S. (1984) Assessing semantic comprehension: Methodological considerations and a new clinical test. *Cognitive Neuropsychology*, 1, 233–243.

Blakeley, R.W. (2000) *Screening Test for Developmental Apraxia of Speech*—2nd ed. Austin, TX: Pro-Ed.

Blank, M., Rose, S.A., and Berlin, L.J. (1978) *Preschool Language Assessment Instrument*. San Antonio, TX: Psychological Corporation.

Bliss, L.S. (1992) Review of Assessing Linguistic Behavior. *11th Mental Measurement Yearbook* (p. 40). Lincoln, NE: University of Nebraska Press.

Bliss, L.S. and Peterson, D.M. (1975) Performance of aphasic and nonaphasic children on a sentence repetition task. *Journal of Communication Disorders*, 8, 207–212.

Blomert, L. (1990) What functional assessment can contribute to setting goals for aphasia therapy. *Aphasiology*, 4, 307–320.

Blomert, L., Kean, M.L., Koster, C., and Schokker, J. (1994) Amsterdam-Nijmegen Everyday Language Test: Construction, reliability, and validity. *Aphasiology*, 8, 381–407.

Blomert, L., Koster, C., Van Mier, H., and Kean, M.L. (1987) Verbal communication abilities of aphasic patients: The everyday language test. *Aphasiology*, 1, 463–474.

Bloom, R.L. (1994) Hemispheric responsibility and discourse production: Contrasting patients with unilateral left and right hemisphere damage. In: R.L. Bloom, L.K. Obler, S. De Santi, and J.S. Ehrlich (Eds.), *Discourse analysis and applications. Studies in adult clinical populations* (pp. 81–94). Hillsdale, NJ: Lawrence Erlbaum.

Bloom, R.L., Borod, J., Obler, L., and Gerstman, L. (1993) Suppression and facilitation of pragmatic performance: Effects of emotional content on discourse following right and left brain damage. *Journal of Speech and Hearing Research*, 36, 1227–1235.

Blumstein, S. (1998) Phonological aspects of aphasia. In: M.T. Sarno (Ed.), *Acquired aphasia*, 3rd ed. (pp. 157–186). San Diego: Academic Press.

Boersma, F., van den Brink, W., Deeg, D.J.H., Eefsting, J.A., and van Tilburg, W. (1999) Survival in a population-based cohort of dementia patients: Predictors and causes of mortality. *International Journal of Geriatric Psychiatry*, 14, 748–753.

Boles, L. (1998) Conversational discourse analysis as a method for evaluating progress in aphasia: A case report. *Journal of Communication Disorders*, 31, 261–274.

Boller, F. and Dennis, M. (1979) *Auditory comprehension: Clinical and experimental studies with the Token Test.* New York: Academic Press.

Boller, F. and Vignolo, L.A. (1966) Latent sensory aphasia in hemisphere-damaged patients: An experimental study with the Token Test. *Brain*, 89, 815–830.

Boone, K.B., Lesser, I.M., Miller, B.L., Wohl, M., Berman, N., Lee, A., Palmer, B., and Back, C. (1995) Cognitive functioning in older depressed outpatients: Relationship of presence and severity of depression to neuropsychological test scores. *Neuropsychology*, 9, 390–398.

Boone, K.B., Ponton, M.O., Gorsuch, R.L., Gonzalez, J.J., and Miller, B.L. (1998) Factor analysis of four measures of prefrontal lobe functioning. *Archives of Clinical Neuropsychology*, 13, 585–595.

Borkowski, J.G., Benton, A.L., and Spreen, O. (1967) Word fluency and brain damage. *Neuropsychologia*, 5, 135–140.

Borod, J.C., Carper, M., Goodglass, H., and Naeser, M. (1984) Aphasic performance on a battery of constructional, visuo-spatial, and quantitative tasks: Factorial structure and CT scan localization. *Journal of Clinical Neuropsychology*, 6, 189–204.

Borod, J.C., Carper, M., Naeser, M., and Goodglass, H. (1985) Left-handed and right-handed aphasics with left hemisphere lesions compared on nonverbal performance measures. *Cortex*, 21, 81–90.

Borod, J.C., Fitzpatrick, P.M., Helm-Estabrooks, N., and Goodglass, H. (1989) The relationship between limb apraxia and the spontaneous use of communicative gestures in aphasia. *Brain and Cognition*, 10, 121–131.

Borod, J.C., Goodglass, H., and Kaplan, E. (1980) Normative data on the Boston Diagnostic Aphasia Examination, Parietal Lobe battery, and the Boston Naming Test. *Journal of Clinical Neuropsychology*, 2, 209–215.

Boyle, M., Coelho, C.A., and Kimbarow, M.L. (1991) Word fluency tasks: A preliminary analysis of variability. *Aphasiology*, 5, 171–182.

Bracken, B.A. and Murray, A.M. (1984) Stability and predictive validity of the PPVT-R over an eleven month interval. *Educational and Psychological Research*, 4, 41–44.

Branconnier, R.J. (1986) A computerized battery for behavioral assessment in Alzheimer's disease. In: L.W. Poon, T. Crook, K.L. Davis, C. Eisdorfer, B.J. Gurland, A.W. Kaszniak, and L.W. Thompson (Eds.), *Handbook for clinical memory assessment of older adults* (pp. 189–196). Washington, D.C.: American Psychological Association.

Brink, T.L., Yesavage, J.A., Owen, L., Heersama, P.H., Adey, M., and Rose, T.L. (1982) Screening tests for geriatric depression. *Clinical Gerontology*, 1, 37–43.

Brookshire, B.L., Chapman, S.B., Song, J., and Levin, H.S. (2000) Cognitive and linguistic correlates of children's discourse after closed head injury: A three-year follow-up. *Journal of the International Neuropsychological Society*, 6, 741–751.

Brookshire, R.H. (1973) *An introduction to aphasia*. Minneapolis, MN: BRK Publishers.

Brookshire, R.H. (1978) A Token Test battery for testing auditory comprehension in brain-injured adults. *Brain and Language*, 6, 149–157.

Brookshire, R.H. (1997) *Introduction to neurogenic communication disorders*, 5th ed. St. Louis: Mosby.

Brookshire, R.H. and Nicholas, L.E. (1984) Comprehension of directly and indirectly stated main ideas and details in discourse by brain-damaged and non-brain-damaged listeners. *Brain and Language*, 21, 21–36.

Brookshire, R.H. and Nicholas, L.E. (1997) *Discourse Comprehension Test: Test manual* (revised edition). Minneapolis, MN: BRK Publishers.

Brown, L., Sherbenou, R., and Johnson, S. (1998) *Test of Nonverbal Intelligence*, 3rd ed. Austin, TX: Pro-Ed.

Brown, S.J., Rourke, B.P., and Cicchetti, D.V. (1989) Reliability of tests and measures used in the neuropsychological assessment of children. *The Clinical Neuropsychologist*, 3, 353–368.

Brownell, H.H. (1988) The neuropsychology of narrative comprehension. *Aphasiology*, 2, 247–250.

Brownell, R. (2000a) *Receptive One-Word Picture Vocabulary Test—2000 edition*. Wilmington, DE: Wide Range.

Brownell, R. (2000b) *Expressive One-Word Picture Vocabulary Test—2000 edition*. Wilmington, DE: Wide Range.

Bryan, J., Luszcz, M.A., and Crawford, J.R. (1997) Verbal knowledge and speed of information processing as mediators of age differences in verbal fluency performance among older adults. *Psychology and Aging*, 12, 473–478.

Bryan, K.L. (1988) Assessment of language deficit after right hemisphere damage. *British Journal of Disorders of Communication*, 23, 111–125.

Bryan, K.L. (1989) *The Right Hemisphere Language Battery*. Kibworth, England: Far Communications.

Bryan, K.L. (1995) *Right Hemisphere Language Battery (2nd edition)*. London: Whurr Publishers.

Bryan, K.L. and Hale, J.B. (2001) Differential effects of left and right cerebral vascular accidents on language competency. *Journal of the International Neuropsychological Society*, 7, 655–664.

Bryan, K.L. and Luszcz, M.A. (2000) Measurement of executive function: Considerations for detecting adult age differences. *Journal of Clinical and Experimental Neuropsychology*, 22, 40–55.

Buffington, D.M., Krantz, P.J., McClannahan, L.E., and Poulson, C.L. (1998) Procedures for teaching appropriate gestural communication skills to children with autism. *Journal of Autism and Developmental Disorders*, 28, 535–545.

Buoyer McDermott, F., Horner, J., and DeLong, E.R. (1996) Evolution of acute aphasia as measured by the Western Aphasia Battery. *Clinical Aphasiology*, 24, 159–172.

Burns, M. (1997) *The Burns Brief Inventory of Communication and Cognition*. San Antonio, TX: Psychological Corporation.

Burns, M.S., Halper, A.S., and Mogil, S.I. (1985) *Clinical management of right hemisphere dysfunction*. Rockville, MD: Aspen.

Butters, N., Granholm, E., Salmon, D.P., Grant, I., and Wolfe, J. (1987) Episodic and semantic memory: A comparison of amnesic and demented patients. *Journal of Clinical and Experimental Neuropsychology*, 9, 479–497.

Butterworth, B., Howard, D., and McLoughlin, P. (1984) The semantic deficit in aphasia: The relationship between semantic errors in auditory comprehension and picture naming. *Neuropsychologia*, 22, 409–426.

Byrd, K.C. (1997) Comparison of language development of upper elementary and secondary students with unilateral hearing loss and with normal hearing. *Dissertation Abstracts International*, 58 (6-A), 2157.

Bzoch, K.R. and Leage, R. (1991) *Receptive-Expressive Emergent Language Test*, 2nd ed. Austin, TX: Pro-Ed.

Cacace, T. and McFarland, D.J. (1998) Central auditory processing disorders in school-age children: A critical review. *Journal of Speech, Language, and Hearing Research*, 41, 355–373.

Cahn, D.A., Salmon, D.P., Butters, N., Wiederholt, W.C., Corey-Bloom, J., Edelstein, S.L., and Barrett-Connor, E. (1995) Detection of dementia of the Alzheimer type in a population-based sample: Neuropsychological test performance. *Journal of the International Neuropsychological Society*, 1, 252–260.

Caldognetto, E.M. and Poggi, I. (1995) Creative iconic gestures: Some evidence from aphasia. In: R. Simone (Ed.), *Iconicity in language*. Amsterdam: John Benjamins Publishing.

Canadian Study of Health and Aging Working Group (1994) Canadian study of health and aging: Study methods and prevalence of dementia. *Canadian Medical Association Journal*, 150, 899–913.

Caplan, D. (1987) Discrimination of normal and aphasic subjects on a test of syntactic comprehension. *Neuropsychologia*, 25, 173–184.

Caplan, D. (1992) *Language: Structure, processing, and disorders*. Cambridge, MA: The MIT Press.

Carrow, E. (1972) Auditory comprehension of English by monolingual and bilingual preschool children. *Journal of Speech and Hearing Research*, 15, 407–412.

Carrow, E. (1973, 1998) *Test for Auditory Comprehension of Language (TACL)*. English/Spanish. 3rd ed. Boston: Teaching Research Corporation.

Carrow-Woolfolk, E. (1990) *CASL: Comprehensive Assessment of Spoken Language*. Circle Pines, MN: American Guidance Service.

Carrow-Woolfolk, E. (1996a) *Oral and Written Language Scales (OWLS)*. Circle Pines, MN: American Guidance Service.

Carrow-Woolfolk, E. (1996b) *Carrow Elicited Language Inventory (CELI)*. Circle Pines, MN: American Guidance Service.

Carrow-Woolfolk, E. (1988) *Theory, assessment and intervention in language disorders: An integrative approach*. Philadelphia: Grune & Stratton.

Carvajal, H., Gerber, J., and Smith, P.D. (1987) Relationship between scores of young adults on Stanford-Binet IV and Peabody Picture Vocabulary Test-Revised. *Perceptual and Motor Skills*, 65, 721–722.

Ceccaldi, M., Joanette, Y., Tikhomirof, F., and Macia, M. (1996) The effects of age-induced changes in communicative abilities on the type of aphasia. *Brain and Language*, 54, 75–85.

Chapey, R. (Ed.) (2001) *Language intervention strategies in aphasia and related neurogenic communication disorders*, 4th ed. Philadelphia: Lippincott Williams & Wilkins.

Chapman, R.S., Schwartz, S.E., and Kay-Raining-Bird, E. (1991) Language skills of children and adolescents with Down's syndrome: I. Comprehension. *Journal of Speech and Hearing Research*, 34, 1106–1120.

Chapman, S.B., Highley, A.P., and Thompson, J.L. (1998) Discourse in fluent aphasia and Alzheimer's disease: Linguistic and pragmatic considerations. *Journal of Neurolinguistics*, 11, 55–78.

Chenery, H.J., Murdoch, B.E., and Ingram, J.C.L. (1996) An investigation of confrontation naming performance in Alzheimer's dementia as a function of disease severity. *Aphasiology*, 10, 423–441.

Cherlow, D.G. and Serafetinides, E.A. (1976) Speech and memory assessment in psychomotor epileptics. *Cortex*, 12, 21–26.

Cherney, L.R. and Canter, G.J. (1993) Informational content in the discourse of patients with probable Alzheimer's disease and patients with right brain damage. *Clinical Aphasiology*, 21, 123–133.

Cherney, L.R. and Halper, A.S. (2000) Assessment and treatment of functional communication following right hemisphere damage. In: L.E. Worrall and C.M. Frattali (Eds.), *Neurogenic communication disorders: A functional approach* (pp. 276–292). New York: Thieme.

Cherry, R.S. (1980) *Selective Auditory Attention Test*. St. Louis: Auditec.

Cicerone, K.D., Dahlberg, C., Kalmar, K., Langenbahn, D.M., Malec, J.F., Bergquist, T.F., et al. (2000) Evidence-based cognitive rehabilitation: Recommendations for clinical practice. *Archives of Physical Medicine and Rehabilitation*, 81, 1596–1615.

Clark, C., Crockett, D.J., and Klonoff, H. (1979a) Factor analysis of the Porch Index of Communication Ability. *Brain and Language*, 7, 1–7.

Clark, C., Crockett, D.J., and Klonoff, H. (1979b) Empirically derived groups in the assessment of recovery from aphasia. *Brain and Language*, 7, 240–251.

Cohen, M.J. and Stanczak, D.E. (2000) On the reliability, validity, and cognitive structure of the Thurstone Word Fluency test. *Archives of Clinical Neuropsychology*, 15, 267–279.

Cohen, R., Gutbrod, K., Meier, E., and Romer, P. (1987) Visual search processes in the Token Test performance of aphasics. *Neuropsychologia*, 25, 983–987.

Cohen, R. et al. (1977a) Validity of the Sklar Aphasia Scale. *Journal of Speech and Hearing Research*, 20, 146–164.

Cohen, R., Kelter, S., and Shaefer, B. (1977b) Zum Einfluss des Sprachverständnisses auf die Leistungen im Token Test. *Zeitschrift für klinische Psychologie*, 6, 1–14.

Cohen, R., Lutzweiler, W., and Woll, G. (1980) Zur Konstruktvalidität des Token Tests. *Nervenarzt*, 51, 30–35.

Cohen, S.R., Hassan, S.A., Lapointe, B.J., and Mount, B.M. (1996) Quality of life in HIV disease as measured by the McGill Quality of Life Questionnaire. *AIDS*, 10, 1421–1427.

Cole, K.N., Dale, P.S., Mills, P.E., and Jenkins, J.R. (1993) Interaction between early intervention curricula and student characteristics. *Exceptional Children*, 60, 17–28.

Cole, K.N. and Fewell, R.R. (1983) A quick language screening test for young children: The Token Test. *Journal of Psychoeducational Assessment*, 1, 149–153.

Cornish, K.M. and Munir, F. (1998) Receptive and expressive language skills in children with cri-du-chat syndrome. *Journal of Communication Disorders*, 31, 73–81.

Correia, L., Brookshire, R.H., and Nicholas, L.E. (1990) Aphasic and non-brain-damaged adults' description of aphasia test pictures and gender-biased pictures. *Journal of Speech and Hearing Disorders*, 55, 713–720.

Cranberg, L.D., Filley, C.M., Edward, J.H., and Alexander, M.P. (1987) Acquired aphasia in childhood: Clinical and CT investigations. *Neurology*, 37, 1165–1172.

Crary, M.A. and Rothi, L.J. (1989) Predicting the Western Aphasia Battery Aphasia Quotient. *Journal of Speech and Hearing Disorders*, 54, 163–166.

Crary, M.A., Wertz, R.T., and Deal, J.L. (1992) Classifying aphasias: Cluster analysis of Western Aphasia Battery and Boston Diagnostic Aphasia Examination. *Aphasiology*, 6, 29–36.

Crewe, N.M. and Dijkers, M. (1995) Functional assessment. In: L.A. Cushman and M.J. Scherer (Eds.), *Psychological assessment in medical rehabilitation. Measurement and instrumentation in psychology.* Washington, D.C.: American Psychological Association.

Crocker, L. (1989) Review of the Sklar Aphasia Scale. In: J.C. Conoley and J.J. Kramer (Eds.), *The 10th mental measurements yearbook.* Lincoln, NE: Buros Institute.

Crockett, D.J. (1972) A multivariate comparison of Schuell's, Howes', Weisenberg and McBride's, and Wepman's types of aphasia. Unpublished doctoral dissertation. University of Victoria.

Crockett, D.J. (1974) Component analysis of within correlations of language-skill tests in normal children. *Journal of Special Education*, 8, 361–375.

Crockett, D.J. (1976) Multivariate comparison of Howes' and Weisenburg and McBride's models of aphasia on the Neurosensory Center Comprehensive Examination for Aphasia. *Perceptual and Motor Skills*, 43, 795–806.

Crockett, D.J. (1977) A comparison of empirically derived groups of aphasic patients on the Neurosensory Center Comprehensive Examination for Aphasia. *Journal of Clinical Psychology*, 33, 194–198.

Crockett, D.J., Spreen, O., and Vernon-Wilkinson, R. (2001) The factor analytic structure of the controlled oral association task. *Archives of Clinical Neuropsychology*, 16, 818–819 (abstract).

Crockford, C. and Lesser, R. (1994) Assessing functional communication in aphasia: Clinical utility and time demands of three methods. *European Journal of Disorders of Communication*, 29, 165–182.

Crofoot, M.J. and Bennett, T.S. (1980) A comparison of three screening tests and the WISC-R in special education evaluations. *Psychology in the Schools*, 17, 474–478.

Crossley, M., D'Arcy, C., and Rawson, N.S.B. (1997) Letter and category fluency in community-dwelling Canadian seniors: A comparison of normal participants to those with dementia of the Alzheimer or vascular type. *Journal of Clinical and Experimental Neuropsychology*, 19, 52–62.

Crosson, B. (1996) Assessment of subtle language deficits in neuropsychological batteries: Strategies and implications. In: R.J. Sbordonne and C.J. Long (Eds.), *Ecological validity of neuropsychological testing* (pp. 243–259). Delray Beach, FL: GR St. Lucie Press.

Crosson, B., Cooper, P.V., Lincoln, R.K., Bauer, R.M., and Velozo, C.A. (1993)

Relationship between verbal memory and language performance after blunt head injury. *The Clinical Neuropsychologist*, 7, 250–267.

Cruice, M.N., Worrall, L.E., and Hickson, L.M.H. (2000) Boston Naming Test results for healthy older Australians: A longitudinal and cross-sectional study. *Aphasiology*, 14, 143–155.

Culatta, B. and Young, C. (1992) Linguistic performance as a function of abstract task demands in children with spina bifida. *Developmental Medicine and Child Neurology*, 34, 434–440.

Culbert, J.P., Hamer, R., and Klinge, V. (1989) Factor structure of the Wechsler Intelligence Scale for Children-Revised, Peabody Picture Vocabulary Test, and the Peabody Individual Achievement Test in a psychiatric sample. *Psychology in the Schools*, 26, 331–336.

Cummings, J.L., Houlihan, J.P., and Hill, M.A. (1986) The pattern of reading deterioration in dementia of the Alzheimer type: Observations and implications. *Brain and Language*, 29, 315–323.

Cunningham, R., Farrow, V., Davies, C., and Lincoln, N. (1995) Reliability of the assessment of communicative effectiveness in severe aphasia. *European Journal of Disorders of Communication*, 30, 1–16.

Damasio, A.R. and Tranel, D. (1993) Nouns and verbs are retrieved with differently distributed neural systems. *Proceedings of the National Academy of Sciences of the USA*, 90, 4957–4960.

Damasio, H. (1991) Neuroanatomical correlates of the aphasias. In: M.T. Sarno (Ed.), *Acquired aphasia* (2nd ed.) (pp. 43–70). New York: Academic Press.

D'Amato, R.C., Gray, J.W., and Dean, R.S. (1987) Concurrent validity of the PPVT-R with the K-ABC for learning problem children. *Psychology in the Schools*, 24, 35–39.

Damico, J.S. (1985) Clinical Discourse Analysis: A functional approach to language assessment. In: C.S. Simon (Ed.), *Communication skills and classroom success* (pp. 165–203). London: Taylor & Francis.

Damico, J.S., Oelschlaeger, M., and Simmons-Mackie, N. (1999) Qualitative methods in aphasia research: Conversation analysis. *Aphasiology*, 13, 667–679.

D'Arcy, R.C.N. and Connolly, J.F. (1999) An event-related brain potential study of receptive speech comprehension using a modified Token Test. *Neuropsychologia*, 37, 1477–1489.

Darley, F.L. (Ed.) (1979) *Evaluation of appraisal techniques in speech and language pathology*. Reading, MA: Addison-Wesley.

Das, J.P., Kirby, J.R., and Jarman, R.F. (1979) *Simultaneous and successive cognitive processes*. New York: Academic Press.

Das, J.P., Mishra, R.K., Davison, M., and Naglieri, J.A. (1995) Measurement of dementia in individuals with mental retardation: Comparison based on PPVT and Dementia Rating Scale. *The Clinical Neuropsychologist*, 9, 32–37.

David, R.M. and Skilbeck, C.E. (1984) Raven IQ and language recovery following stroke. *Journal of Clinical Neuropsychology*, 6, 302–308.

Davidoff, M. and Katz, R. (1985) Automated telephone therapy for improving comprehension in aphasic adults. *Cognitive Rehabilitation*, 3, 26–28.

Davis, G.A. (1993) *A survey of adult aphasia and related language disorders*, 2nd ed. Englewood Cliffs, NJ: Prentice Hall.

Davis, L., Foldi, N.S., Gardner, H., and Zurif, E.B. (1978) Repetition in the transcortical aphasias. *Brain and Language*, 6, 226–238.

Dean, R.S. (1980) The use of the Peabody Picture Vocabulary Test with emotionally disturbed adolescents. *Journal of School Psychology*, 18, 172–175.

DeAvila, E.A. and Duncan, S.E. (1986) *Scoring and interpretation manual for the Language Assessment Scales*, 5th ed. San Rafael, CA: Linguametrics Group.

DeBettignies, B.H. and Mahurin, R.K. (1989) Assessment of independent living skills in geriatric populations. *Clinics in Geriatric Medicine*, 5, 461–475.

De Bleser, R., Denes, G.F., Luzzatti, C., and Mazzucchi, A. (1986) L'Aachener Aphasia Test (AAT): I. Problemi esoluzioni per una versione italiana del Test e per uno studio crosslinguistico dei disturbi afasici. *Archivio di Psicologia, Neurologia e Psichiatria*, 47, 209–237.

Dehaene, S., Dupoux, E., Mehler, J., Cohen, L., Paulesu, E., Perani, D., van de Mootele, P.F., Lehericy, S., and Bihan, D. (1997) Anatomical variability in the cortical representation of first and second language. *Neuroreport*, 8, 3809–3815.

Delis, D.C., Kaplan, E., and Kramer, J.H. (2001) *Delis-Kaplan Executive Function System*. San Antonio, TX: Psychological Corporation.

Denes, G., Semenza, C., and Calgognetto, E.M. (1999) Phonological disorders in aphasia. In: G. Denes and L. Pizzamiglio (Eds.), *Handbook of clinical and experimental neuropsychology*. Hove, East Sussex, UK: Psychology Press.

Dennis, M. and Barnes, M.A. (1990) Knowing the meaning, getting the point, bridging the gap, and carrying the message: Aspects of discourse following closed head injury in childhood and adolescence. *Brain and Language*, 39, 428–446.

Dennis, M., Purvis, K., Barnes, M.A., Wilkinson, M., and Winner, E. (2001) Understanding of literal truth, ironic criticism, and deceptive praise following childhood head injury. *Brain and Language*, 78, 1–16.

De Renzi, E. (1980) The Token Test and the Reporter's Test: A measure of verbal input and a measure of verbal output. In: M.T. Sarno and O. Hook (Eds.), *Aphasia: assessment and treatment*. Stockholm: Almqvist & Wiksell, New York: Masson.

De Renzi, E. and Faglioni, P. (1978) Development of a shortened version of the Token Test. *Cortex*, 14, 41–49.

De Renzi, E. and Ferrari, C. (1979) The Reporter's Test: A sensitive test to detect expressive disturbances in aphasics. *Cortex*, 15, 279–291.

De Renzi, E. and Vignolo, L.A. (1962) The Token Test: A sensitive test to detect receptive disturbances in aphasics. *Brain*, 85, 665–678.

Diamond, K.E. (1990) Effectiveness of the Revised Denver Developmental Screening Test in identifying children at risk for learning problems. *Journal of Educational Research*, 83, 152–157.

Diamond, K.E. and le Furgy, W.G. (1988) Screening for developmental handicaps: Outcomes from an early childhood screening program. *Physical and Occupational Therapy in Pediatrics*, 8, 43–59.

Dikmen, S.S., Heaton, R.K., Grant, I., and Temkin, N.R. (1999) Test-retest reliability and practice effects of expanded Halstead-Reitan neuropsychological test battery. *Journal of the International Neuropsychological Society*, 5, 346–356.

DiSimoni, F.G. (1978) *The Token Test for Children: Manual*. Bingham, MA: Teaching Resources Corporation.

DiSimoni, F.G. and Keith, R.L. (1983) "Tuning in" and "fading out": Performance of aphasic patients on ordered PICA subtests. *Journal of Communication Disorders*, 16, 31–40.

DiSimoni, F.G., Keith, R.L., and Darley, F.L. (1980) Prediction of PICA overall score by short versions of the test. *Journal of Speech and Hearing Research*, 23, 511–516.

DiSimoni, F.G., Keith, R.L., Holt, D.L., and Darley, F.L. (1975) Practicality of shortening the Porch Index of Communicative Ability. *Journal of Speech and Hearing Research*, 18, 491–497.

Divenyi, P.L. and Robinson, A.J. (1989) Nonlinguistic auditory capabilities in aphasia. *Brain and Language*, 37, 290–326.

Docking, K., Jordan, F.M., and Murdoch, B.E. (1999) Interpretation and comprehension of linguistic humour by adolescents with head injury: A case-by-case analysis. *Brain Injury*, 13, 953–972.

Docking, K., Murdoch, B.E., and Jordan, F.M. (2000) Interpretation and comprehension of linguistic humour by adolescents with head injury: A group analysis. *Brain Injury*, 14, 89–108.

Domitz, D.M. and Schow, R.L. (2000) The new CAPD Battery—Multiple Auditory Processing Assessment: Factor analysis and comparisons with SCAN. *American Journal of Audiology*, 9, 31–45.

Douglas, J., O'Flaherty, C., and Snow, P. (2000) Measuring perception of communicative ability: The development and evaluation of the La Trobe Communication Questionnaire. *Aphasiology*, 14, 251–268.

Ducarne de Ribaucourt, B., Foulgoc, V., Francois, F., and Thomas, D. (1982) Essai d'analyse de la communication non verbale dans 20 cas d'aphasie. *La Linguistique*, 18, 59–84.

Dunn, L.M. and Dunn, E.S. (1997) *Peabody Picture Vocabulary Test—III*. Circle Pines, MN: American Guidance Service.

Edwards, S., Garman, M., Hughes, A., Letts, C., and Sinka, I. (1999) Assessing the comprehension and production of language in young children: An account of the Reynolds Developmental Language Scales. *International Journal of Language and Communication Disorders*, 34, 151–171.

Ehrlich, J.S. (1994) Studies of discourse production in adults with Alzheimer's disease. In: R.L. Bloom, L.K. Obler, S. De Santi, and J.S. Ehrlich (Eds.), *Discourse analysis and applications. Studies in adult clinical populations* (pp. 149–160). Hillsdale, NJ: Lawrence Erlbaum.

Eisenson, J. (1954) *Examining for aphasia: A manual for the examination of aphasia and related disturbances*, 3rd ed., 1993. San Antonio, TX: Psychological Corporation.

Eisenson, J. (1972) *Aphasia in children*. New York: Harper.

Elias, M.F., Elias, P.K., D'Agostino, R.B., Silbershatz, H., and Wolf, P.A. (1997) Role of age, education, and gender on cognitive performance in the Framingham Heart Study: Community-based norms. *Experimental Aging Research*, 23, 201–235.

Eling, P. (Ed.) (1994) *Reader in the history of aphasia. From Gall to Geschwind.* Amsterdam: John Benjamins.

El-Khatib, L.M. (1997) The development of language in children prenatally exposed to drugs. *Dissertation Abstracts International*, 58 A, 0735.

Elliott, L., Hammer, M.A., and Scholl, M.E. (1990) Fine-grained auditory discrimination and performance on tests of receptive vocabulary and receptive language. *Annals of Dyslexia*, 40, 170–179.

Emerick, L. L. (1971). *The Appraisal of Language Disturbance*. Marquette, MI: Northern Michigan University

Emerson, M.F., Crandall, K.K., Seikel, J.A., and Cermak, G.D. (1997) Observations on the use of SCAN to identify children at risk for auditory processing disorder. *Language, Speech, and Hearing Services in the Schools*, 28, 43–49.

Emery, O.B. (1986) Linguistic decrement in normal aging. *Language and Communication*, 6, 47–64.

Emery, B. and Breslau, L.D. (1988) The problem of naming in SDAT: A relative deficit. *Experimental Aging Research*, 14, 181–193.

Emery, B. and Breslau, L.D. (1989) Language deficit in depression: Comparison with SDAT and normal aging. *Journal of Gerontology*, 44, M85–M92.

Enderby, P. (1983) *Frenchay Dysarthria Assessment*. Austin, TX: Pro-Ed.

Enderby, P. and Crow, E. (1996) Frenchay Aphasia Screening Test: Validity and comparability. *Disability and Rehabilitation*, 18, 238–240.

Enderby, P. and John, A. (1999) Therapy outcome measures in speech and language therapy: Comparing performance between different providers. *International Journal of Communication Disorders*, 34, 417–429.

Enderby, P., Wood, V., and Wade, D. (1987a) *Frenchay Aphasia Screening Test*. Windsor, England: NFER-Nelson.

Enderby, P.M, Wood, V.A., Wade, D.T., and Hewer, R.L. (1987b) The Frenchay Aphasia Screening Test: A short, simple test for aphasia appropriate for non-specialists. *International Rehabilitation Medicine*, 8, 166–170.

Engle, R.W., Conway, A.R.A., Tuholski, S.W., and Shisler, R.J. (1995) A resource account of inhibition. *Psychological Science*, 6, 122–125.

Epker, M.O., Lacritz, L.H., and Cullum, C.M. (1999) Comparative analysis of qualitative verbal fluency performance in normal elderly and demented populations. *Journal of Clinical and Experimental Neuropsychology*, 21, 425–434.

Epstein, A.G. (1982) Mastery of language measured by means of a sentence span test. Unpublished manuscript, Lyngby, Denmark.

Ernst, J. (1988) Language, grip strength, sensory-perceptual, and receptive skills in a normal elderly sample. *The Clinical Neuropsychologist*, 2, 30–40.

Eslinger, P.J., Damasio, A.R., Benton, A.L., and Van Allen, M. (1985) Neuropsychologic detection of abnormal mental decline in older persons. *Journal of the American Medical Association*, 253, 670–674.

Evesham, M. (1977) Teaching language skills to children with language disorders. *British Journal of Disorders of Communication*, 12, 23–29.

Ewing-Cobbs, L., Levin, H.S., Eisenberg, H.M., and Fletcher, J.M. (1987) Language functions following closed-head injury in children and adolescents. *Journal of Clinical and Experimental Neuropsychology*, 9, 575–592.

Fagundes, D.D., Haynes, W.O., Haak, N.J., and Moran, M.J. (1998) Task variability on the language test performance of Southern lower socioeconomic class African American and Caucasian five-year-olds. *Language, Speech, and Hearing Services in Schools*, 3, 148–157.

Farver, P.F. and Farver, T.B. (1982) Performance of normal older adults on tests designed to measure parietal lobe function (constructional apraxia, Gerstmann's syndrome, visuospatial organization). *American Journal of Occupational Therapy*, 36, 444–449.

Faust, D.S. and Hollingsworth, J.O. (1991) Concurrent validation of the Wechsler Preschool and Primary Scale of Intelligence-Revised (WPPSI-R) with two criteria of cognitive abilities. *Journal of Psychoeducational Assessment*, 9, 224–229.

Feeney, J. and Bernthal, J. (1996) The efficiency of the Revised Denver Developmental Screening Test as a language screening tool. *Language, Speech, and Hearing Services in the Schools*, 27, 330–332.

Ferguson, A. and Armstrong, E. (1996) The PALPA: A valid investigation of language? *Aphasiology*, 10, 194–197.

Ferman, T.J., Ivnik, R.J., and Lucas, J.A. (1998) Boston Naming Test discontinuation rule: Rigorous versus lenient interpretation. *Assessment*, 5, 13–18.

Ferraro, F.R. and Bercier, B. (1996) Boston Naming Test performance in a sample of Native American elderly adults. *Clinical Gerontologist*, 17, 58–60.

Ferraro, F.R., Bercier, B., and Chelminski, I. (1997) Geriatric Depression Scale—Short Form in Native American elderly adults. *Clinical Gerontologist*, 18, 52–55.

Ferro, J.M. and Kertesz, A. (1987) Comparative classification of aphasic disorders. *Journal of Clinical and Experimental Neuropsychology*, 9, 365–375.

Feyereisen, P., Barter, D., Goossens, M., and Clerebaut, N. (1988) Gestures and speech in referential communication by aphasic subjects: Channel use and efficiency. *Aphasiology*, 2, 21–32.

Fillenbaum, G.G., Huber, M., and Taussig, I.M. (1997) Performance of elderly White and African American community residents on the abbreviated CERAD Boston Naming Test. *Journal of Clinical and Experimental Neuropsychology*, 19, 204–210.

Fillenbaum, G.G., Peterson, B., Welsh-Bohmer, K.S., Kukull, W.A., and Heyman, A. (1998) Progression of Alzheimer's disease in black and white patients: The CERAD experience, Part XVI. *Neurology*, 51, 154–158.

Fink, R.B. and Schwartz, M.F. (2000) Moss Rehab Aphasia Center: A collaborative model for long-term rehabilitation. *Topics in Stroke Rehabilitation*, 7, 32–43.

Fischer, M.A. (1998) Review of Joliet 3-Minute Speech and Language Screen. *The 13th Mental Measurement Yearbook* (pp. 564–565). Lincoln, NE: Buros Institute.

Fisher, J.P. and Glenister, J.M. (1992) *The Hundred Pictures Naming Test*. Victoria, Australia: Australian Council for Educational Research.

Fisher, N.J., Tierney, M.C., Snow, W.G., and Szalai, J.P. (1999) Odd/even short forms of the Boston Naming Test: Preliminary geriatric norms. *The Clinical Neuropsychologist*, 13, 359–364.

Fitch, J.L. (1985) *Computer Managed Screening Test*. Communication Skill Builders.

Flanagan, J.L. and Jackson, S.T. (1997) Test-retest reliability of three aphasia tests: Performance on non-brain-damaged older adults. *Journal of Communication Disorders*, 30, 33–42.

Flavell, J.H. (1987) *The development of role taking and communication skills in children*. New York: Krieger Press.

Florance, C.L. (1981) Methods of communication analysis used in family interaction therapy. In: R.H. Brookshire (Ed.), *Clinical aphasiology: Conference proceedings* (pp. 204–211). Minneapolis, MN: BRK Publishers.

Fluharty, N.B. (2000) *Fluharty Preschool Speech and Language Screening Test*, 2nd ed. Austin, TX: Pro-Ed.

Folstein, M.F., Folstein, S.E., and McHugh, P.R. (1975) Mini-Mental State: A practical method for grading the cognitive state of patients for the clinician. *Journal of Psychiatry Research*, 12, 189–198.

Fontanari, J.L. (1989) O' Token Test: Elegancia e concisao na avaliacao de compreensao do afasico: Validatione da versao reduzida de De Renzi para o portugues. *Neurobiologia*, 52, 177–218.

Forns-Santacana, M. and Gomez-Benito, J. (1990) Factor structure of the McCarthy scales. *Psychology in the Schools*, 27, 111–115.

Foster, R., Giddon, J., and Stark, J. (1983) *Assessment of children's language comprehension* (1983 rev.). Palo Alto, CA: Consulting Psychologists Press.

Franenburg, W.K. and Dodds, J.B. (1990) *Denver Developmental Screening Test*, 2nd ed. Denver, CO: Denver Developmental Materials.

Frank, E.M. and Barrineau, S. (1996) Current speech-language assessment protocols for adults with traumatic brain injury. *Journal of Medical Speech Language Pathology*, 4, 81–101.

Franklin, S., Howard, D., and Patterson, K. (1994) Abstract word meaning deafness. *Cognitive Neuropsychology*, 11, 1–34.

Frattali, C.M. (1992) Functional assessment of communication: Merging public policy with clinical views. *Aphasiology*, 6, 63–83.

Frattali, C.M. (1993) Perspectives on functional assessment: Its use for policy making. *Disability and Rehabilitation*, 15, 1–9.

Frattali, C.M. (Ed.) (1998) *Measuring outcomes in speech-language pathology*. New York: Thieme.

Frattali, C.M. and Lynch, C. (1989) Functional assessment: Current issues and future challenges. *American Speech and Hearing Association*, 31, 70–74.

Frattali, C.M., Thompson, C.K., Holland, A., Wohl, C.B., and Ferketic, M.M. (1995) *Functional Assessment of Communication Skills for Adults*. Administra-

tion and scoring manual. Rockville, MD: American Speech-Language-Hearing Association.

Freedman, L., Snow, W.G., and Millikin, C. (1995) Anomia in Alzheimer's disease. *Journal of the International Neuropsychological Society*, 1, 386 (abstract).

Fressola, D.R., Cipponeri, S., Hoerchler, J.S., McDannold, S.B., Meyer, J., and McCarney, S.B. (1990) *Speech and Language Evaluation Scale*. Columbia, MO: Hawthorne Educational Services.

Friedland, D. and Miller, N. (1998) Conversation analysis of communication breakdown after closed head injury. *Brain Injury*, 12, 1–14.

Froeschels, E., Dittrich, O., and Wilhelm, I. (1932) *Psychological elements in speech* (E. Ferre, transl.). Boston: Expression.

Fromm, D., Greenhouse, J.B., Holland, A.L., and Swindell, C.S. (1986) An application of exploratory statistical methods to language pathology: Analysis of the Western Aphasia Battery's cortical quotient in acute stroke patients. *Journal of Speech and Hearing Research*, 29, 135–142.

Fromm, D. and Holland, A.L. (1989) Functional communication in Alzheimer's disease. *Journal of Speech and Hearing Disorders*, 54, 535–540.

Gaddes, W.H. and Crockett, D.J. (1975) The Spreen-Benton aphasia tests: Normative data as a measure of normal language development. *Brain and Language*, 2, 257–280.

Gallaher, A.J. (1979) Temporal reliability of aphasic performance on the Token Test. *Brain and Language*, 7, 34–41.

Ganguli, M., Ratcliff, G., Huff, F.J., Belle, S., Kancel, M.J., Fischer, L., Seaberg, E.C., and Kuller, L.H. (1991) Effects of age, gender, and education on cognitive tests in a rural elderly community sample: Norms from the Monongahela Valley independent elderly survey. *Neuroepidemiology*, 10, 42–52.

Ganguli, M., Seaburg, E.C., Ratcliff, G.G., Belle, S.H., and DeKosky, S.T. (1996) Cognitive stability over 2 years in a rural elderly population: The MoVIES project. *Neuroepidemiology*, 15, 42–50.

Garcia, L.J. and Joanette, I. (1994) Conversational topic-shifting analysis in dementia. In: R.L. Bloom, L.K. Obler, S. De Santi, and J.S. Ehrlich (Eds.), *Discourse analysis and applications. Studies in adult clinical populations* (pp. 161–184). Hillsdale, NJ: Lawrence Erlbaum.

Garcia-Albea, J.E., Sanchez-Bernardos, M.L., and del Viso-Pabon, S. (1986) Test de Boston parael diagnostico de la afasia: Adaptacion Espagnola. In: H. Goodglass and E. Kaplan (Eds.), *La Evolacion de la Afasio y de Transtornos Relacionados*, 2nd ed. (Translated by Carlos Wernicke). Madrid: Editorial Medical Panamericana.

Gardner, H., Zurif, E., Berry, T., and Baker, E. (1976) Visual communication in aphasia. *Neuropsychologia*, 14, 275–292.

Gardner, M.F. (1998) *Test of Auditory Perceptual Skills—Revised*. Novato, CA: Academic Therapy Publications.

Gass, C.S. and Russell, A.W. (1986) Minnesota Multiphasic Personality Inventory correlates of lateralized cerebral lesions and aphasic deficits. *Journal of Consulting and Clinical Psychology*, 54, 359–363.

Gentry, B., Hayes, B.T., Dancer, J., and Davis, P. (1997) Language and motor skills of preschool children with sickle-cell disease. *Perceptual and Motor Skills*, 84, 486.

Gerber, S. and Gurland, G.B. (1989) Applied pragmatics in the assessment of aphasia. *Seminars in Speech and Language*, 10, 263–281.

Gernsbacher, M.A. (Ed.) (1994) *Handbook of psycholinguistics*. San Diego: Academic Press.

Gerstmann, J. (1930) Zur Symptomatologie der Hirnläsionen im Übergangsgebiet der unteren Parietal- und mittleren Okzipitalwindung. *Nervenarzt*, 3, 691–695.

Geschwind, N. (1971) Current concepts: Aphasia. *New England Journal of Medicine*, 284, 654–656.

Geschwind, N. and Kaplan, E. (1962) A human cerebral disconnection syndrome. *Neurology*, 12, 675–685.

Gibson, L., MacLennan, W.J., Gray, C., and Pentland, B. (1991) Evaluation of a comprehensive assessment battery for stroke patients. *International Journal of Rehabilitation Research*, 14, 93–100.

Gillon, G. and Dodd, B.J. (1994) A prospective study of the relationship between phonological, semantic and syntactic skills and specific reading disability. *Reading and Writing*, 6, 321–345.

Giovannetti, T., Lamar, M., Cloud, B.S., Swenson, R., et al. (2001) Different underlying mechanisms for deficits in concept formation in dementia. *Archives of Clinical Neuropsychology*, 16, 547–560.

Giovannetti-Carew, T., Lamar, M., Cloud, B.S., Grossman, M., and Libon, D.J. (1997) Impairment in category fluency in ischemic vascular dementia. *Neuropsychology*, 11, 400–412.

Glosser, G. and Deser, T. (1990) Patterns of discourse production among neurological patients with fluent language disorders. *Brain and Language*, 40, 67–88.

Glosser, G. and Donofrio, N. (2001). Differences between nouns and verbs after anterior temporal lobectomy. *Neuropsychology*, 15, 39–47.

Glosser, G., Wiley, M.J., and Barnoski, E.J. (1998) Gestural communication in Alzheimer's disease. *Journal of Clinical and Experimental Neuropsychology*, 20, 1–13.

Golden, C., Hammeke, T., and Purish, A. (1980) *Manual for the Luria-Nebraska Neuropsychological Battery*. Los Angeles: Western Psychological Services.

Goldin-Meadow, S. (1999) The role of gesture in communication and thinking. *Trends in Cognitive Sciences*, 3, 419–429.

Goldstein, B.C., Harris, K.C., and Klein, M.D. (1993) Assessment of oral story telling abilities in Latino junior high school students with learning handicaps. *Journal of Learning Disabilities*, 26, 138–143.

Goldstein, D.S. and Pliskin, N.H. (2002) The influence of demographics and dementia on Boston Naming Test errors. *The Clinical Neuropsychologist* (In press).

Goldstein, F.C., Levin, H.S., Roberts, V.J., et al. (1996) Neuropsychological effects of closed head injury in older adults: A comparison with Alzheimer's disease. *Neuropsychology*, 10, 147–154.

Goldstein, G. and Shelly, C. (1984) Relationship between language skills as assessed by the Halstead-Reitan battery and the Luria-Nebraska language-related factor scales in a non-aphasic patient population. *Journal of Clinical Neuropsychology*, 6, 143–156.

Gonzales-Rothi, L.J. and Heilman, K.M. (1984) Acquisition and retention of gestures by aphasic patients. *Brain and Cognition*, 3, 426–437.

Goodglass, H., Kaplan, E., and Barresi, B. (2000) *Boston Diagnostic Aphasia Examination*, 3rd ed. Philadelphia: Lippincott Williams & Wilkins.

Goodglass, H. and Blumstein, S. (1973) *Psycholinguistics and aphasia*. Baltimore: Johns Hopkins Press.

Goodglass, H. and Kaplan, E. (1972) *The assessment of aphasia and related disorders*. Malvern, PA: Lea & Febiger.

Goodglass, H. and Kaplan, E. (1983) *The assessment of aphasia and related disorders*. 2nd ed. Malvern, PA: Lea & Febiger.

Goodglass, H. and Kaplan, E. (1986) *La evaluacion de la afasia y de transfornos relacionados*, 2nd ed. Madrid: Editorial Medical Panamericana.

Goodglass, H. and Kaplan, E. (2000) *Boston Naming Test*. Philadelphia: Lippincott Williams and Wilkins.

Goodglass, H., Kaplan, E., and Weintraub, S. (1983) *Boston Diagnostic Aphasia Examination*. Philadelphia: Lea & Febiger.

Goodglass, H. and Wingfield, A. (1995) The changing relationship between anatomic and cognitive explanation in the neuropsychology of language. *Journal of Psycholinguistic Research*, 27, 147–165.

Goodglass, H., Wingfield, A., Hyde, M.R., Gleason, J.B., Bowles, N.L., and Gallagher, R.E. (1997) The importance of word-initial phonology: Error patterns in prolonged naming efforts by aphasic patients. *Journal of the International Neuropsychological Society*, 3, 128–138.

Goodglass, H., Wingfield, A., and Ward (1999) Decision latencies for phonological and semantic information in object identification. *Brain and Language*, 66, 294–305.

Gordon, W.A., Hibbard, M.R., Egelko, S., Diller, L., et al., (1984) Evaluation of the deficits associated with right brain damage: Normative data on the Institute of Rehabilitation Test Battery. New York: New York University Medical Center.

Gorelick, P.B., Brody, J., Cohen, D., and Freels, S. (1993) Risk factors for dementia associated with multiple cerebral infarcts: A case-control analysis in predominantly African-American hospital-based patients. *Archives of Neurology*, 50, 714–720.

Goren, A.R., Tucker, G., and Ginsberg, G.M. (1996) Language dysfunction in schizophrenia. *European Journal of Disorders of Communication*, 31, 153–170.

Goulet, P., Ska, B., and Kahn, H.J. (1994) Is there a decline in picture naming with advancing age? *Journal of Speech and Hearing Research*, 37, 629–644.

Gourovitch, M.L., Kirkby, B.S., Goldberg, T.E., Weinberger, D.R., et al. (2000) A comparison of rCBF patterns during letter and semantic fluency. *Neuropsychology*, 14, 353–360.

Graetz, P., De Bleser, R., and Willmes, K. (1992) *Akense Afasie Test.* Lisse, Netherlands: Swets & Zeitlinger.

Gray, S.A. (1996) The effects of the caregiving environment on the development of canonical babbling and phonology in prenatally crack cocaine/polydrug-exposed infants and toddlers. *Dissertation Abstracts International,* B., 56, 5449.

Grayson, E., Hilton, R., and Franklin, S. (1997) Early intervention in a case of jargon aphasia: Efficacy of language comprehension therapy. *European Journal of Disorders of Communication,* 32, 257–276.

Greer, S., Bauchner, H., and Zuckerman, B. (1989) The Denver Developmental Screening Test: How good is its predictive validity? *Developmental Medicine and Child Neurology,* 31, 774–781.

Gregory, R.J. (2000) *Psychological testing: History, principles, and applications* (3rd edition). Boston: Allyn & Bacon.

Grice, H.P. (1975) Logic in conversation. In: P. Cole and P. Morgan (Eds.), *Studies in syntax and semantics, Volume 3* (pp. 41–58). New York: Academic Press.

Grieve, R. and Campbell, R. (1999) Ancient and medieval experiments on child language: A comment on Bonvillian, Garber and Dell. *First Language,* 19, 91–98.

Grosjean, F. and Hirt, C. (1996) Using prosody to predict the end of sentences in English and French: Normal and brain-damaged subjects. *Language and Cognitive Processes,* 11, 107–134.

Gruen, A.K., Frankle, B.C., and Schwartz, R. (1990) Word fluency generation skills of head-injured patients in an acute trauma center. *Journal of Communication Disorders,* 23, 163–170.

Gunther, I.A. (1981) Uma tentativa de adaptacao do Indice Porch de Habilitade Communicativa para Criancas, para uso no Brasil. *Archivos Brasilieiros de Psicologia,* 33, 71–86.

Guruje, O., Unverzagt, F.W., Osuntokun, B.O., Hendrie, H.C., Baiyewu, O., Ogunniyi, A., and Hali, K.S. (1995) The CERAD neuropsychological test battery: Norms from a Yoruba-speaking Nigerian sample. *West African Journal of Medicine,* 14, 29–33.

Gutbrod, K., Mager, B., Meier, E., and Cohen, R. (1985) Cognitive processing of tokens and their description in aphasia. *Brain and Language,* 25, 37–51.

Gutbrod, K. and Michel, M. (1986) Zur klinischen Validität des Token Tests bei hirngeschädigten Kindern mit und ohne Aphasia. *Diagnostica,* 32, 118–128.

Hachisuka, K., Okazaki, T., and Ogata, H. (1997) Self-rating Barthel index compatible with the original Barthel Index and the Functional Independence Measure motor score. *Japanese Journal of Rehabilitaion Medicine,* 19, 107–121.

Hagen, C. (1981) Language disorders secondary to closed head injury: Diagnosis and treatment. *Topics in Language Disorders,* 5, 73–87.

Hagtvet, K.A. and Hagtvet, B.E. (1990) The discriminant predictive validity of the Reynell Developmental Language Scales. *Scandinavian Journal of Educational Research,* 34, 77–88.

Haley, S.M., Coster, W.J., Ludlow, L.H., Haltiwanger, J.T., and Andrellos, P.J. (1992) *Pediatric Evaluation of Disability Inventory (PEDI)*. Boston: New England Medical Center Hospitals.

Hall, P.K. (1995) Review of Speech and Language Evaluation Scale. In: J.C. Conoley and J.C. Impara (Eds.), *The 12th Mental Measurement Yearbook*. Lincoln, NE: University of Nebraska Press.

Hall, P.K. and Jordan, L.S. (1985) The Token and Reporter's Tests using two scoring conventions: A normative study with 286 grade and junior high students. *Language, Speech, and Hearing Services in Schools*, 16, 227–243.

Hall, P.K. and Jordan, L.S. (1988) An attempt to revise scoring conventions for the Token and Reporter's Tests. *Language, Speech, and Hearing Services in Schools*, 19, 227–234.

Hall, P.K., Jordan, L.S., and Robin, D.A. (1993) *Developmental apraxia of speech: Theory and clinical practice*. Austin, TX: Pro-Ed.

Halper, A.S., Cherney, L.R., and Burns, M.S. (1996) *Clinical management of right hemisphere dysfunction (2nd edition)*. Gaithersburg, MD: Aspen Publishers.

Halper, A.S., Cherney, L.R., and Miller, T.K. (1991) *Clinical management of communication problems in adults with traumatic brain injury*. Gaithersburg, MD: Aspen Publishers.

Hamberger, M.J. and Seidel, W.T. (2001) Subjective word finding complaints: Unexpected relationships with visual naming and semantic fluency. *Archives of Clinical Neuropsychology*, 16, 860 (abstract).

Hamilton, B.B., Granger, C.V., Sherwin, F.S., et al. (1987) A uniform national data system for medical rehabilitation. In: M.J. Fuhrer (Ed.), *Rehabilitation outcome: Analysis and measurement* (pp. 137–147). Baltimore: Paul H. Brooks.

Hamilton, M. (1960) A rating scale for depression. *Journal of Neurology, Neurosurgery, and Psychiatry*, 12, 189–198.

Hammill, D.D. and Larsen, S.C. (1996) *TOWL-3: Test of Written Language*, 3rd ed. Circle Pines, MN: American Guidance Service.

Hammill, D.D., Mather, N., and Roberts, R. (2002) *Illinois Test of Psycholinguistic Abilities—3 (IPTA-3)*. Los Angeles: Western Psychological Services.

Hammill, D.D., Pearson, N.A., and Wiederholt, J.L. (1996) *C-TONI: Test of Nonverbal Intelligence—Computer version*. Wilmington, DE: Wide Range.

Hamsher, K. (1980) *Percentile rank norms for children on the NCCEA*. Milwaukee: University of Wisconsin Medical School, Department of Neurology.

Handleman, J.S., Harris, S.L., Kristoff, B., and Fuentes, F. (1991) A specialized program for preschool children with autism. *Language, Speech, and Hearing Services in Schools*, 22, 107–110.

Hanson, W.R. and Riege, W.H. (1982) Factor-derived categories of chronic aphasia. *Brain and Language*, 15, 369–380.

Haravon, A., Obler, L.K., and Sarno, M.T. (1994) A method for microanalysis of discourse in brain-damaged patients. In: R.L. Bloom, L.K. Obler, S. De Santi, and J.S. Ehrlich (Eds.), *Discourse analysis and applications. Studies in adult clinical populations* (pp. 47–80). Hillsdale, NJ: Lawrence Erlbaum.

Harris, S.L., Handleman, J.S., Gordon, R., and Kristoff, B. (1991) Changes in cognitive and language functioning in preschool children with autism. *Journal of Autism and Developmental Disorders*, 21, 281–290.

Harris, S.R. and Langkamp, D.L. (1994) Predictive value of the Bayley Mental Scale in the early detection of cognitive delay in high-risk infants. *Journal of Perinatology*, 14, 275–279.

Hartley, L.L. and Jensen, P.J. (1992) Three discourse profiles of closed-head-injury speakers: Theoretical and clinical implications. *Brain Injury*, 6, 271–282.

Haveman, A.P. (1994) On prosody in Broca's aphasia. *Gothenburg Papers in Theoretical Linguistics*, 72, 95–104.

Hawkins, K.A., Sledge, W.H., Orleans, J.F., Quinland, D.M., Rakfeldt, J., and Hoffman, R.E. (1993) Normative implications of the relationship between reading vocabulary and Boston Naming Test performance. *Archives of Clinical Neuropsychology*, 8, 525–537.

Haynes, S.D. and Bennett, T.L. (1990) Cognitive impairment in adults with complex partial seizures. *International Journal of Clinical Neuropsychology*, 12, 74–81.

Head, H. (1926) *Aphasia and kindred disorders of speech*. New York: Macmillan.

Heaton, R.K., Avitable, N., Grant, I., and Matthews, C.G. (1999) Further cross validation of regression-based neuropsychological norms with an update for the Boston Naming Test. *Journal of Clinical and Experimental Neuropsychology*, 21, 571–582.

Heaton, R.K., Grant, I., and Matthews, C.G. (1991) *Comprehensive norms for an expanded Halstead-Reitan Battery: Demographic corrections, research findings, and clinical applications*. Odessa, FL: Psychological Assessment Resources.

Hecaen, H., DeAgostini, M., and Monzon-Montes, A. (1981) Cerebral organization in lefthanders. *Brain and Language*, 12, 261–284.

Heilman, K.M., Bowers, D., Speedie, L., and Coslett, H.B. (1984) Comprehension of affective and non-affective prosody. *Neurology*, 34, 917–921.

Helm-Estabrooks, N. (1992a) *Aphasia Diagnostic Profiles*. Chicago: Riverside Publishing.

Helm-Estabrooks, N. (1992b) *Test of Oral and Limb Apraxia*. Chicago: Riverside Publishing.

Helm-Estabrooks, N. and Hotz, G. (1990) *Brief Test of Head Injury*. San Antonio, TX: Special Press.

Helm-Estabrooks, N. and Ramsberger, G. (1986) Treatment of agrammatism in long-term Broca's aphasia. *British Journal of Disorders of Communication*, 21, 39–45.

Helm-Estabrooks, N., Ramsberger, G., Moyan, A.L., and Nicholas, M. (1989) *Boston Assessment of Severe Aphasia*. Chicago: Riverside Publishing.

Henderson, L.W., Frank, E.M., Pigatt, T., Abramson, R.K., and Houston, M. (1998) Race, gender, and educational effects on the Boston Naming Test scores. *Aphasiology*, 12, 901–911.

Henderson, V.W., Mack, W., Freed, D.M., Kemper, D., and Andersen, E.S. (1990) Naming consistency in Alzheimer's disease. *Brain and Language*, 39, 530–538.

Hermann, B.P., Seidenberg, M., Haltiner, A., and Wyler, A.R. (1992) Adequacy of language function and verbal memory performance in unilateral temporal lobe epilepsy. *Cortex*, 28, 423–433.

Hermann, B.P. and Wyler, A.R. (1988) Effects of anterior temporal lobectomy on language function. *Annals of Neurology*, 23, 585–588.

Herrmann, M., Britz, A., Bartels, C., and Wallesch, C.W. (1995) The impact of aphasia on the patient and family in the first year poststroke. *Topics in Stroke Rehabilitation*, 2, 5–19.

Herrmann, M. and Wallesch, C-W. (1989) Psychosocial changes and psychosocial adjustment with chronic and severe nonfluent aphasia. *Aphasiology*, 3, 513–526.

Hershberger, P. (1996) The relationship of medical and family characteristics to language development skills of low birthweight children at three years of age. *Infant and Toddler Intervention*, 6, 75–85.

Hestad, K., Dybing, E., Haugen, P.K., and Klove, H. (1998) Sprakforstyrrelser hos demente pasienter undersokt med Boston Naming Test. *Tidsskrift for Norsk Psykologforening*, 35, 322–327.

Hill, C.D., Stoudemire, A., Morris, R., Martino-Saltzman, D., Markwalter, H.R., and Lewison, B.J. (1992) Dysnomia in the differential diagnosis of major depression, depression-related cognitive dysfunction, and dementia. *Journal of Neuropsychiatry and Clinical Neuroscience*, 4, 64–69.

Hilton, L.M. and Mumma, K. (1991) Screening rural and suburban children with the Preschool Language Scale. *Journal of Communication Disorders*, 24, 111–122.

Hinchliffe, F.J., Murdoch, B.E., Chenery, H.J., Baglioni Jr., A.J., and Harding-Clark, J. (1998) Cognitive-linguistic subgroups in closed-head injury. *Brain Injury*, 12, 369–398.

Hinton, G.G. and Knights, R.M. (1971) Children with learning problems. Academic history, academic prediction, and adjustment three years after assessment. *Exceptional Children*, 37, 513–519.

Hodson, B. (1986) *The Assessment of Phonological Processes—Revised* (APP-R). Austin, TX: Pro-Ed.

Holland, A. (1980) *Communicative Abilities in Daily Living: Manual*. Austin, TX: Pro-Ed.

Holland, A.L. (1982) Observing functional communication of aphasic adults. *Journal of Speech and Hearing Disorders*, 47, 50–56.

Holland, A.L., Boller, F., and Bourgeois, M. (1986) Repetition in Alzheimer's disease: A longitudinal study. *Journal of Neurolinguistics*, 2, 163–177.

Holland, A., Frattali, C., and Fromm, D. (1998) *Communication Abilities in Daily Living*, 2nd ed. (CADL-2). Austin, TX: Pro-Ed.

Holland, A. and Sonderman, J.C. (1974) Effects of a program based on the Token Test for teaching comprehension skills to aphasics. *Journal of Speech and Hearing Research*, 17, 589–598.

Holland, A.L. and Thompson, C.K. (1998) Outcome measurement in aphasia. In:

C.M. Frattali (Ed.), *Measuring outcomes in speech-language pathology* (pp. 245–266). New York: Thieme.

Hollinger, C.L. and Sarvis, P.A. (1984) Interpretation of the PPVT-R: A pure measure of verbal comprehension? *Psychology in the Schools*, 21, 34–41.

Horner, J., Dawson, D.V., Eller, M.A., Buoyer, F.G., Crowder, J.L., and Reus, C.M. (1995) Prognosis for improvement during acute rehabilitation as measured by the Western Aphasia Battery. *Clinical Aphasiology*, 23, 141–154.

Horner, J., Dawson, D.V., Heyman, A., and McGorman-Fish, A. (1992) The usefulness of the Western Aphasia Battery for differential diagnosis of Alzheimer dementia and focal stroke syndromes: Preliminary evidence. *Brain and Language*, 42, 77–88.

Hough, M.S. and Pierce, R.S. (1994) Pragmatics and treatment. In: R. Chapey (Ed.), *Language intervention strategies in adult aphasia (3rd edition)* (pp. 246–268). Baltimore: Williams & Wilkins.

Houghton, P.M., Pettit, J.M., and Towey, M.P. (1982) Measuring communication competence in global aphasia. In: R.H. Brookshire (Ed.), *Clinical aphasiology: Conference proceedings* (pp. 28–39). Minneapolis, MN: BRK Publishers.

Howard, M.R. and Hulit, L.M. (1992) Response patterns to central auditory tests and the Clinical Evaluation of Language Fundamentals-Revised: A pilot study. *Perceptual and Motor Skills*, 74, 120–122.

Howes, D. (1964) Application of the word-frequency concept to aphasia. In: A.V.S. de Rueck and M. O'Connor (Eds.), *Disorders of language*. Boston: Little, Brown.

Howes, D. (1966) A word count of spoken English. *Journal of Verbal Learning and Verbal Behavior*, 5, 572–606.

Howes, D. (1967) Some experimental investigations of language in aphasia. In: K. Salzinger and S. Salzinger (Eds.), *Research in verbal behavior and some neuropsychological implications*. New York: Academic Press.

Howes, D. and Geschwind, N. (1964) Quantitative studies of aphasic language. In: D.M.K. Rioch and E.A. Weinstein (Eds.), *Disorders of communication*. Baltimore: Williams & Wilkins.

Hresko, W.P., Reid, D.K., and Hammill, D.D. (1999) *Test of Early Language Development—Third Edition (TELD-3)*. Austin, TX: Pro-Ed.

Hua, M.S., Chang, S.H., and Chen, S.T. (1997) Factor structure and age effects with an aphasia test battery in normal Taiwanese adults. *Neuropsychology*, 11, 156–162.

Huber, W., Poeck, K., Weniger, D., and Willmes, K. (1983) *Der Aachener Aphasie-Test (AAT)*. Goettingen: Hogrefe.

Huber, W., Poeck, K., and Willmes, K. (1984) The Aachen Aphasia Test. In: F.C. Rose (Ed.), *Advances of Neurology, 42: Progress in Aphasiology*, 291–303.

Huff, F.J., Collins, C., Corkin, S., and Rosen, T.J. (1986) Equivalent forms of the Boston Naming Test. *Journal of Clinical and Experimental Neuropsychology*, 8, 556–562.

Hughlings Jackson, J. (1915) On the physiology of language. *Medical Times and Gazette*, 2, 275 (Reprinted in *Brain*, 1968, 38, 59–64).

Huntley, R.A. and Helfer, K.S. (Eds.) (1995) *Communication in later life*. Boston: Butterworth-Heinemann.

Inglis, J. and Lawson, J.S. (1981) Sex differences in the effects of unilateral brain damage on intelligence. *Science*, 212, 693–695.

Isaacs, B. and Kennie, A.T. (1973) The Set Test as an aid to the detection of dementia in old people. *British Journal of Psychiatry*, 123, 467–470.

Isaki, E. and Plante, E. (1997) Short-term and working memory differences in language/learning disabled and normal adults. *Journal of Communication Disorders*, 30, 427–437.

Iverson, G.L., Franzen, M.D., and Lovell, M.R. (1999) Normative comparisons for the Controlled Oral Word Association test following acute traumatic brain injury. *The Clinical Neuropsychologist*, 13, 437–441.

Ivnik, R., Malec, J.F., Smith, G.E., Tangelos, E.G., and Petersen, R.C. (1996) Neuropsychological tests' norms above age 55: COWAT, BNT, MAE Token, WRAT-R Reading, AMNART, Stroop, TMT, and JLO. *The Clinical Neuropsychologist*, 10, 262–278.

Jackson, S.T. and Tompkins, C.A. (1991) Supplemental aphasia tests: Frequency of use and psychometric properties. *Clinical Aphasiology*, 20, 91–99.

Jacobs, D.M., Sano, M., Dooneief, G., Marder, K., Bell, K.L., and Stern, Y. (1995) Neuropsychological detection and characterization of preclinical Alzheimer's disease. *Neurology*, 45, 957–962.

James, D., Van Steenbrugge, W., and Chiveralls, K. (1994) Underlying deficits in language-disordered children with central auditory processing difficulties. *Applied Psycholinguistics*, 15, 311–328.

Joanette, Y. and Goulet, P. (1990) Narrative discourse in right-brain-damaged right-handers. In: Y. Joanette and H.H. Brownell (Eds.), *Discourse ability and brain damage: Theoretical and empirical perspectives* (pp. 131–153). New York: Springer-Verlag.

Joanisse, M.F. and Seidenberg, M.S. (1998) Specific language impairment: A deficit in grammar or processing? *Trends in Cognitive Sciences*, 2, 240–247.

Johnson, C.J., Taback, N., Escobar, M., Wilson, B., and Beitchman, J.H. (1999) Local norming of the Test of Adolescent and Adult Language in the Ottawa Speech and Language Study. *Journal of Speech, Language, and Hearing Research*, 42, 761–766.

Johnson, F. and Stansfield, J. (1997) Expressive pragmatic skills in pre-school children with and without Down's syndrome. *Journal of Intellectual Disability Research*, 41, 19–29.

Jones, R.D. and Benton, A.L. (1995) Use of the Multilingual Aphasia Examination in the detection of language disorders. *Journal of the International Neuropsychological Society*, 1, 364 (abstract).

Jones-Gotman, M. and Milner, B. (1977) Design fluency: The invention of nonsense drawings after focal cortical lesions. *Neuropsychologia*, 15, 653–674.

Jordan, F.M. and Ashton, R. (1996) Language performance of severely closed head injured children. *Brain Injury*, 10, 91–97.

Jordan, F.M., Cremona-Meteyard, S., and King, A. (1996) High-level linguistic disturbances subsequent to childhood closed head injury. *Brain Injury*, 10, 729–738.

Jordan, F.M., Ozanne, A.E., and Murdoch, B.E. (1988) Long-term speech and language disorders subsequent to closed head injury in children. *Brain Injury*, 2, 179–185.

Jordan, F.M. and Murdoch, B.E. (1990) Linguistic status following closed head injury in children: A follow-up study. *Brain Injury*, 4, 147–154.

Jordan, F.M. and Murdoch, B.E. (1994) Severe closed-head injury in childhood: Linguistic outcomes into adulthood. *Brain Injury*, 8, 501–508.

Jordan, F., Ward, K., and Cremona-Meteyard, S. (1997) Word-finding in the conversational discourse of children with closed head injury. *Aphasiology*, 11, 877–888.

Joynt, R.J. (1964) Paul Pierre Broca: His contribution to the knowledge of aphasia. *Cortex*, 1, 206–213.

Juncos-Rabadan, O. (1994) The assessment of bilingualism in normal aging with the Bilingual Aphasia Test. *Journal of Neurolinguistics*, 8, 67–73.

Juncos-Rabadan, O. and Iglesias, F.J. (1994) Decline in the elderly language: Evidence from cross-linguistic data. *Journal of Neurolinguistics*, 8, 183–190.

Jurado, M.A., Mataro, M., Verger, K., Bartumeus, F., and Junque, C. (2000) Phonemic and semantic fluencies in traumatic brain injury patients with focal frontal lesions. *Brain Injury*, 14, 789–795.

Kacker, S.K., Pandit, R., and Dua, D. (1991) Reliability and validity studies of examination for aphasia test in Hindi. *Indian Journal of Disability and Rehabilitation*, 5, 13–19.

Kamphaus, R.W. and Lozano, R. (1984) Developing local norms for individually administered tests. *School Psychology Review*, 13, 491–498.

Kaplan, E. (1988) A process approach to neuropsychological assessment. In: T. Boll and B.K. Bryant (Eds.), *Clinical neuropsychology and brain function: Research, measurement, and practice* (pp. 125–167). Washington, D.C.: American Psychological Association.

Kaplan, E.F. and Goodglass (1983) *The Boston Naming Test*, 2nd ed. Philadelphia: Lippincott Williams & Wilkins.

Kaplan, E.F., Goodglass, H., and Weintraub, S. (1978) *The Boston Naming Test*. Experimental ed. Philadelphia: Lea & Febiger.

Karbe, H., Kertesz, A., and Polk, M. (1993) Profiles of language impairment in primary progressive aphasia. *Archives of Neurology*, 50, 193–201.

Karbe, H., Kessler, J., Herholz, K., Fink, G.R., and Heiss, W.D. (1995) Long-term prognosis of post-stroke aphasia studied with positron emission tomography. *Archives of Neurology*, 52, 186–190.

Kasher, A., Batori, G., Soroker, N., Graves, D., and Zaidel, E. (1999) Effects of right and left hemisphere damage on understanding conversational implicatures. *Brain and Language*, 68, 566–590.

Katsuki-Nakamura, J., Brookshire, R.H., and Nicholas, L.E. (1988) Comprehension of monologues and dialogues by aphasic listeners. *Journal of Speech and Hearing Disorders*, 53, 408–415.

Katz, S., Ford, A.B., Moskowitz, R.W., Jackson, B.A., and Jaffee, M.W. (1963) Studies of illness in the aged. The index of ADL: A standardized measure of biological and psychosocial functioning. *Journal of the American Medical Association*, 185, 94–108.

Kaufman, A.S. and Kaufman, N. (1993) *Kaufman Survey of Early Academic and Language Skills* (K-SEALS). Odessa, FL: Psychological Assessment Resources.

Kaufman, A.S. and Kaufman, N. (1995) *Kaufman Assessment Battery for Children*. Los Angeles: Western Psychological Services.

Kay, J., Lesser, R., and Coltheart, M. (1996) Psycholinguistic assessments of language processing in aphasia (PALPA): An introduction. *Aphasiology*, 10, 159–180.

Kay, J., Lesser, R., and Coltheart, R.M. (1992) *Psycholinguistic Assessment of Language Performance in Aphasia*. Hove, East Sussex, UK: Lawrence Erlbaum.

Kazniak, A.W., Bayles, K.A., Tomoeda, C.K., and Slauson, T. (1988) Assessing linguistic communicative functioning in Alzheimer's dementia: A theoretically motivated approach. *Journal of Clinical and Experimental Neuropsychology*, 10, 53 (abstract).

Kearns, K.P. (2000) Single-subject experimental designs in aphasia. In: S.E. Nadeau, L.J. Gonzales Rothi, and B. Crosson (Eds.), *Aphasia and language. Theory and practice*. New York: Guilford Press.

Keenan, J.S. and Brassell, E.G. (1975) *Aphasia Language Performance Scales* (Spanish version). Murfreesboro, TN: Pinnacle Press.

Keith, R.W. (1994) *SCAN-A: A screening test for auditory processing disorders*. San Antonio, TX: Psychological Corporation.

Keith, R.W. (1999) *SCAN-C Test for Auditory Processing Disorders in Children-Revised*. San Antonio, TX: Psychological Corporation.

Kempen, J.H., Krichevsky, M., and Feldman, S.T. (1994) Effect of visual impairment on neuropsychological test performance. *Journal of Clinical and Experimental Neuropsychology*, 16, 223–231.

Kempler, D., Teng, E.L., Dick, M., Taussig, I.M., and Davis, D.S. (1998) The effects of age, education, and ethnicity on verbal fluency. *Journal of the International Neuropsychological Society*, 4, 531–538.

Kenin, M. and Swisher, L.P. (1972) A study of patterns of recovery in aphasia. *Cortex*, 8, 56–68.

Kerschensteiner, M., Poeck, K., and Brunner, E. (1972) The fluency-nonfluency dimension in the classification of aphasic speech. *Cortex*, 8, 233–247.

Kertesz, A. (1979) *Aphasia and associated disorders: Taxonomy, localization, and recovery*. New York: Grune & Stratton.

Kertesz, A. (1981) Evolution of aphasia syndromes. *Topics in Language Disorders*, 1, 15–27.

Kertesz, A. (1982) *Western Aphasia Battery*. New York: Grune & Stratton.

Kertesz, A. (1988) Is there a need for standardized aphasia tests? Why, how, what and when to test aphasics. *Aphasiology*, 2, 313–318.

Kertesz, A. (1994) Neuropsychological evaluation of language. *Journal of Clinical Neurophysiology*, 11, 205–215.

Kertesz, A. and Hooper, P. (1982) Praxis and language: The extent and variety of apraxia in aphasia. *Neuropsychologia*, 20, 275–286.

Kertesz, A. and McCabe, P. (1975) Intelligence and aphasia: Performance of aphasics on Raven's Coloured Progressive Matrices (RCPM). *Brain and Language*, 2, 387–395.

Kertesz, A. and Phipps, J. (1980) The numerical taxonomy of acute and chronic aphasic syndromes. *Psychological Research*, 41, 179–198.

Kertesz, A. and Poole, E. (1974) The aphasia quotient: The taxonomic approach to measurement of aphasic disability. *Canadian Journal of Neurological Science*, 1, 7–16.

Kiernan, J. (1986) Visual presentation of the Revised Token Test: Some normative data and use in modality independence testing. *Folia Phoniatrica*, 38, 25–30.

Killgore, W.D.S. and Adams, R.L. (1999) Prediction of Boston Naming Test performance from vocabulary scores: Preliminary guidelines for interpretation. *Perceptual and Motor Skills*, 89, 327–337.

Kim, H. and Na, D.L. (1999) Normative data on a Korean version of the Boston Naming Test. *Journal of Clinical and Experimental Neuropsychology*, 21, 127–133.

King, D.A., Caine, E.D., Conwell, Y., and Cox, C. (1991) Predicting severity of depression in the elderly at six-months follow-up: A neuropsychological study. *Journal of Neuropsychiatry and Clinical Neuroscience*, 3, 64–66.

Kinzler, M.C. (1993) *Joliet 3-Minute Preschool Speech and Language Screen*. San Antonio, TX: Psychological Corporation.

Kinzler, M.C. and Johnson, C.C. (1993) *Joliet 3-Minute Speech and Language Screen* (Revised). San Antonio, TX: Psychological Corporation.

Kirk, A. and Kertesz, A. (1994) Cortical and subcortical aphasias compared to clinicoanatomical correlation or unifying features of language. *Aphasiology*, 8, 65–82.

Kirk, S.A., McCarthy, J., and Kirk, W. (1968) *The Illinois Test of Psycholinguistic Abilities* (rev. ed.) Urbana: Illinois University Press.

Kirshner, H.S. (1982) Language disorders in dementia. In: F. Freeman and H.S. Kirshner (Eds.), *Neurolinguistics. Vol. 12. Neurology of aphasia*. Amsterdam: Swets & Zeitlinger.

Kirshner, H.S. (1986) *Behavioral neurology: A practical approach*. New York: Churchill Livingstone.

Kirshner, H.S. (1995) Introduction to aphasia. In: H.S. Kirshner (Ed.), *Handbook of neurological speech and language disorders* (pp. 1–21). New York: Marcel Dekker.

Kitchens, H. (1995) Review of Examining For Aphasia, 3rd ed. In: J.C. Conoley and J.C. Impara (Eds.), *The 12th mental measurement yearbook*. Lincoln, NE: University of Nebraska Press.

Knesevich, J.W., LaBarge, E., and Edwards, D. (1986) Predictive value of the Boston

Naming Test in mild senile dementia of the Alzheimer type. *Psychiatry Research*, 19, 155–161.

Knopman, D.S., Selnes, O.A., Niccum, N., and Rubens, A. (1984) Recovery of naming in aphasia: Relationship to fluency, comprehension, and CT findings. *Neurology*, 34, 1461–1470.

Kohn, S.E., Smith, K.L., and Arsenault, J.K. (1990) The remediation of conduction aphasia via sentence repetition: A case study. *British Journal of Communication Disorders*, 25, 45–60.

Kohnert, K.J., Hernandez, A.E., and Bates, E. (1998) Bilingual performance on the Boston Naming Test: Preliminary norms in Spanish and English. *Brain and Language*, 65, 422–440.

Korkman, M., Barron-Linnankoski, S., and Lahti-Nuuttila, P. (1999) Effects of age and duration of reading instruction on the development of phonological awareness. *Developmental Neuropsychology*, 16, 415–431.

Korkman, M. and Haekkinen-Rihu, P. (1994) A new classification of developmental language disorders (DLD). *Brain and Language*, 47, 96–116.

Korkman, M., Kirk, U., and Kemp, S. (1997) *NEPSY: A developmental neuropsychological assessment.* San Antonio, TX: Psychological Corporation.

Korkman, M., Liikanen, A., and Fellman, V. (1996) Neuropsychological consequences of very low birthweight and asphyxia at term: Follow-up until school age. *Journal of Clinical and Experimental Neuropsychology*, 18, 220–233.

Kostrin, R.K. and Schwartz, M.F. (1986) Reconstructing from a degraded trace: A study of sentence repetition in agrammatism. *Brain and Language*, 28, 328–345.

Kreutzer, J.S., Gordon, W.A., Rosenthal, M., and Marwitz, J. (1993) Neuropsychological characteristics of patients with brain injury: Preliminary findings from a multicenter investigation. *Journal of Head Trauma Rehabilitation*, 8, 47–59.

Kronfol, Z., Hamsher, K., Digre, K., and Waziri, R. (1978) Depression and hemispheric function changes associated with unilateral ECT. *British Journal of Psychiatry*, 132, 560–567.

Krug, R.S. (1971) Antecedent probabilities, cost efficiency, and differential prediction of patients with cerebral organic conditions or psychiatric disturbances by means of a short test for aphasia. *Journal of Clinical Psychology*, 27, 468–471.

Krull, K.R., Scott, J.G., and Scherer, M. (1995) Estimation of premorbid intelligence from combined performance and demographic variables. *The Clinical Neuropsychologist*, 9, 83–88.

Kunik, M.E., Champagne, L., Harper, R.G., and Chacko, R.C. (1994) Cognitive functioning in elderly depressed patients with and without psychosis. *International Journal of Geriatric Psychiatry*, 9, 871–874.

Kusunoki, T. (1985) A study on scaling of Standard Language Test of Aphasia (SLTA): A practical scale based on a three-factor structure. *Japanese Journal of Behaviormetrics*, 12 (23), 8–12.

Kutas, M. and Hillyard, S.A. (1980) Reading senseless sentences: Brain potentials reflect semantic incongruity. *Science*, 207, 203–205.

Kynette, D. and Kemper, S. (1986) Aging and the loss of grammatical forms: A cross-sectional study of language performance. *Language and Communication*, 6, 65–72.

LaBarge, E., Balota, D.A., Storandt, M., and Smith, D. (1992b) An analysis of confrontation naming errors in senile dementia of the Alzheimer type. *Neuropsychology*, 6, 77–95.

LaBarge, E., Edwards, D., and Knesevich, J.W. (1986) Performance of normal elderly on the Boston Naming Test. *Brain and Language*, 27, 380–384.

LaBarge, E., Smith, D.S., Dick, L., and Storandt, M. (1992a) Agraphia in dementia of the Alzheimer type. *Archives of Neurology*, 49, 1151–1156.

Laine, M., Koivuselkä-Sallinen, P., Hänninen, R., and Niemi, J. (1993) *Bostonin Nimentätestin Suomenkielinen Versio*. Helsinki: Psykologien Kustannus.

Landre, N.A. and Taylor, M.A. (1995) Formal thought disorder in schizophrenia: Linguistic, attentional, and intellectual correlates. *Journal of Nervous and Mental Disease*, 183, 673–680.

Landre, N.A., Taylor, M.A., and Kearns, K.P. (1992) Language functioning in schizophrenic and aphasic patients. *Neuropsychiatry, Neuropsychology, and Behavioral Neurology*, 5, 7–14.

Lansing, A.E., Ivnick, R.J., Cullum, C.M., and Randolph, C. (1999) An empirically derived short form of the Boston Naming Test. *Archives of Clinical Neuropsychology*, 14, 481–487.

LaPointe, L.L. and Horner, J. (1979) *Reading Comprehension Battery for Aphasia*. Tegoid, OR: C.C. Publications.

LaPointe, L.L. and Horner, J. (1999) *Reading Comprehension Battery for Aphasia–2*. Austin, TX: Pro-Ed.

Larkins, B.M., Worrall, L.E., and Hickson, L.M.H. (2000) Functional communication in cognitive communication disorders following traumatic brain injury. In: L.E. Worrall and C.M. Frattali (Eds.), *Neurogenic communication disorders: A functional approach* (pp. 206–219). New York: Thieme.

La Rue, A., Swan, G.E., and Carmelli, D. (1995) Cognition and depression in a cohort of aging men: Results from the Western Collaborative Group Study. *Psychology and Aging*, 10, 30–33.

Lawriw, I. (1976) A test of the predictive validity and a cross-validation of the Neurosensory Center Comprehensive Examination for Aphasia. Unpublished Master's thesis, University of Victoria.

Lecours, A.R., Mehler, J., Parente, M.S., Aguiar, L.R., da Silva, A.B., Caetano, M., Camarotti, H., Castro, M.J., Dehaut, F., and Dumais, C. (1987) Illiteracy and brain damage. 2: Manifestations of unilateral neglect in testing "auditory comprehension" with iconographic material. *Brain and Cognition*, 6, 243–265.

Lecours, A.R., Mehler, J., Parente, M.A., and Beltrami, M.C. (1988) Illiteracy and brain damage. III: A contribution to the study of speech and language disorders in illiterates with unilateral brain damage. *Neuropsychologia*, 26, 575–589.

Le Dorze, G. and Bedard, C. (1998) Effects of age and education on the lexico-semantic content of connected speech in adults. *Journal of Communication Disorders*, 31, 53–71.

Le Dorze, G., Croteau, C., Brassard, C., and Michallet, B. (1999) Research considerations guiding interventions for families affected by aphasia. *Aphasiology*, 13, 922–927.

Le Dorze, G. and Durocher, J. (1992) The effects of age, education, and stimulus length on naming in normal subjects. *Journal of Speech and Language Pathology and Audiology*, 16, 21–29.

Le Dorze, G., Julien, M., Brassard, C., Durocher, J., and Boivin, G. (1994) An analysis of the communication of adult residents of a long-term care hospital as perceived by their caregivers. *European Journal of Disorders of Communication*, 29, 241–267.

Lee, G.P. and Hamsher, K. (1988) Neuropsychological findings in toxicometabolic confusional states. *Journal of Clinical and Experimental Neuropsychology*, 10, 769–778.

Lee, L.L. (1970) A screening test for syntax development. *Journal of Speech and Hearing Disorders*, 35, 103–112.

Lees, J. (1999) From 'which pig is not outside the field?' to 'which horse is not outside the field?': Commentary on the Reynell Developmental Language Scales III (RDLS III). *International Journal of Language and Communication Disorders*, 34, 174–180.

Lees, J., Cass, H., Waring, M., Burch, V., and Neville, B.G.R. (1998) Monitoring response to pharmacological treatment in children with acquired epileptic aphasias (Landau-Kleffner syndrome). *Developmental Medicine and Child Neurology*, 39, Suppl. 77, 9.

Leikin, M. and Aharon-Peretz, J. (1998) An aspect of auditory word and sentence comprehension in Alzheimer's disease. *Journal of Medical Speech-Language Pathology*, 6, 115–122.

Lendrem, W. and Lincoln, N.B. (1985) Spontaneous recovery of language in patients with aphasia between 4 and 34 weeks after stroke. *Journal of Neurology, Neurosurgery, and Psychiatry*, 48, 743–748.

Lendrem, W. and McGuirk, E. (1988) Factors affecting language recovery in aphasic stroke patient receiving speech therapy. *Journal of Neurology, Neurosurgery, and Psychiatry*, 51, 1103–1104.

Lenneberg, E.H. (1967) *Biological foundation of language*. New York: Wiley.

Leonard, L.B. (1997) *Children with specific language impairment*. Cambridge, MA: MIT Press.

Lesser, R. (1976) Verbal and non-verbal memory components in the Token Test. *Neuropsychologia*, 14, 79–85.

Lesser, R., Bryan, K., Anderson, J., and Hilton, R. (1986) Involving relatives in aphasia: An application of language enrichment therapy. *International Journal of Rehabilitation Research*, 9, 259–267.

Levin, H., Grossman, R.G., and Kelly, P.J. (1976) Aphasic disorders in patients with closed head injury. *Journal of Neurology, Neurosurgery, and Psychiatry*, 39, 1062–1070.

Levin, H., Grossman, R.G., Sarwar, M., and Meyers, C.A. (1981) Linguistic recovery after closed head injury. *Brain and Language*, 12, 360–374.

Lezak, M.D. (1995) *Neuropsychological assessment*, 3rd ed. New York: Oxford University Press.

Lezak, M.D., Whitham, R., and Bourdette, D. (1990) Emotional impact of cognitive insufficiencies in multiple sclerosis (MS). *Journal of Clinical and Experimental Neuropsychology*, 12, 50 (abstract).

Li, E.C. and Williams, S.E. (1990) Repetition deficits in three aphasic syndromes. *Journal of Communication Disorders*, 23, 77–88.

Lichtenberg, P.A. (Ed.) (1999) *Handbook of assessment in clinical gerontology*. New York: Wiley.

Lichtenberg, P.A., Ross, T., and Christensen, B. (1994) Preliminary normative data on the Boston Naming Test for an older urban population. *The Clinical Neuropsychologist*, 8, 109–111.

Lincoln, N.B. and McGuirk, E. (1986) Prediction of language recovery in aphasic stroke victims using the Porch Index of Communicative Ability. *British Journal of Disorders of Communication*, 21, 83–88.

Lincoln, N.B. and Pickersgill, M.J. (1981) Is the Porch Index of Communicative Abilities an equal interval scale? *British Journal of Disorders of Communication*, 16, 185–191.

Lincoln, R.K., Crosson, B., Bauer, R.M., Cooper, P.V., and Velozo, C.A. (1994) Relationship between WAIS-R subtests and language measures after blunt head injury. *The Clinical Neuropsychologist*, 8, 140–152.

Lindamood, C. and Lindamood, P. (1998) *Lindamood Auditory Conceptualization Test* (LAC). Odessa, FL: Psychological Assessment Resources.

Lindman, K.K. (1996) Gender differences in dementia of the Alzheimer's type: Evidence for differential semantic memory degradation. Paper presented at the Meeting of the International Neuropsychological Society, Chicago.

Linebaugh, C.W., Kryzer, K.M., Oden, S.E., and Myers, P.S. (1982) Reapportionment of communicative burden in aphasia. In: R.H. Brookshire (Ed.), *Clinical aphasiology: Conference proceedings*. Minneapolis, MN: BRK Publishers.

Lipowski, Z.J. (1980) *Delirium: Acute brain failure in man*. Springfield, IL: CC Thomas.

Lippke, B.A., Dickey, S.E., Selmar, J.W., and Soder, A.L. (1997) *Photo Articulation Test*, 3rd ed. Austin, TX: Pro-Ed.

Livingston, R.B., Gray, R.M., and Haak, R.A. (1999) Internal consistency of three tests from the Halstead-Reitan Neuropsychological Battery for Older Children. *Assessment*, 6, 93–100.

Loewenstein, D.A., Rubert, M.P., Berkowitz-Zimmer, N., Guterman, A., Morgan, R., and Hayden, S. (1992) Neuropsychological test performance and prediction of functional capacities in dementia. *Behavior, Health, and Aging*, 2, 149–158.

Lomas, J., Pickard, L., Bester, S., Elbard, H., Finlayson, A., and Zochaib, C. (1989) The Communicative Effectiveness Index. *Journal of Speech and Hearing Disorders*, 54, 113–124.

Ludlow, C.L. (1977) Recovery from aphasia: A foundation for treatment. In: M. Sullivan and M.S. Kommers (Eds.), *Rationale for adult aphasia therapy*. Omaha: University of Nebraska Medical Center.

Luick, A.H., Agranowitz, A., Kirk, S.A., and Busby, R. (1982) Profiles of children with severe oral language disorders. *Journal of Speech and Hearing Disorders*, 47, 88–92.

Luotonen, M., Uhari, M., Aitola, L., Lukkaroinen, A.M., Luotonen, J., Uhari, M., and Korkeamaki, R.L. (1996) Recurrent otitis media during infancy and linguistic skills at the age of nine years. *Pediatric Infectious Diseases Journal*, 15, 854–858.

Luria, A.R. (1966) *Higher cortical functions in man*. New York: Basic Books.

Luzzatti, C. (1999) Language disorders in dementia. In: G. Denes and L. Pizzamiglio (Eds.), *Handbook of clinical and experimental neuropsychology* (pp. 809–846). Hove, England: Psychology Press/Erlbaum.

Luzzatti, C., Willmes, K., and de Bleser, R. (1992) *Aachener Aphasie Test: Versione Italiana*. Firenze: Organizazzioni Speciali.

Lyon, J.G. and Helm-Estabrooks, N. (1987) Drawing: Its communicative significance for expressively restricted aphasic adults. *Topics in Language Disorders*, 8, 61–71.

Lyytinen, P., Lari, N., Lausvaara, A., and Poikkeus, A.M. (1994) Assessment of early lexical and communicative development. *Psykologia*, 29, 244–252.

Lyytinen, P., Poikkeus, A.M., and Laakso, M.L. (1997) Language and symbolic play in toddlers. *International Journal of Behavioral Development*, 21, 289–302.

Mack, W.J., Freed, D.M., Williams, B.W., and Henderson, V.W. (1992) Boston Naming Test: Shortened version for use in Alzheimer's disease. *Journal of Gerontology*, 47, 164–158.

Mackenzie, C., Begg, T., Brady, M., and Lees, K.R. (1997) The effects on verbal communication skills of right hemisphere stroke patients. *Aphasiology*, 11, 929–945.

Macleod, A.D. and Whitehead, L.E. (1997) Dysgraphia and terminal delirium. *Palliative Medicine*, 11, 127–132.

Manly, J.J., Miller, S.W., Heaton, R.K., Byrd, D., Reilly, J., Velasquez, R.J., Saccuzzo, D.P., and Grant, I. (1998) The effect of African-American acculturation on neuropsychological test performance in normal and HIV-positive individuals. *Journal of the International Neuropsychological Society*, 4, 291–302.

Mann, L., Ramsberger, G., and Helm-Estabrooks, N. (1994) A linguistic communication measure for aphasic narratives. *Aphasiology*, 8, 343–359.

Manochiopinig, S., Sheard, C., and Reed, V.A. (1992) Pragmatic assessment in adult aphasia: A clinical review. *Aphasiology*, 6, 519–533.

Margolin, D.I., Pate, D.S., Friedrich, F.J., and Elia, E. (1990) Dysnomia in dementia and in stroke patients: Different underlying cognitive deficits. *Journal of Clinical and Experimental Neuropsychology*, 12, 597–612.

Marie, P. (1883) De l'aphasie, cecite verbal, surdite verbale, aphasie motire, agraphie. *Revue Medicale*, 3, 693–703.

Marien, P., Engelborghs, S., Fabbro, F., and De Deyn, P.P. (2001) The lateralized linguistic cerebellum: A review and a new hypothesis. *Brain and Language*, 79, 580–600.

Marien, P., Mampaey, E., Vervaet, A., Saerens, J., and De Deyn, P.P. (1998) Normative data for the Boston Naming Test in native Dutch-speaking Belgian elderly. *Brain and Language*, 65, 447–467.

Marinac, J.V. and Ozanne, A.E. (1999) Comprehension strategies: The bridge between literal discourse and discourse understanding. *Child Language Teaching and Therapy*, 15, 233–246.

Mark, V.W. and Thomas, B.E. (1992) Factors associated with improvement in global aphasia. *Aphasiology*, 6, 121–134.

Marquardt, T.P., Stoll, J., and Sussman, H. (1988) Disorders of communication in acquired cerebral trauma. *Journal of Learning Disabilities*, 21, 340–351.

Marshall, J. (1996) The PALPA: A commentary and consideration of the clinical implications. *Aphasiology*, 10, 197–202.

Marshall, J.C. (1986) The description and interpretation of aphasic language disorder. *Neuropsychologia*, 24, 5–24.

Marshall, R.C. and Neuberger, S.I. (1994) Verbal self-correction and improvement in treated aphasia clients. *Aphasiology*, 8, 535–547.

Marshall, R.C. and Tompkins, C.A. (1983) Improvement in treated aphasia: Examination of selected prognostic factors. *Folia Phoniatrica*, 34, 305–315.

Martin, A.D. (1977) Aphasia testing: A second look at the Porch Index of Communicative Ability. *Journal of Speech and Hearing Disorders*, 42, 547–561.

Martin, C.W. (1992) Review of Oral Speech Mechanism Screening Examination—Revised. *11th mental measurement yearbook* (pp. 629–632). Lincoln, NE: University of Nebraska Press.

Martin, L. and Bench, L. (1997) Some observations on the use of conjunctions when using the CELF-R with hearing-impaired children. *Child Language Teaching and Therapy*, 13, 73–88.

Martin, P., Manning, L., Munoz, P., and Montero, I. (1990) Communicative Abilities in Daily Living: Spanish standardization. *Evaluacion Psicologica*, 6, 369–384.

Martin, R.C., Loring, D.W., Meador, K.J., and Lee, G.P. (1990) The effects of lateralized temporal lobe dysfunction on formal and semantic word fluency. *Neuropsychologia*, 28, 823–829.

Martino, A.A., Pizzamiglio, L., and Razzano, C. (1976) A new version of the Token Test for aphasics: A concrete objects form. *Journal of Communication Disorders*, 9, 1–15.

Martins, I.O. (1997) Childhood aphasias clinical neuroscience. *Language Disorders*, 4, 73–77.

Martins, I.O. and Ferro, J.M. (1991) Types of aphasia and lesion localization. In: I.P. Martins, H.R. Castro-Caldas, and A.V. Van Dongen (Eds.), *Acquired aphasia in children—Acquisition and breakdown of language in the developing brain*. Dordrecht, Netherlands: Kluwer.

Martins, I.O. and Ferro, J.M. (1992) Recovery of aphasia in children. *Aphasiology*, 6, 431–448.

Martins, I.O. and Ferro, J.M. (1993) Acquired childhood aphasias: A clinical radiological study of 11 stroke patients. *Aphasiology*, 7, 489–495.

Matarazzo, J.D. (1990) Psychological assessment vs. psychological testing: Validation from Binet to the school, clinic and courtroom. *American Psychologist*, 45, 991–1017.

Mattis, S. (1976) Mental status examination for organic mental syndrome in the elderly patient. In: L. Bellack and T.B. Karasu (Eds.), *Geriatric psychiatry* (pp. 77–121). New York: Grune & Stratton.

Mattis, S. (1991) *Dementia Rating Scales: Professional Manual*. Odessa, FL: PAR.

Mattis, S., Jurica, P.J., and Leitten, C.L. (2001) *Dementia Rating Scale–2*. San Antonio, TX: Psychological Corporation.

Mazaux, J.M. and Orgogozo, J.M. (1985) *Echelle d'evaluation de l'aphasie*. Paris: Editions Scientifiques et Psychologiques.

McClenehan, R., Johnston, M., and Densham, Y. (1992) Factors influencing accuracy of estimation of comprehension problems in patients following CVA by doctors, nurses, and relatives. *European Journal of Disorders of Communication*, 27, 209–219.

McConnell, S.R. (2000) Assessment in early intervention and early childhood special education: Building on the past to project into the future. *Topics in Early Childhood Special Education*, 20, 43–48.

McConnell, S.R., Priest, J.S., Davis, S.D., and McEvoy, M.A. (2001) Best practices in measuring growth and development for preschool children. In: A. Thomas and J. Grimes (Eds.), *Best practices in school psychology IV*. Washington, D.C.: National Association of School Psychologists.

McDonald, S. (1993) Pragmatic language loss following closed head injury: Inability to meet the informational needs of the listener. *Brain and Language*, 44, 28–46.

McDonald, S. and Pearce, S. (1995) The 'dice' game: A new test of pragmatic language skills after closed-head injury. *Brain Injury*, 9, 255–271.

McNamara I.P., Obler, L.K., Au, R., Durso, R., and Albert, M.L. (1992) Speech monitoring skills in Alzeheimer's disease, Parkinson's disease, and normal aging. *Brain and Language*, 42, 38–51.

McNeil, M.R. (1979) Porch Index of Communicative Ability. In: F.L. Darley (Ed.), *Evaluation of appraisal techniques in speech and language pathology*. Reading, MA: Addison-Wesley.

McNeil, M.R. and Campbell, T.F. (1998) Review of Joliet 3-Minute Speech and Language Screen (Revised). In: J.C. Impara and B.S. Plake (Eds.), *The 13th mental measurement yearbook* (pp. 565–568). Lincoln, NE: Buros Institute.

McNeil, M.R. and Prescott, T.E. (1978) *Revised Token Test*. Baltimore: University Park Press.

McNeill-Brown, D. and Douglas, J. (1997) Perceptions of communication skills in severely brain-injured adults. In: J. Ponsford, V. Anderson, and P. Snow (Eds.), International Perspectives on Traumatic Brain Injury: Proceedings of the Fifth International Association for the Study of Traumatic Brain Injury Conference, Melbourne, Australia (pp. 247–250). Brisbane, Australia: Australian Academic Press.

Mcneilly, L.G.J. (1999) A descriptive analysis of the receptive and expressive language skills of young children born to mothers with Human Immunodeficiency Virus infection. *Dissertation Abstracts International*, 60 B, 1053.

Mecham, M.J., Jex, J.L., and Jones, J.D. (1967) *Utah Test of Language Development*, rev. ed. Salt Lake City, UT: Communication Research Associates.

Meffer, E. and Jeffrey, K. (1984) Correlations of glucose matabolism and structural damage to language functions in aphasia. *Brain and Language*, 21, 187–207.

Mega, M.S. and Alexander, M.P. (1994) Subcortical aphasia: The core profile of capsulostriatal infarction. *Neurology*, 44, 1824–1829.

Mendez, M.F. and Ashla-Mendez, M. (1991) Differences between multi-infarct dementia and Alzheimer's disease on unstructured neuropsychological tasks. *Journal of Clinical and Experimental Neuropsychology*, 13, 923–932.

Merriman, W.J., Barnett, B.E., and Isenberg, D. (1995) A preliminary investigation of the relationship between language and gross motor skills in preschool children. *Perceptual and Motor Skills*, 81, 1211–1216.

Messick, S. (1980) The validity and ethics of assessment. *American Psychologist*, 35, 1012–1027.

Mesulam, M-M. (2001) Primary progressive aphasia. *Annals of Neurology*, 49, 425–432.

Mesulam, M-M. and Weintraub (1992) The spectrum of primary progressive aphasia. In: M.N. Rossor (Ed.), *Unusual dementias*. London: Balliere Tindall.

Metter, E.J., Hanson, W.R., Jackson, C.A., Kempler, D., van Lancker, D., Mazziotta, J.C., and Phelps, M.E. (1990) Temporoparietal cortex in aphasia: Evidence from positron emission tomography. *Archives of Neurology*, 47, 1235–1238.

Metter, E.J. and Jackson, C.A. (1992) Temporoparietal cortex and the recovery of language comprehension in aphasia. *Aphasiology*, 6, 349–358.

Meyers, J.E., Volkert, K., and Diep, A. (2000) Sentence repetition test: Updated norms and clinical utility. *Applied Neuropsychology*, 7, 154–159.

Miceli, G. (1999) Grammatical deficit in aphasia. In: G. Denes and L. Pizzamiglio (Eds.), *Handbook of clinical and experimental neuropsychology*. Hove, East Sussex, UK: Psychology Press.

Miller, E. and Hague, F. (1975) Some characteristics of verbal behavior in presenile dementia. *Psychological Medicine*, 5, 255–259.

Miller, G.E. (1991) *The science of words*. New York: Freeman.

Miller, N. (1989) Strategies of language use in assessment and therapy for acquired dysphasia. In: P. Grunwell and A. James (Eds.), *Functional evaluation of language disorders*. London: Groom Helm.

Miller, N., De Bleser, R., and Willmes, K. (1998) The English language version of the Aachen Aphasia Test. In: W. Ziegler and K. Deger (Eds.), *Clinical phonetics and linguistics* (pp. 253–261). London: Whurr Publishers.

Miller, N., Willmes, K., and De Bleser, R. (2000) The psychometric properties of the English language version of the Aachen Aphasia Test (EAAT). *Aphasiology*, 14, 683–722.

Miller, N., Willmes, K., and De Bleser, R. (In press) *Aachen Aphasia Test* (English Version). Goettingen: Hogrefe.

Millis, S.R., Rosenthal, M., Novack, T.A., Sherer, M., Nick, T.G., Kreutzer, J.S.,

High, Jr., W.M., and Ricker, J.H. (2001) Long-term neuropsychological outcome after traumatic brain injury. *Journal of Head Trauma Rehabilitation*, 16, 343–355.

Milner, B. (1964) Some effects of frontal lobectomy in man. In: J.M. Warren and K. Akert (Eds.), *The frontal granular cortex and behavior*. New York: McGraw-Hill.

Milton, S.B., Prutting, C.A., and Binder, G.M. (1984) Appraisal of communicative competence in head injured adults. In: R. H. Brookshire (Ed.), *Clinical aphasiology: Proceedings of the conference 1984* (pp. 114–123). Minneapolis, MN: BRK Publishers.

Miniutti, A.M. (1991) Language deficiencies in inner-city children with learning and behavior problems. *Language, Speech, and Hearing Services in Schools*, 22, 31–38.

Mitchell-Person, C. (2001) Review of the Bedside Evaluation Screening Test, 2nd ed. In: B.S. Plake and J.C. Impara (Eds.), *The 14th mental measurements yearbook*. Lincoln, NE: Buros Institute.

Mitrushina, M.N., Boone, K.B., and D'Elia, L.F. (1999) *Handbook of normative data for neuropsychological assessment*. New York: Oxford University Press.

Mitrushina, M. and Satz, P. (1989) Differential decline of specific memory components in normal aging. *Brain Dysfunction*, 2, 330–335.

Mitrushina, M. and Satz, P. (1995) Repeated testing of normal elderly with the Boston Naming Test. *Aging*, 7, 123–127.

Moly, P. (1988) La Gestualite chez l'aphasique. *Revue de Phonetique Appliquee*, 87–89, 177–198.

Monsch, A.U., Bondi, M.W., Butters, N., and Salmon, D.P. (1992) Comparison of verbal fluency tasks in the detection of dementia of the Alzheimer type. *Archives of Neurology*, 49, 1253–1258.

Monsch, A.U., Bondi, M.W., Butters, N., Paulsen, J.S., Salmon, D.P., Brugger, P., and Swenson, M.R. (1994) A comparison of category and letter fluency in Alzheimer's disease and Huntington's disease. *Neuropsychologia*, 8, 25–30.

Montgomery, K.M. (1982) A normative study of neuropsychological test performance of a normal elderly sample. M.A. thesis, University of Victoria.

Morales, P. (2001) Review of the Bedside Evaluation Screening Test, 2nd ed. In: B.S. Plake and J.C. Impara (Eds.), *The 14th mental measurements yearbook*. Lincoln, NE: Buros Institute.

Moran, B.M. (1989) Removing communication barriers from language tests. *Language, Speech and Hearing Services in Schools*, 20, 431–432.

Morford, J.P. (1996) Insights to language from the study of gesture: A review of research on the gestural communication of non-signing deaf people. *Language and Communication*, 16, 165–178.

Morgan, H., and Murray, H.A. (1943) *Thematic Apperception Test: Manual*. Cambridge, MA: Harvard University Press.

Morgan, R.L., Dawson, B., and Kirby, D. (1992) The performance of preschoolers with speech/language disorders on the McCarthy Scales of Children's Abilities. *Psychology in the Schools*, 29, 11–17.

Morgan-Berry, R. (1988) *The Auditory Discrimination and Attention Test*. Windsor, England: NFER-Nelson.

Morley, G.K., Lundgren, S., and Haxby, J. (1979) Comparison and clinical applicability of auditory comprehension scores on the behavioral neurology deficit evaluation, Boston Diagnostic Aphasia Examination, Porch Index of Communicative Ability, and Token Test. *Journal of Clinical Neuropsychology*, 1, 249–258.

Morris, J.C., Heyman, A., Mohs, R.C., Hughes, J.P., van Belle, G., Fillenbaum, G., Mellits, E.D., and Clark, C. (1989) The Consortium to Establish a Registry for Alzheimer's Disease. Part 1: Clinical and neuropsychological assessment of Alzheimer's disease. *Neurology*, 39, 1159–1165.

Morrison, L.E., Smith, L.A., and Sarazin, F.F-A. (1996) Boston Naming Test: A French-Canadian normative study (preliminary analyses). *Journal of the International Neuropsychological Society*, 2, 4 (abstract).

Müller, D.J. and Code, C. (1983) Interpersonal perceptions of psychosocial adjustment to aphasia. In: C. Code and D.J. Müller (Eds.), *Aphasia therapy* (pp. 101–112). London: Edward Arnold.

Munoz-Sandoval, A.F., Cummins, J., Alvarado, C.G., and Ruef, M.L. (1998) *Bilingual Verbal Abilitiy Test*. Chicago: Riverside Publishing.

Murdoch, B.E., Chenery, H.J., Wilks, V., and Boyle, R.S. (1987) Language disorders in dementia of the Alzheimer type. *Brain and Language*, 31, 122–137.

Murray, L.L. and Chapey, R. (2001) Assessment of language disorders in adults. In: R. Chapey (Ed.), *Language intervention strategies in aphasia and related neurogenic communication disorders*, 4th ed. (pp. 55–126). Philadelphia: Lippincott Williams & Wilkins.

Murray, L.L. and Stout, J.C. (1999) Discourse comprehension in Huntington's and Parkinson's diseases. *American Journal of Speech Language Pathology*, 8, 137–148.

Musiek, F.E. (1983) Assessment of central auditory asymmetry: The dichotic digit test revisited. *Ear and Hearing*, 4, 79–83.

Musso, M., Weiller, C., Kiebel, S., Muller, S.P., Bulau, P., and Rijntjes, M. (1999) Training-induced brain plasticity in aphasia. *Brain*, 122, 1781–1790.

Myers, P.S. (1978) Analysis of right hemisphere communication deficits: Implications for speech pathology. In: R.H. Brookshire (Ed.), *Clinical aphasiology: Conference proceedings* (pp. 49–57). Minneapolis, MN: BRK Publishers.

Myers, P.S. (1979) Profiles of communication deficits in patients with right cerebral hemisphere damage. In: R.H. Brookshire (Ed.), *Clinical aphasiology: Conference proceedings* (pp. 38–46). Minneapolis, MN: BRK Publishers.

Myers, P.S. (1997) Right hemisphere syndrome. In: L.L. LaPointe (Ed.), *Aphasia and related neurogenic language disorders*, 2nd ed. (pp. 201–225). New York: Thieme.

Myers, P.S. (1999) *Right hemisphere damage: Disorders of communication and cognition*. San Diego: Singular Publishing.

Myers, P.S. (2001) Communication disorders associated with right hemisphere damage. In: R. Chapey (Ed.), *Language intervention strategies in aphasia and related neurogenic communication disorders*, 4th ed. (pp. 809–828). Philadelphia: Lippincott Williams & Wilkins.

Naeser, M.A. and Hayward, R.W. (1978) Lesion localization in aphasia with cranial computed tomography and the Boston Diagnostic Aphasia Exam. *Neurology*, 28, 545–551.

Naeser, M.A., Hayward, R.W., Laughlin, S.A., and Zatz, L.M. (1981) Quantitative CT scan studies in aphasia: I. Infarct size and CT numbers. *Brain and Language*, 12, 140–164.

Naeser, M.A., Mazurski, P., Goodglass, H., and Peraino, M. (1987) Auditory syntactic comprehension in nine aphasia groups (with CT scans) and children: Differences in degree but not order of difficulty observed. *Cortex*, 23, 359–380.

Naglieri, J.A. (1981) Concurrent validity of the revised Peabody Picture Vocabulary Test. *Psychology in the Schools*, 18, 286–289.

Naglieri, J.A. and Pfeiffer, S.I. (1983) Stability, concurrent and predictive validity of the PPVT-R. *Journal of Clinical Psychology*, 39, 965–967.

Natalicio, D.S. (1977) Sentence repetition as a language assessment technique: Some issues and applications. *Bilingual Review*, 4, 107–112.

Naylor, M.W., Staskowski, M., Kenney, M.C., and King, C.A. (1994) Language disorders and learning disabilities in school-refusing adolescents. *Journal of the American Academy of Child and Adolescent Psychiatry*, 33, 1331–1337.

Neils, J., Baris, J.M., Carter, C., Dell'aira, A.L., Nordloh, S.J., Weiler, E., and Weisiger, B. (1995) Effects of age, education, and living environment on Boston Naming Test performance. *Journal of Speech and Hearing Research*, 38, 1143–1149.

Newborg, J., Stock, J.R., and Wnek, L. (1984) *Battelle Developmental Inventory*. Chicago: Riverside Publishing.

Newcomer, P.L. and Hammill, D.D. (1999a) *Test of Language Development (Primary)–3rd Edition*. Novato, CA: Academic Therapy Publications.

Newcomer, P.L. and Hammill, D.D. (1999b) *Test of Language Development (Intermediate)–3rd Edition*. Novato, CA: Academic Therapy Publications.

Newton, D.P. (1994) Pictorial support for discourse comprehension. *British Journal of Educational Psychology*, 64, 221–229.

Nicholas, L.E. and Brookshire, R.H. (1993) A system for quantifying the information and efficiency of the connected speech of adults with aphasia. *Journal of Speech and Hearing Research*, 36, 338–350.

Nicholas, L.E. and Brookshire, R.H. (1995a) Presence, completeness, and accuracy of main concepts in the connected speech on non-brain-damaged adults and adults with aphasia. *Journal of Speech and Hearing Research*, 38, 145–157.

Nicholas, L.E. and Brookshire, R.H. (1995b) Comprehension of spoken narrative discourse by adults with aphasia, right-hemisphere brain damage, or traumatic brain injury. *American Journal of Speech-Language Pathology*, 4, 69–81.

Nicholas, L.E., Brookshire, R.H., MacLennan, D.L., Schumacher, J.G., and Porrazzo, S.A. (1989) Revised administration and scoring procedures for the Boston Naming Test and norms for non-brain-damaged adults. *Aphasiology*, 3, 569–580.

Nicholas, L.E., MacLennan, D.L., and Brookshire, R.H. (1986) Validity of multiple sentence reading of comprehension tests for aphasic adults. *Journal of Speech and Hearing Disorders*, 51, 82–87.

Nicholas, M., Connor, L.T., Obler, L.K., and Albert, M.L. (1998) Aging, language, and language disorders. In: M.T. Sarno (Ed.), *Acquired aphasia* (3rd ed.) (pp. 413–449). San Diego: Academic Press.

Nicholas, M.L., Helm-Estabrooks, N., Ward-Lonergan, J., and Morgan, A.R. (1993) Evolution of severe aphasia in the first two years post onset. *Archives of Physical Medicine and Rehabilitation*, 74, 830–836.

Nicholas, M., Obler, L.K., Au, R., and Albert, M.L. (1996) On the nature of naming errors in aging and dementia: A study of semantic relatedness. *Brain and Language*, 54, 184–195.

Nicholas, M., Obler, L., Albert, M., and Goodglass, H. (1995) Lexical retrieval in healthy aging. *Cortex*, 21, 595–606.

Nippold, M.A., Schwarz, I.E., and Jescheniak, J.D. (1991) Narrative ability in school-age stuttering boys: A preliminary investigation. *Journal of Fluency Disorders*, 16, 289–308.

Norris, J.A. (1998) Review of Preschool Language Scale—3. In: J.C. Impara and B.S. Plake (Eds.), *The 13th mental measurement yearbook* (pp. 784–786). Lincoln, NE: Buros Institute.

Obler, L.K. and Albert, M.L. (1982) *Action Naming Test*. Boston: VA Medical Center.

Obler, L.K., Au, R., and Albert, M.L. (1995) Language and aging. In: R.A. Huntley and K.S. Helfer (Eds.), *Communication in later life* (pp. 85–97). Boston: Butterworth-Heinemann.

Obler, L.K., Nicholas, M., Albert, M.L., and Woodward, S. (1985) On comprehension across the adult lifespan. *Cortex*, 21, 273–280.

Oelschlaeger, M.L. and Thorn, J.C. (1999) Application of the Correct Information Unit analysis to the naturally occurring conversations of a person with aphasia. *Journal of Speech, Language, and Hearing Research*, 42, 636–648.

O'Flaherty, C.A. and Douglas, J.M. (1997) Living with cognitive-communicative difficulties following traumatic brain injury: Using a model of interpersonal communication to characterize the subjective experience. *Aphasiology*, 11, 889–911.

Ogden, J.A. (1966) Phonological dyslexia and phonological dysgraphia following left and right hemispherectomy. *Neuropsychologia*, 34, 905–918.

Ohyama, M., Senda, M., Kitamura, S., Ishi, K., Mishina, M., and Terashi, A. (1996) Role of the nondominant hemisphere and undamaged area during word repetition in poststroke aphasics. *Stroke*, 27, 897–903.

Olswang, L.B., Stoel-Gammon, C., Coggins, T.E., and Carpenter, R.L. (1987) *Assessing linguistic behaviors: Assessing prelinguistic and early linguistic behaviors in developmentally young children*. Seattle: University of Washington Press.

O'Neill, P.A., Cheadle, B., Wyatt, R., McGuffog, J., et al. (1990) The value of the Frenchay Aphasia Screening Test in screening for dysphasia: Better than the clinician? *Clinical Rehabilitation*, 4, 123–128.

Orgass, B. (1986) *Der Token Test*. Weinheim: Beltz.

Orgass, B. and Poeck, K. (1966) Clinical validation of a new test for aphasia: An experimental study of the Token Test. *Cortex*, 2, 222–243.

Orgogozo, J.M. (1999) Piracetam in the treatment of acute stroke. *Pharmacopsychiatry*, 32, 25–37.

Orzeck, A.Z. (1964) *The Orzeck Aphasia Evaluation*. Los Angeles: Western Psychological Services.

Paradis, M. and Libben, G. (1987) *The assessment of bilingual aphasia*. Hillsdale, NJ: Lawrence Erlbaum.

Paradis, M. and Libben, G. (1993) *La Evaluacion de la Afasie en los Bilingues*. Barcelona: Masson.

Park, G.H., McNeil, M.R., and Tompkins, C.A. (2000) Reliability of the Five-Item Revised Token Test for individuals with aphasia. *Aphasiology*, 14, 527–535.

Parkin, A.J. (1993) Progressive aphasia without dementia: A clinical and cognitive neuropsychological analysis. *Brain and Language*, 44, 201–220.

Paul, R. and Cohen, D.J. (1984) Outcome of severe disorders of language acquisition. *Journal of Autism and Developmental Disorders*, 14, 405–421.

Pearsall, T.S., O'Neill, D., and Wilcox, G.K. (1995) Use of the Mini-Mental State Examination to determine the usefulness of subsequent cognitive assessment in moderately to severely demented subjects. *International Journal of Geriatric Psychiatry*, 10, 975–980.

Peck, E.A., Mitchell, S.A., Burke, E.A., and Schwartz, S.M. (1992) *Post head injury normative data for selected Benton neuropsychological tests*. Paper presented at the annual meeting of the American Psychological Association, Washington, D.C.

Pell, M.D. (1998) Recognition of prosody following unilateral brain lesions: Influence of functional and structural attributes of prosodic contours. *Neuropsychologia*, 36, 701–715.

Pendleton, M.G., Heaton, R.K., Lehman, R.A.W., and Hulihan, D. (1982) Diagnostic utility of the Thurstone Word Fluency test in neuropsychological evaluations. *Journal of Clinical Neuropsychology*, 4, 307–317.

Penn, C. (1983) Syntactic and pragmatic aspects of aphasic language. Unpublished Ph.D. dissertation: University of Witwatersrand.

Penn, C. (1988) The profiling of syntax and pragmatics in aphasia. *Clinical Linguistics and Phonetics*, 2, 179–207.

Penn, C. and Cleary, J. (1988) Compensatory strategies in the language of closed head injured patients. *Brain Injury*, 2, 3–17.

Penn, C., Milner, K., and Fridjhon, P. (1992) The Communicative Effectiveness Index: Its use with South African stroke patients. *South African Journal of Communication Disorders*, 39, 74–82.

Peterson, L.N. and Kirshner, H.S. (1981) Gestural impairment and gestural ability in aphasia: A review. *Brain and Language*, 14, 333–348.

Petheram, B. (1998) A survey of speech and language therapists' practice in the assessment of aphasia. *International Journal of Language and Communication Disorders*, 33, 180–182.

Petrick, J.D., Kunkle, J., and Franzen, M.D. (1992) Confrontational and productive naming in depression and dementia. *The Clinical Neuropsychologist*, 6, 323 (abstract).

Petrie, I. (1975) Characteristics and progress of a group of language disordered children with severe receptive difficulties. *British Journal of Disorders of Communication*, 10, 123–133.

Phelps, L. and Cottone, J.W. (1999) Long-term developmental outcomes of prenatal cocaine exposure. *Journal of Psychoeducational Assessment*, 17, 343–353.

Phelps, L., Wallace, N.V., and Bontrager, A. (1997) Risk factors in early child development: Is prenatal cocaine/polydrug exposure a key variable? *Psychology in the Schools*, 34, 245–252.

Phelps-Terasaki, D. and Phelps-Gunn, T. (1994) *Test of Pragmatic Language*. Austin, TX: Pro-Ed.

Piatt, A.L., Fields, J.A., Paolo, A.M., Koller, W.C., and Troster, A.I. (1999) Lexical, semantic, and action verbal fluency in Parkinson's disease with and without dementia. *Journal of Clinical and Experimental Neuropsychology*, 21, 435–443.

Pick, A. (1913) Die agrammatischen Sprachstörungen. Studien zur psychologischen Grundlegung der Aphasielehre. Part 1. In: A. Alzheimer and M. Lewandowsky (Eds.), *Monographien aus dem Gesamtgebiet der Neurologie und Psychiatrie (Volume 7)*. Berlin: Springer.

Pimental, P.A. and Kingsbury, N.A. (1989a) *Neuropsychological aspects of right brain injury*. Austin, TX: Pro-Ed.

Pimental, P.A. and Kingsbury, N.A. (1989b) *Mini Inventory of Right Brain Injury*. Austin, TX: Pro-Ed.

Pineda, D.A., Rosselli, M., Ardila, A., Mejia, S.E., Romero, M.G., and Perez, C. (2000) The Boston Diagnostic Aphasia Examination—Spanish version: The influence of demographic variables. *Journal of the International Neuropsychological Society*, 6, 802–814.

Pinheiro, M.L. (1977) Test of central auditory function in children with learning disabilities. In: R. Keith (Ed.), *Central auditory dysfunction* (pp. 223–256). New York: Grune & Stratton.

Pizzamiglio, L., Laicardi, C., Appicciafuoco, A., Gentili, P., Judica, A., Luglio, L., Margheriti, M., and Razzano, C. (1984) Capacita communicative di pazienti afasici in situationi di vita quotidiana: addatamento italiano. *Archivio di psicologia neurologia e psichiatria*, 45, 187–210.

Poeck, K. (1974) *Neurologie*, 3rd ed. Berlin: Springer.

Poeck, K., Kerschensteiner, M., and Hartje, W. (1972) A quantitative study on language understanding in fluent and nonfluent aphasia. *Cortex*, 8, 299–304.

Pollock, K.E. (1991) The identification of vowel errors using traditional articulation or phonological process test stimuli. *Language, Speech, and Hearing Services in the Schools*, 22, 39–50.

Ponton, M.O., Gonzalez, J.J., Hernandez, I., Herrara, L., and Higareda, I. (2000) Factor analysis of the Neuropsychological Screening Battery for Hispanics (NeSBHIS). *Applied Neuropsychology*, 7, 32–39.

Ponton, M.O., Satz, P., Herrera, L., Young, R. Ortiz, F., d'Elia, L., Furst, C., and Namerow, N. (1992) A modified Spanish version of the Boston Naming Test. *The Clinical Neuropsychologist*, 6, 334 (abstract).

Porch, B.E. (1967) *Porch Index of Communicative Ability: Theory and development* (*Volume 1*). Palo Alto, CA: Consulting Psychologists Press.

Porch, B.E. (1973) *Porch Index of Communicative Ability: Administration and Interpretation* (*Volume 2*). Palo Alto, CA: Consulting Psychologists Press.

Porch, B.E. (1981) *Porch Index of Communicative Ability in Children: Theory and development* (*Volume 1*). Chicago: Riverside Publishing.

Porch, B.E. (2001) Treatment of aphasia subsequent to the Porch Index of Communicative Ability. In: R. Chapey (Ed.), *Language intervention strategies in aphasia and related neurogenic communication disorders* (4th Ed.) (pp. 663–674). Philadelphia: Lippincott Williams & Wilkins.

Porch, B.E., Collins, M., Wertz, R.T., and Friden, T.P. (1980) Statistical prediction of change in aphasia. *Journal of Speech and Hearing Research*, 23, 312–321.

Poreh, A.M. (2000) The quantified process approach: An emerging methodology to neuropsychological assessment. *The Clinical Neuropsychologist*, 14, 212–222.

Powell, G.E., Bayley, S., and Clark, E. (1980) A very short form of the Minnesota Aphasia Test. *British Journal of Social and Clinical Psychology*, 19, 189–194.

Powell, T.W. and Germani, M.J. (1993) Linguistic, intellectual, and adaptive skills in a sample of children with communication disorders. *Journal of Psychoeducational Assessment*, 11, 158–172.

Pracharitpukdee, N., Phanthumchinda, K., Huber, W., and Willmes, K. (1998) The Thai version of the German Aachen Aphasia Test (AAT): Description of the test and performance of normal subjects. *Journal of the Medical Association of Thailand*, 81, 402–412.

Prather, E.M., Breecher, S.V.A., Stafford, L., and Wallace, E.M. (2000) *Screening Test of Adolescent Language*. Los Angeles: Western Psychological Services.

Price, D.R., Herbert, D.A., Walsh, M.L., and Law, J.G. (1990) Study of the WAIS-R, Quick Test and PPVT IQs for neuropsychiatric patients. *Perceptual and Motor Skills*, 70, 1320–1322.

Prigatano, G. P. (1999) *Principles of neuropsychological rehabilitation*. New York: Oxford University Press.

Prins, R.S., Snow, C.E., and Wagenaar, E. (1978) Recovery from aphasia: Spontaneous speech vs. language comprehension. *Brain and Language*, 5, 192–211.

Proctor, R.W. and van Zandt, T. (1994) *Human factors in simple and complex systems*. Boston: Allyn & Bacon.

Prutting, C.A. and Kirchner, D.M. (1987) A clinical appraisal of the pragmatic aspects of language. *Journal of Speech and Hearing Disorders*, 52, 105–119.

Quattrochi, M.M. and Golden, C.J. (1983) Peabody Picture Vocabulary Test-Revised and Luria-Nebraska Neuropsychological Battery for Children: Intercorrelations for normal youngsters. *Perceptual and Motor Skills*, 56, 632–634.

Randolph, C., Lansing, A., Ivnick, R.J., Cullum, C.M., and Hermann, B.P. (1999) Determinants of confrontation naming performance. *Archives of Clinical Neuropsychology*, 14, 489–496.

Rao, P. (1990) Functional communication assessment of the elderly. In: E. Cherov (Ed.), *Proceedings of the Research Symposium on Communication Sciences and Disorders and Aging* (pp. 28–34). Rockville, MD: American Speech and Hearing Association.

Rapcsak, S.Z., Arthur, S.A., Bliklen, D.A., and Rubens, A.B. (1989) Lexical agraphia in Alzheimer's disease. *Archives of Neurology*, 46, 65–68.

Rapp, B.C. and Caramazza, A. (1998) Lexical deficits. In: M.T. Sarno (Ed.), *Acquired aphasia*, 3rd ed. (pp. 187–228). San Diego: Academic Press.

Raven, J.C. (1938) *Progressive Matrices. A perceptual test of intelligence*. London: H.K. Lewis.

Read, D.E. and Spreen, O. (1986) Neuropsychological assessment of memory in early dementia. Normative data for a battery of memory tests. Unpublished manuscript. University of Victoria.

Rebok, G., Brandt, J., and Folstein, J. (1990) Longitudinal cognitive decline in patients with Alzheimer's disease. *Journal of Geriatric Psychiatry and Neurology*, 3, 91–97.

Records, N.L. (1994) A measure of the contribution of a gesture to the perception of speech in listeners with aphasia. *Journal of Speech and Hearing Research*, 37, 1086–1099.

Records, N.L., Tomblin, J.B., and Buckwalter, P.R. (1995) Auditory verbal learning in young adults with specific language impairment. *The Clinical Neuropsychologist*, 9, 187–193.

Reed, J.C. (1998) Review of Minnesota Test for Differential Diagnosis of Aphasia. In: J.C. Impara and B.S. Plake (Eds.), *The 13th mental measurements yearbook*. Lincoln, NE: Buros Institute.

Regard, M., Strauss, E., and Knapp, P. (1982) Children's production of verbal and nonverbal fluency tasks. *Perceptual and Motor Skills*, 55, 839–844.

Reinvang, I. (1985) *Aphasia and brain organization*. New York: Plenum.

Reinvang, I. and Graves, R. (1975) A basic aphasia examination: Description with discussion of first results. *Scandinavian Journal of Rehabilitation Medicine*, 7, 129–135.

Reisberg, B., Ferris, S.H., de Leon, M.J., and Crook, T. (1982) The global deterioration scale (GDS). An instrument for the assessment of primary degenerative dementia (PDD). *American Journal of Psychiatry*, 139, 1136–1139.

Reitan, R.M. (1991) *Aphasia Screening Test*. Tuscon, AZ: Reitan Neuropsychology Laboratory.

Reitan, R.M. and Wolfson, D. (1985) *The Halstead-Reitan Neuropsychological Test Battery: Theory and clinical interpretation*. Tucson, AZ: Neuropsychology Press.

Reitan, R.M. and Wolfson, D. (1992) A short screening examination for impaired brain function in school-age children. *The Clinical Neuropsychologist*, 6, 287–294.

Rey, G.J. and Benton, A.L. (1991) *Examen de afasia multilingue: Manual de instrucciones*. Iowa City: AJA Associates.

Rey, G.J., Feldman, E., Hernandez, D., Levin, B.E., Rivas-Vazquez, R., Nedd, K.J., and Benton, A.L. (2001) Application of the Multilingual Aphasia Examination

—Spanish in the evaluation of Hispanic patients post closed-head trauma. *The Clinical Neuropsychologist*, 15, 13–18.

Rey, G.J., Feldman, E., Rivas-Vazquez, R., Levin, B.E., and Benton, A. (1999) Neuropsychological test development and normative data on Hispanics. *Archives of Clinical Neuropsychology*, 14, 593–601.

Reynell, J.K. and Gruber, C.P. (1990) *Reynell Developmental Language Scales*-III. Los Angeles: Western Psychological Services.

Reynell, J.K. and Huntley, R.M. (1971) New scales for the assessment of language development in young children. *Journal of Learning Disabilities*, 4, 549–557.

Rich, J.B. (1993) Pictorial and verbal implicit and recognition memory in aging and Alzheimer's disease: A transfer-appropriate processing account. Ph.D. dissertation. University of Victoria.

Richards, R.A. (1998) Test of Adolescent and Adult Language, 3rd ed.—Review. In: J.C. Impala and B.S. Plake (Eds.), *The 13th mental measurement yearbook* (pp. 1019–1021). Lincoln, NE: University of Nebraska Press.

Riedel, K. and Studdert-Kennedy, M. (1985) Extending formant transition may not improve aphasic's perception of stop consonant place of articulation. *Brain and Language*, 24, 223–232.

Ripich, D.N., Carpenter, B., and Ziol, E. (1997) Comparison of African-American and white persons with Alzheimer's disease on language measures. *Neurology*, 48, 781–783.

Riva, D., Nichelli, F., and Devoti, M. (2000) Developmental aspects of verbal fluency and confrontation naming in children. *Brain and Language*, 71, 267–284.

Rizzo, J.M. and Stephens, M.I. (1981) Performance of children with normal and impaired oral language production on a set of auditory comprehension tests. *Journal of Speech and Hearing Disorders*, 46, 150–159.

Robert, P.H., Lafont, V., Medecin, I., Berthet, L., Thauby, S., Baudu, C., and Darcourt, G. (1998) Clustering and switching strategies in verbal fluency tasks: Comparison between schizophrenics and healthy adults. *Journal of the International Neuropsychological Society*, 4, 539–546.

Roberts, J.E., Burchinal, M., and Footo, M.M. (1990) Phonological process decline from 2;12 to 8 years. *Journal of Communication Disorders*, 23, 205–217.

Roberts, P.M. and Le Dorze, G. (1998) Bilingual aphasia: Semantic organization, strategy use, and productivity in semantic verbal fluency. *Brain and Language*, 65, 287–312.

Roberts, R.J. and Hamsher, K. (1984) Effects of minority status on facial recognition and naming performance. *Journal of Clinical Psychology*, 40, 539–545.

Rome-Flanders, T. and Cronk, C. (1998) Stability and usefulness of language test results under two years of age. *Journal of Speech/Language Pathology and Audiology*, 2 (June) 74–80.

Rosen, W.G. (1980) Verbal fluency in aging and dementia. *Journal of Clinical Neuropsychology*, 2, 135–146.

Rosenthal, R., Hall, J.A., DiMatteo, M.R., Rogers, P.L., and Archer, D. (1979) *Sensitivity to nonverbal communication: The PONS test*. Baltimore: Johns Hopkins University Press.

Rosner, J. (1999) *Test of Auditory Analysis Skills*. Novato, CA: Academic Therapy Publications.

Ross, D.G. (1986) *Ross Information Processing Assessment*. Austin, TX: Pro-Ed.

Ross, E.D. (1980) The aprosodias: The functional-anatomic organization of the prosodic elements of language in the right hemisphere. *Neurology*, 30, 391.

Ross, K.B. and Wertz, R.T. (2001) Possible demographic influences on differentiating normal from aphasic performance. *Journal of Communication Disorders*, 34, 115–130.

Ross, T.P. and Lichtenberg, P.A. (1998) Expanded normative data for the Boston Naming Test for use with urban, elderly medical patients. *The Clinical Neuropsychologist*, 12, 475–481.

Ross, T.P., Lichtenberg, P.A., and Christensen, K. (1995) Normative data on the Boston Naming Test for elderly adults in a demographically diverse medical sample. *The Clinical Neuropsychologist*, 9, 321–325.

Rosselli, M., Ardila, A., Araujo, K., Weekes, V., Caracciolo, V., Padilla, M., and Ostrosky-Solis, P. (2000) Verbal fluency and repetition skills in healthy older Spanish-English bilinguals. *Applied Neuropsychology*, 7, 17–24.

Rosselli, M., Ardila, A., Florez, A., and Castro, C. (1990) Normative data on the Boston Diagnostic Aphasia Examination in a Spanish-speaking population. *Journal of Clinical and Experimental Neuropsychology*, 12, 313–322.

Rourke, B.P. (1978) Reading, spelling, arithmetic disability: A neuropsychological perspective. In: H.R. Myklebust (Ed.), *Progress in learning disabilities, Volume IV*. New York: Wiley.

Rudd, A.G., Wolfe, C.D., Tilling, K., and Beech, R. (1997) Randomised controlled trial to evaluate early discharge scheme for patients with stroke. *British Medical Journal*, 315, 1039–1044.

Ruff, R.M., Light, R.H., Parker, S.B., and Levin, H.S. (1996) Benton Controlled Oral Word Association test: Reliability and updated norms. *Archives of Clinical Neuropsychology*, 11, 329–338.

Ruff, R.M., Light, R.H., Parker, S.B., and Levin, H.S. (1997) The psychological construct of word fluency. *Brain and Language*, 57, 394–405.

Ruhl, K.L., Hughes, C.A., and Camarata, S.M. (1992) Analysis of expressive and receptive language characteristics of emotionally handicapped students served in public school settings. *Journal of Childhood Communication Disorders*, 14, 165–176.

Russell, E.W. and Starkey, R.I. (1993) *Halstead Russell Neuropsychological Evaluation System*. Los Angeles: Western Psychological Services.

Ryan, J.J., Farage, C.M., Mittenberg, W., and Kasprisin, A. (1988) Validity of the Luria-Nebraska Language Scales in aphasia. *International Journal of Neuroscience*, 43, 75–80.

Sacchett, C. and Marshall, J. (1992) Functional assessment of communication: Implications for the rehabilitation of aphasic people: Reply to Carol Frattali. *Aphasiology*, 6, 95–100.

Safi-Stagni, S. (1991) Agrammatism in Arabic. In: B. Comrie and M. Eid (Eds.),

Perspectives on Arabic linguistics III (pp. 251–270). Amsterdam: John Benjamins Publishing.

Salmon, D.P., Jin, H., Zhang, M., Grant, I., and Yu, E. (1995) Neuropsychological assessment of Chinese elderly in the Shanghai Dementia Survey. *The Clinical Neuropsychologist*, 9, 159–168.

Sands, E., Sarno, M.T., and Shankweiler, D. (1969) Long-term assessment of language function in aphasia due to stroke. *Archives of Physical Medicine and Rehabilitation*, 50, 202–222.

Sandson, J. and Albert, M.L. (1987) Varieties of perseveration. *Neuropsychologia*, 22, 715–732.

Sanger, D.D., Creswell, J.W., Dworak, J., and Schulz, L. (2000) Cultural analysis of communication behaviors among juveniles in a correctional facility. *Journal of Communication Disorders*, 33, 31–57.

Santiago, R.L. (1995) The interdependence between linguistic and cognitive performance among bilingual preschoolers with differing home language environments. *Proceedings of the Annual Boston University Conference on Language Development*, 19, 511–520.

Sarno, J.E. and Gainotti, G. (1998) The psychological and social sequelae of aphasia. In: M.T. Sarno (Ed.), *Acquired aphasia*, 3rd ed. San Diego: Academic Press.

Sarno, J.E., Sarno, M.T., and Levita, E. (1973) The functional life scale. *Archives of Physical Medicine and Rehabilitation*, 54, 214–220.

Sarno, M.T. (1969) *Functional Communication Profile*. New York: Institute of Rehabilitation Medicine.

Sarno, M.T. (1984a) Functional measurement in verbal impairment secondary to brain damage. In: C.V. Granger and G.E. Gresham (Eds.), *Functional assessment in rehabilitation medicine* (pp. 210–222). Baltimore: Williams & Wilkins.

Sarno, M.T. (1984b) Verbal impairment after closed head injury: Report of a replication study. *Journal of Nervous and Mental Disease*, 172, 476–479.

Sarno, M.T. (1986) Verbal impairment in head injury. *Archives of Physical and Medical Rehabilitation*, 67, 399–405.

Sarno, M.T. (1997) Quality of life in aphasia in the first post-stroke year. *Aphasiology*, 11, 665–679.

Sarno, M.T., Buonaguro, A., and Levita, E. (1985) Gender and recovery from aphasia after stroke. *Journal of Nervous and Mental Disease*, 173, 605–609.

Sarno, M.T., Buonaguro, A., and Levita, E. (1986) Characteristics of verbal impairment in closed head injured patients. *Archives of Physical Medicine and Rehabilitation*, 67, 400–405.

Sarno, M.T., Buonaguro, A., and Levita, E. (1987) Aphasia in closed head injury and stroke. *Aphasiology*, 1, 331–338.

Sarno, M.T. and Levita, E. (1979) Recovery in treated aphasia in the first year post-stroke. *Stroke*, 10, 663–670.

Sarno, M.T. and Levita, E. (1981) Some observations on the nature of recovery in global aphasia after stroke. *Brain and Language*, 13, 1–12.

Sasanuma, S. (1991) Aphasia rehabilitation in Japan. In: M.T. Sarno and D.E.

Woods (Eds.), *Aphasia rehabilitation: Views from the Asian-Pacific region*. New York: Academic Press.

Sattler, J.M. (1988) *Assessment of children*, 3rd ed. San Diego: J.M. Sattler.

Satz, P. and Fletcher, J. (1982) *Manual for the Florida Kindergarten Screening Battery*. Odessa, FL: Psychological Assessment Resources.

Sawrie, S.M., Chelune, G.J., Naugle, R.I., and Luders, H.O. (1996) Empirical methods for assessing meaningful change following epilepsy surgery. *Journal of the International Neuropsychological Society*, 2, 556–564.

Schetz, K.F. (1994) The examination of software used with enhancement for preschool discourse skill improvement. *Journal of Educational Computing Research*, 11, 51–71.

Schlenk, K.J., Huber, W., and Willmes, K. (1987) Prepairs and repairs: Different monitoring functions in aphasic language production. *Brain and Language*, 30, 226–244.

Schmitter-Edgecombe, M., Vesneski, M., and Jones, D.W.R. (2000) Aging and word-finding: A comparison of spontaneous and constrained naming tests. *Archives of Clinical Neuropsychology*, 15, 479–493.

Schuell, H. (1957) *Minnesota Test for Differential Diagnosis of Aphasia*. Minneapolis: University of Minnesota Press.

Schuell, H. (1957) A short examination for aphasia. *Neurology*, 7, 625–634.

Schuell, H. (1965) *Differential diagnosis of aphasia with the Minnesota test*. Minneapolis: University of Minnesota Press.

Schuell, H. (1966) A re-evaluation of the short examination for aphasia. *Journal of Speech and Hearing Disorders*, 31, 137–147.

Schuell, H. (1973) *Differential diagnosis of aphasia with the Minnesota test*, 2nd ed. Minneapolis: University of Minnesota Press.

Schuell, H. (1974a) Diagnosis and prognosis in aphasia. In: L.F. Sies (Ed.), *Aphasia, theory and therapy*. Baltimore: University Park Press.

Schuell, H. (1974b) A theoretical framework for aphasia. In: L.F. Sies (Ed.), *Aphasia, theory and therapy*. Baltimore: University Park Press.

Schuell, H. and Jenkins, J.J. (1959) The nature of language deficit in aphasia. *Psychological Review*, 66, 45–67.

Schuell, H., Jenkins, J.J., and Carroll, J.B. (1962) A factor analysis of the Minnesota Test for Differential Diagnosis of Aphasia. *Journal of Speech and Hearing Research*, 5, 350–369.

Schuell, H., Jenkins, J.J., and Jiminez-Pabon, E. (1964) *Aphasia in adults: Diagnosis, prognosis, and treatment*. New York: Harper.

Schum, R.L. and Sivan, A.B. (1997) Verbal abilities in healthy elderly adults. *Applied Neuropsychology*, 4, 130–134.

Schum, R.L., Sivan, A.B., and Benton, A.L. (1989) Multilingual Aphasia Examination: Norms for children. *The Clinical Neuropsychologist*, 3, 375–383.

Schwartz, G.E. (1983) Development of validation of the Geriatric Evaluation of Relative's Rating Instrument (GERRI). *Psychological Reports*, 53, 479–488.

Schwartz, J., Kaplan, E., and Schwartz, A. (1981) Childhood dyscalculia and

Gerstmann syndrome. Paper presented at the American Academy of Neurology, Toronto.

Secada, W.G. (1991) Degree of bilingualism and arithmetic problem solving in Hispanic first graders. *Elementary School Journal*, 92, 213–231.

Selnes, O.A., Niccum, N.E., Knopman, D.S., and Rubens, A.B. (1984) Recovery of single word comprehension: CT-scan correlates. *Brain and Language*, 21, 72–84.

Semel, E., Wiig, E.H., and Secord, W. (1987, 1995) *Clinical Evaluation of Language Fundamentals, 3rd ed.* San Antonio, TX: Psychological Corporation.

Semenza, C. (1999) Lexical-semantic disorders in aphasia. In: G. Denes and L. Pizzamiglio (Eds.), *Handbook of clinical and experimental neuropsychology*. Hove, East Sussex, UK: Psychology Press.

Seron, X., van der Kaas, R.A., and van der Linden, M. (1979) Pantomime interpretation and aphasia. *Neuropsychologia*, 17, 661–668.

Servaes, P., Draper, B., Conroy, P., and Bowring, G. (1999) Informal carers of aphasic stroke patients: Stresses and interventions. *Aphasiology*, 13, 889–900.

Shah, S., Vanclay, F., and Cooper, B. (1989) Improving the sensitivity of the Barthel Index for stroke rehabilitation. *Journal of Clinical Epidemiology*, 42, 703–709.

Shapiro, L.P., McNamara, P., Zurif, E., Lanzoni, S., and Cermak, L. (1992) Processing complexity and sentence memory: Evidence from amnesia. *Brain and Language*, 42, 431–453.

Sherman, A.M. and Massman, P.J. (1999) Prevalence and correlates of category versus letter fluency discrepancies in Alzheimer's disease. *Archives of Clinical Neuropsychology*, 14, 411–418.

Sherman, T. and Shulman, B.B. (1999) Specificity and sensitivity ratios of the Pediatric Language Acquisition Screening Tool for Early Referral-Revised. *Infant and Toddler Intervention*, 9, 315–330.

Sherratt, S.M. and Penn, C. (1990) Discourse in a right-hemisphere brain-damaged subject. *Aphasiology*, 4, 539–560.

Shewan, C.M. (1980) *Auditory Comprehension Test for Sentences*. Chicago: Biolinguistics Clinical Institutes.

Shewan, C.M. (1986) The language quotient (LQ): A new measure of the Western Aphasia Battery (WAB). *Journal of Communication Disorders*, 19, 427–439.

Shewan, C.M. (1988) The Shewan Spontaneous Language Analysis (SSLA) system for aphasic adults: Description, reliability, and validity. *Journal of Communication Disorders*, 103–138.

Shewan, C.M. and Donner, A.P. (1988) A comparison of three methods to evaluate change in the spontaneous language of aphasic individuals. *Journal of Communication Disorders*, 21, 171–176.

Shewan, C.M. and Kertesz, A. (1980) Reliability and validity characteristics of the Western Aphasia Battery (WAB). *Journal of Speech and Hearing Disorders*, 45, 308–324.

Shewan, C.M. and Kertesz, A. (1984) Effects of speech and language treatment on recovery from aphasia. *Brain and Language*, 23, 272–299.

Shriberg, L.D. (1993) Four new speech and prosody-voice measures for genetics research and other studies in developmental phonological disorders. *Journal of Speech and Hearing Research*, 36, 105–140.

Shriberg, L.D., Kwiatkowski, J., and Rasmussen, C. (1990) *Prosody-Voice Screening Profile*. Tucson, AZ: Communication Skill Builders.

Shulman, B.B. and Sherman, T. (1996) The Pediatric Language Acquisition Screening Tool for Early Referral—Revised. *Brain Injury*, 10, 329–345.

Siegel, L., Cooper, D.C., Fitzhardinge, P.M., and Ash, A.J. (1995) The use of the mental development index of the Bayley Scale to diagnose language delay in 2-year-old high-risk infants. *Infant Behavior and Development*, 18, 493–496.

Silveri, M., Leggio, M., and Molinari, M. (1994) The cerebellum contributes to linguistic production: A case of agrammatic speech following a right cerebellar lesion. *Neurology*, 44, 2047–2050.

Simmons-Mackie, N.N. (2000) Social approaches to the management of aphasia. In: L.E. Worrall and C.M. Frattali (Eds.), *Neurogenic communication disorders: A functional approach* (pp. 162–187). New York: Thieme.

Skarakis-Doyle, E., Yovetich, W., Strauss, K., Storie, A., Fisk, L.L., and Torrie, D. (1998) A Canadian normative sample for the Preschool Language Assessment Instrument. *Journal of Speech-Language Pathology and Audiology*, 22, 126–132.

Skenes, L.L. and McCauley, R.J. (1985) Psychometric review of nine aphasia tests. *Journal of Communication Disorders*, 18, 461–474.

Sklar, M. (1983) *Sklar Aphasia Scale-Revised*. Los Angeles: Western Psychological Services.

Small, J.A., Kemper, S., and Lyons, K. (2000) Sentence repetition and processing resources in Alzheimer's disease. *Brain and Language*, 75, 232–258.

Snow, P.C. and Douglas, A.M. (2000) Conceptual and methodological challenges in discourse assessment with TBI speakers: Towards an understanding. *Brain Injury*, 14, 397–415.

Snow, P., Douglas, J., and Ponsford, J. (1997) Conversational assessment following traumatic brain injury: A comparison across two control groups. *Brain Injury*, 11, 409–429.

Snow, P., Douglas, J., and Ponsford, J. (1998) Conversational discourse abilities following severe traumatic brain injury: A follow-up study. *Brain Injury*, 12, 911–935.

Snow, W.G. (1987) Aphasia Screening Test performance in patients with lateralized brain damage. *Journal of Clinical Psychology*, 43, 266–271.

Snow, W.G. and Tierney, M. (1988) One-year test-retest reliability of selected neuropsychological tests in older adults. Paper presented at the meeting of the International Neuropsychological Society, New Orleans, LA.

Sohlberg, M.M. and Mateer, C.A. (2001) *Cognitive rehabilitation: An integrative neuropsychological approach*. New York: Guilford Press.

Sommers, R.K., Kozarevich, M., and Michaels, C. (1994) Word skills of children normal and impaired in communication skills and measures of language and speech development. *Journal of Communication Disorders*, 27, 223–240.

Sorin-Peters, R. and Behrmann, M. (1995) Change in perception of communicative abilities of aphasic patients and their relatives. *Aphasiology*, 9, 565–575.

Sparrow, S.S., Balla, D.A., and Cicchetti, D.V. (1984) *Vineland Adaptive Behavior Scales*. Circle Pines, MN: American Guidance Service.

Spellacy, F.J. and Brown, W.G. (1984) Prediction of recidivism in young offenders after brief institutionalization. *Journal of Clinical Psychology*, 40, 1070–1074.

Spellacy, F.J. and Spreen, O. (1969) A short form of the Token Test. *Cortex*, 5, 390–397.

Spiegel, D.K., Jones, L.V., and Wepman, J.M. (1965) Test responses as predictors of free-speech characteristics in aphasia patients. *Journal of Speech and Hearing Research*, 8, 349–362.

Spreen, O. (1968) Psycholinguistic aspects of aphasia. *Journal of Speech and Hearing Research*, 11, 467–477.

Spreen, O. (1973) Psycholinguistics and aphasia: The contribution of Arnold Pick. In: H. Goodglass and S. Blumstein (Eds.), *Psycholinguistics and aphasia* (pp. 141–170). Baltimore: Johns Hopkins University Press.

Spreen, O. (1988) *Learning disabled children growing up*. New York: Oxford University Press.

Spreen, O. and Benton, A.L. (1966) Reliability of the Sentence Repetition Test. Iowa City, IA: Unpublished paper.

Spreen, O. and Benton, A.L. (1965) Comparative studies of some psychological tests for cerebral damage. *Journal of Nervous and Mental Disease*, 140, 323–333.

Spreen, O. and Benton, A.L. (1974) *Sound Recognition Test*. Victoria, B.C.: University of Victoria.

Spreen, O. and Benton, A.L. (1969, 1977) *Neurosensory Center Comprehensive Examination for Aphasia* (1977 rev.). Victoria, B.C.: University of Victoria, Neuropsychology Laboratory.

Spreen, O. and Strauss, E. (1998) *A compendium of neuropsychological tests*, 2nd ed. New York: Oxford University Press.

Spreen, O. and Wachal, R.S. (1973) Psycholinguistic analysis of aphasic language: Theoretical foundations and procedures. *Language and Speech*, 16, 130–146.

State University of New York at Buffalo Research Foundation (1993) *Guide for use of the Uniform Data Set for medical rehabilitation: Functional Independence Measure*. Buffalo, NY.

Still, C.N., Goldschmidt, T.J., and Mallin, R. (1983) Mini-Object-Test: A new brief clinical assessment for aphasia-apraxia-agnosia. *Southern Medical Journal*, 76, 52–54.

St. Louis, K.O. and Ruscello, D.M. (2000) *Oral Speech Mechanism Screening Examination*, 3rd ed. Austin, TX: Pro-Ed.

Stokes, S.F. and Wong, A.M.Y. (1996) Validation of a Cantonese version of the Preschool Language Assessment Instrument. *Asia Pacific Journal of Speech, Language, and Hearing*, 1, 75–90.

Stone, B.J., Gray, J.W., Dean, R.S., and Strom, D.A. (1989) Neuropsychological constructs of the PPVT with learning-disabled children: Printed stimulus cards versus oral administration. *Developmental Neuropsychology*, 5, 61–67.

Stoner, S.B. (1981) Alternate form reliability of the revised Peabody Picture Vocabulary Test for Head Start children. *Psychological Reports*, 49, 628.

Stothard, S.E., Snowling, M.J., Bishop, D.V.M., Chipchase, B.B., and Kaplan, C.A. (1998) Language-impaired preschoolers: A follow-up into adolescence. *Journal of Speech, Language, and Hearing Research*, 41, 407–418.

Strauss, E., Spreen, O., and Hunter, M. (2000) Implications of test revisions for research. *Psychological Assessment*, 12, 237–244.

Strub, R.L. and Black, F.W. (1993) *The mental status examination in neurology*, 3rd ed. Philadelphia: F.A. Davis.

Sturner, R.A., Funk, S.G., and Green, J.A. (1996) Preschool speech and language screening: Further validation of the sentence repetition test. *Journal of Developmental and Behavioral Pediatrics*, 17, 405–413.

Sturner, R.A., Heller, J.H., Funk, S.G., and Layton, T.L. (1993) The Fluharty Preschool Speech and Language Screening Test: A population-based validation study using sample-independent decision rules. *Journal of Speech and Hearing Research*, 36, 738–745.

Sturner, R.A., Kunze, L., Funk, S.G., and Green, J.A. (1993) Elicited imitation: Its effectiveness for speech and language screening. *Developmental Medicine and Child Neurology*, 35, 715–726.

Stuss, D.T., Alexander, M.P., Hamer, L., Palumbo, C., et al. (1998) The effects of focal anterior and posterior brain lesions on verbal fluency. *Journal of the International Neuropsychological Society*, 4, 265–278.

Sugishita, M. (1988) *WAB aphasia test in Japanese*. Tokyo: Igaku Shoin.

Suhr, J.A. and Jones, R.D. (1998) Letter and semantic fluency in Alzheimer's, Huntington's, and Parkinson's dementias. *Archives of Clinical Neuropsychology*, 13, 447–454.

Sundet, K. and Engvik, H. (1985) The validity of aphasia subtypes. *Scandinavian Journal of Psychology*, 26, 219–226.

Sussman, H., Marquardt, T., Hutchinson, J., and MacNeilage, P. (1986) Compensatory articulation in Broca's aphasia. *Brain and Language*, 27, 56–74.

Sutcliff, L.M. and Lincoln, N.B. (1998) The assessment of depression in aphasic stroke patients: The development of the Stroke Aphasic Depression Questionnaire. *Clinical Rehabilitation*, 12, 506–513.

Swaab, T.Y., Brown, C., and Hagoort, P. (1998) Understanding ambiguous words in sentence contexts: Electrophysiological evidence for delayed contextual selection in Broca's aphasia. *Neuropsychologia*, 36, 737–761.

Sweeney, T., Sheahan, N., Rice, I., Malone, J., et al. (1993) Communication disorders in a hospital elderly population. *Clinical Rehabilitation*, 7, 113–117.

Swihart, A.A. and Panisset, M. (1989) The Token Test: Validity and diagnostic power in Alzheimer's disease. *Developmental Neuropsychology*, 5, 69–78.

Swisher, L.P. and Sarno, M.T. (1969) Token Test scores of three matched patient groups: Left brain-damaged with aphasia, right brain-damaged without aphasia, non-brain-damaged. *Cortex*, 5, 264–273.

Tallal, P., Stark, R.E., and Mellits, D. (1985) The relationship between auditory temporal analysis and receptive language disorder: Evidence from studies of developmental language disorders. *Neuropsychologia*, 23, 527–534.

Tamura, A., Shichijo, F., and Matsumoto, K. (1996) A study on simplification of the Standard Test of Aphasia (SLTA). *Tokushima Journal of Experimental Medicine*, 43, 39–46.

Taussig, I.M., Henderson, V.W., and Mack, W. (1988) Spanish translation and validation of a neuropsychological battery: Performance of Spanish- and English-speaking Alzheimer's disease patients and normal comparison subjects. Paper presented at the meeting of the Gerontological Society of America, San Francisco.

Taylor, L.J. (1975) The Peabody Picture Vocabulary Test: What does it Measure? *Perceptual and Motor Skills*, 41, 777–778.

Taylor, M.L. (1965) A measurement of functional communication in aphasia. *Archives of Physical Medicine and Rehabilitation*, 46, 101–107.

Tedeschi, M.J. (1995) Stanford-Binet Fourth Edition and language development: Relationships for a group of referred/delayed preschoolers. *Dissertation Abstracts International*, 56 B, 2907.

Terrell, B. and Ripich, D. (1989) Discourse competence as a variable in intervention. *Seminars in Speech and Language: Aphasia and Pragmatics*, 10, 282–297.

Tesak, J. (2001) *Geschichte der Aphasie*. Idstein: Schulz-Kirchner Verlag.

Theml, T., Heldmann, B., and Jahn, T. (2001) Der Beitrag der Neuropsychologie zum Problem der differentialdiagnose Depression versus Demenz. *Zeitschrift für Neuropsychologie*, 12, 302–313.

Theriault-Wahlen, C. and Beaudichon, J. (1997) De la difficulte a traduire et exporter des tests de vocabulaire. *Bulletin de Psychologie*, 50, 112–114.

Thommessen, B., Thoresen, G.E., Bautz-Holter, E., and Laake, K. (1999) Screening by nurses for aphasia in stroke—The Ullevaal Aphasia Screening (UAS) test. *Disability and Rehabilitation*, 21, 110–115.

Thompson, L.L. and Heaton, R.K. (1989) Comparison of different versions of the Boston Naming Test. *The Clinical Neuropsychologist*, 3, 184–192.

Thorndike, R.L., Hagen, E., and Sattler, J. (1996) *Stanford-Binet Intelligence Scale (4th Ed.)*. Itasca, IL: Riverside Publishing.

Thurstone, L.L. (1938) *Primary mental abilities*. Chicago: University of Chicago.

Tillinghast, B.S., Morrow, J.E., and Uhlig, G.E. (1983) Retest and alternate form reliability of the PPVT-R with fourth, fifth, and sixth grade pupils. *Journal of Educational Research*, 76, 243–244.

Tombaugh, T.N. and Hubley, A. (1997) The 60-item Boston Naming Test: Norms for cognitively intact adults aged 25 to 88 years. *Journal of Clinical and Experimental Neuropsychology*, 19, 922–932.

Tombaugh, T.N., Kozak, J., and Rees, L. (1999) Normative data stratified by age and education for two measures of verbal fluency: FAS and animal naming. *Archives of Clinical Neuropsychology*, 14, 167–177.

Tompkins, C.A. (1995) *Right hemisphere communication disorders: Theory and management*. San Diego: Singular Publishing.

Tompkins, C.A., Bloise, C.G., Timko, M.L., and Baumgaertner, A. (1994) Working memory and inference revision in brain-damaged and normally aging adults. *Journal of Speech and Hearing Research*, 37, 896–912.

Tompkins, C.A., Spencer, K.A., and Schulz, R. (1999) Evaluating stresses and interventions for informal carers of aphasic adults: Taking a broader perspective. A commentary on Servaes, Draper, Conroy, and Bowring. *Aphasiology*, 13, 902–907.

Toner, J., Gurland, B., and Gasquoine, P. (1984) Measuring depressive symptomatology in a psychogeriatric inpatient population. *The Gerontologist*, 24, 196.

Toner, J., Gurland, B., and Leung, M. (1990) Chronic mental illness and functional communication disorders in the elderly. In: Cherov (Ed.), *Proceedings of the Research Symposium on Communication Sciences and Disorders and Aging*. Rockville, MD: American Speech and Hearing Association.

Torgesen, J.K. and Bryant, B.R. (1994) *Test of Phonological Awareness*. Austin, TX: Pro-Ed.

Towne, R.L. (1995a) Frenchay Aphasia Screening Test. In: J.C. Conoley and J.C. Impara (Eds.), *The 12th mental measurement yearbook*. Lincoln, NE: University of Nebraska Press.

Towne, R.L. (1995b) Boston Assessment of Severe Aphasia. In: J.C. Conoley and J.C. Impara (Eds.), *The 12th mental measurement yearbook*. Lincoln, NE: University of Nebraska Press.

Tramontana, M.G. and Boyd, T.A. (1986) Psychometric screening of neuropsychological abnormality in older children. *International Journal of Clinical Neuropsychology*, 8, 53–59.

Tranel, D. (1992) Functional neuroanatomy: Neuropsychological correlates of cortical and subcortical changes. In: S.C. Yudofsky and R.E. Hales (Eds.), *Textbook of neuropsychiatry* (pp. 57–88). Washington, D.C.: American Psychiatric Press.

Tranel, D., Anderson, S.W., and Benton, A. (1994) Development of the concept of 'executive function' and its relationship to the frontal lobes. In: F. Boller and J. Grafman (Eds.), *Handbook of neuropsychology, Volume 9* (pp. 125–148). Amsterdam: Elsevier Science.

Trenerry, M.R., Cascino, G.D., Jack, C.R., Sharbrough, F.W., So, F.L., and Lagerlund, T.D. (1995) Boston Naming Test performance after temporal lobectomy is not associated with lateral of cortical resection. *Archives of Clinical Neuropsychology*, 10, 399 (abstract).

Tröster, A.I., Fields, J.A., Testa, J.A., Paul, R.H., et al. (1998) Cortical and subcortical influences on clustering and switching in the performance of verbal fluency tasks. *Neuropsychologia*, 36, 295–304.

Troyer, A.K. (2000) Normative data for clustering and switching on verbal fluency tasks. *Journal of Clinical and Experimental Neuropsychology*, 22, 370–378.

Troyer, A.K., Moscovitch, M., and Winocur, G. (1997) Clustering and switching as two components of verbal fluency: Evidence from younger and older healthy adults. *Neuropsychology*, 11, 138–146.

Tucha, O., Smely, C., and Lange, K.W. (1999) Verbal and figural fluency in patients with mass lesions of the left or right frontal lobes. *Journal of Clinical and Experimental Neuropsychology*, 21, 229–236.

Tuokko, H. (1985) *Normative data for elderly subjects*. Unpublished manuscript. Vancouver, B.C.: University of British Columbia.

Turkstra, L.S. (1999) Language testing in adolescents with brain injury: A consideration of the CELF-3. *Language, Speech, and Hearing Services in the Schools*, 30, 132–140.

Turkstra, L.S., McDonald, S., and Kaufman, P.M. (1995) Assessment of pragmatic communication skills in adolescents after traumatic brain injury. *Brain Injury*, 10, 329–345.

Turton, L.J. (1989) Review of the Sklar Aphasia Scale. In: J.C. Conoley and J.J. Kramer (Eds.), *The 10th mental measurements yearbook*. Lincoln, NE: Buros Institute.

Ulatowska, H.K., Allard, L., Reyes, B., and Ford, J. (1992) Conversational discourse in aphasia. *Aphasiology*, 6, 325–331.

Ulatowska, H.K. and Chapman, S.B. (1994) Discourse macrostructure in aphasia. In: R.L. Bloom, L.K. Obler, S. De Santi, and J.S. Ehrlich (Eds.), *Discourse analysis and applications. Studies in adult clinical populations* (pp. 29–46). Hillsdale, NJ: Lawrence Erlbaum.

Unverzagt, F.W., Hall, K.S., Torke, A.M., Rediger, J.D., Mercado, N., Gureje, O., Osuntokun, B.O., and Hendrie, H.C. (1996) Effects of age, education, and gender on CERAD neuropsychological test performance in an African American sample. *The Clinical Neuropsychologist*, 10, 180–190.

Unverzagt, F.W., Morgan, O.S., Thesiger, C.H., Eldemire, D.A., Luseko, J., Pokuri, S., Hui, S.L., Hall, K., and Hendrie, H.C. (1999) The clinical utility of CERAD neuropsychological battery in elderly Jamaicans. *Journal of the International Neuropsychological Society*, 5, 255–259.

van Demark, A.A., Lemmer, E.C.J., and Drake, M.L. (1982) Measurement of reading comprehension in aphasia with the RCBA. *Journal of Speech and Hearing Disorders*, 47, 288–291.

Van Dongen, H.R., Paquier, P.F., Creten, W.L., Van Borsel, J., and Catsman-Berrevoets, C.E. (2001) Clinical evaluation of conversational speech fluency in the acute phase of acquired childhood aphasia: Does a fluency/nonfluency dichotomy exist? *Journal of Child Neurology*, 16, 345–351.

van Gorp, W.G. (1998) Review of Aphasia Diagnostic Profiles. In: J.C. Impara and B.S. Plake (Eds.), *The 13th mental measurements yearbook*. Lincoln, NE: Buros Institute.

van Gorp, W.G., Satz, P., Kiersch, M.E., and Henry, R. (1986) Normative data on the Boston Naming Test for a group of normal older adults. *Journal of Clinical and Experimental Neuropsychology*, 8, 702–705.

Van Harskamp, F. and Van Dongen, H.R. (1977) Construction and validation of different short forms of the Token Test. *Neuropsychologia*, 15, 467–470.

Van Kleek, A., Gillam, R.B., Hamilton, L., and McGrath, C. (1997) The relationship between middle-class parents' book-sharing discussion and their preschooler's abstract language development. *Journal of Speech, Language, and Hearing Research*, 40, 1261–1271.

Van Mourik, M., Verschaeve, M., Boon, P., Paquiers, P., and Van Harskamp, F. (1992) Cognition in global aphasia: Indicators for therapy. *Aphasiology*, 6, 491–499.

van Spaendonck, K.P.M., Berger, H.J.C., Horstink, M.W.I.M., Buytenhuijs, E.L. et al. (1996) Executive functions and disease characteristics in Parkinson's disease. *Neuropsychologia*, 34, 617–626.

Vargo, M.E. and Black, F.W. (1984) Normative data for the Spreen-Benton Sentence Repetition Test: Its relationship to age, intelligence, and memory. *Cortex*, 20, 585–590.

Varney, N.R. (1978) Linguistic correlates of pantomime recognition in aphasic patients. *Journal of Neurology, Neurosurgery, and Psychiatry*, 41, 564–568.

Varney, N.R. (1980) Sound recognition in relation to aural language comprehension in aphasic patients. *Journal of Neurology, Neurosurgery, and Psychiatry*, 43, 71–75.

Varney, N.R. (1984a) Phonemic imperception in aphasia. *Brain and Language*, 21, 85–94.

Varney, N.R. (1984b) The prognostic significance of sound recognition in receptive aphasia. *Archives of Neurology*, 41, 181–182.

Varney, N.R. and Benton, A.L. (1979) Phonemic discrimination and aural comprehension among aphasic patients. *Journal of Clinical Neuropsychology*, 1, 65–73.

Varney, N.R. and Damasio, H. (1986) CT scan correlates of sound recognition defect in aphasia. *Cortex*, 22, 483–486.

Vena, N.R. (1982) Revised Token Test in Kannada. *Journal of the All-India Institute of Speech and Hearing*, 13, 192–204.

Villardita, C., Cultrera, S., Cupone, V., and Meija, R. (1985) Neuropsychological test performances and normal aging. *Archives of Gerontology and Geriatrics*, 4, 311–319.

Voinescu, I., Mihailescu, L., and Lugoji, G. (1987) Communication value of a standard interview. A functional subtest to assess progress in treated aphasics. *Neurologie et Psychiatrie*, 25, 221–237.

Wachal, R.S. and Spreen, O. (1973) Some measures of lexical diversity in aphasic and normal language performance. *Language and Speech*, 16, 169–181.

Wagner, R., Torgesen, J.K., and Rashotte, C. (1999) *Comprehensive Test of Phonological Processing (CTOPP)*. Longmont, CO: Sopris West.

Walker, K.C. (1994) Review of Preschool Language Scale-3 (PLS-3). *Journal of Psychoeducational Assessment*, 12, 92–97.

Wallace, G. and Hammill, D.D. (1994) *Comprehensive Receptive and Expressive Vocabulary Test*. Austin, TX: Pro-Ed.

Wallace, G.L. and Holmes, S. (1993) Cognitive-linguistic assessment of individuals with multiple sclerosis. *Archives of Physical Medicine and Rehabilitation*, 74, 637–643.

Wang, P.L., Ennis, K.E., and Copland, S.L. (1986) *The Cognitive Competency Test: Manual*. Toronto: Mount Sinai Medical Centre.

Ward, G., Macauley, F., Jagger, C., and Harper, W. (1998) Standardized assessment: A comparison of the community dependency index and the Barthel index with an elderly hip fracture population. *British Journal of Occupational Therapy*, 61, 121–126.

Watamori, T., Takauechi, M.I., Fukasako, Y., Suzuki, K., Takahashi, M., and Sasanuma, S. (1987) Development and standardization of Communication Abilities in Daily Living (CADL) test for Japanese aphasic patients. *Japanese Journal of Rehabilitation Medicine*, 24, 103–112.

Webster, J.S., Godlewski, M.C., Hanley, G.L., and Sowa, M.V. (1992) A scoring method for logical memory that is sensitive to right-hemisphere dysfunction. *Journal of Clinical and Experimental Neuropsychology*, 14, 222–238.

Webster, P.E. and Plante, A.S. (1995) Productive phonology and phonological awareness in preschool children. *Applied Linguistics*, 16, 43–57.

Wechsler, D. (1991) *Wechsler Adult Intelligence Scale-III*. San Antonio, TX: Psychological Corporation.

Wechsler, D. (1996) *Wechsler Intelligence Scale for Children-III*. San Antonio, TX: Psychological Corporation.

Weintraub, S. and Mesulam, M-M. (1985) Mental state assessment of young and elderly adults in behavioral neurology. In: M-M. Mesulam (Ed.), *Principles of behavioral neurology* (pp. 71–124). Philadelphia: F.A. Davis.

Weisenburg, T.H. and McBride, K.E. (1935) *Aphasia*. New York: Commonwealth Fund.

Welch, L.W., Doineau, D., Johnson, S., and King, D. (1996) Educational and gender normative data for the Boston Naming Test in a group of older adults. *Brain and Language*, 53, 260–266.

Welsh, K.A., Butters, N., Mohs, R.C., Beekly, D., Edland, S., Fillenbaum, G., and Heyman, A. (1994) The Consortium to Establish a Registry for Alzheimer's Disease (CERAD). Part V: A normative study of the neuropsychological battery. *Neurology*, 44, 609–614.

Welsh, K.A., Fillenbaum, G., Wilkinson, W., et al. (1995a) Neuropsychological test performance in African-American and white patients with Alzheimer's disease. *Neurology*, 45, 2207–2211.

Welsh, K.A., Watson, M., Hoffman, J.M., Lowe, V., Earl, N., and Rubin, D.C. (1995b) The neural basis of visual naming errors in Alzheimer's disease: A positron emission tomography study. *Archives of Clinical Neuropsychology*, 10, 403 (abstract).

Wepman, J.M. (1951) *Recovery from aphasia*. New York: Ronald Press.

Wepman, J.M. (1961) *Language Modalities Test for Aphasia*. Chicago: Education Industry Service.

Wepman, J.M., Bock, R.D., Jones, L.V., and Van Pelt, D. (1956) Psycholinguistic study of aphasia. *Journal of Speech and Hearing Disorders*, 21, 468–477.

Wepman, J.W., Bock, R.D., Jones, L.V., and Van Pelt, D. (1973) Psycholinguistic study of aphasia: A revision of the concept of anomia. In: H. Goodglass and S. Blumstein (Eds.), *Psycholinguistics and aphasia* (pp. 219–229). Baltimore: Johns Hopkins University Press.

Wepman, J.M. and Jones, L.V. (1964) Five aphasias: A commentary on aphasia as a regressive linguistic phenomenon. In: D.M. Rioch and E.A. Weinstein (Eds.), *Disorders of communication*. Baltimore: Williams & Wilkins.

Wepman, J.M. and Reynolds, W.M. (1998) *Wepman's Auditory Discrimination Test (ADT)—2nd Edition*. Los Angeles: Western Psychological Services.

Werner, M.H., Ernst, J., Townes, B.D., Peel, J., and Preston, M. (1987) Relationship between IQ and neuropsychological measures in neuropsychiatric populations: Within-laboratory and cross-cultural replications using WAIS and WAIS-R. *Journal of Clinical and Experimental Neuropsychology*, 9, 545–562.

Wernicke, C. (1908) The symptom complex of aphasia. In: A. Church (Ed.), *Diseases of the nervous system*. New York: Appleton (original work published in 1874).

Wertz, R.T. (1979) Word fluency measure. In: F.L. Darley (Ed.), *Evaluation of appraisal techniques in speech and language pathology*. Reading, MA: Addison-Wesley.

Wertz, R.T. (1996) The PALPA's proof is in the predicting. *Aphasiology*, 10, 180–190.

Wertz, R., LaPointe, L., and Rosenbek, J. (1984) *Apraxia of speech in adults*. Orlando, FL: Grune & Stratton.

Wertz, R.T. and Lemme, M.L. (1974) *Input and output measures with adult aphasics (Final Report)*. Washington, D.C.: Research and Training Center 10, Social Rehabilitation Services.

Wertz, R.T., Weiss, D.G., Aten, J.L., Brookshire, R.H., Garcia-Brunuel, L., Holland, A.L., et al. (1986) Comparison of clinic, home, and deferred language treatment for aphasia: A Veterans Administration cooperative study. *Archives of Neurology*, 43, 653–658.

West, J.A. (1973) Auditory comprehension in aphasic adults: Improvement through training. *Archives of Physical Medicine and Rehabilitation*, 54, 78–86.

West, J.F., Sands, E.S., and Ross-Swain, D. (1998) *Bedside Evaluation Screening Test*, 2nd ed. (BEST-2). Austin, TX: Pro-Ed.

Westbury, C. and Bub, D. (1997) Primary progressive aphasia: A review of 112 cases. *Brain and Language*, 60, 381–406.

Wheeler, L. and Reitan, R.M. (1962) The presence and laterality of brain damage predicted from responses to a short aphasia screening test. *Perceptual and Motor Skills*, 15, 783–799.

Whitworth, R.H. and Larson, C.M. (1989) Differential diagnosis and staging of Alzheimer's disease with an aphasia battery. *Neuropsychiatry, Neuropsychology, and Behavioral Neurology*, 1, 255–265.

Whitworth, A., Perkins, L., and Lesser, R. (1997) *Conversation Analysis Profile for People with Aphasia (CAPPA)*. London: Whurr Publishers.

Whurr, R. (1996) *Aphasia Screening Test (AST)*, 2nd ed. London: Whurr Publishers.

Whurr, R. and Evans, S. (1998) Children's Acquired Aphasia Screening Test (CAAST). *International Journal of Language and Communication Disorders*, 33, Suppl., 343–344.

Wiig, E.H. (1990) *Wiig Criterion Referenced Inventory of Language*. San Antonio, TX: Psychological Corporation.

Wiig, E.H. and Secord, W. (1989) *Test of Language Competence Expanded Edition (TLC-EE)*. San Antonio, TX: Psychological Corporation.

Wiig, E.H., Secord, W.A., and Semel, E. (1992) *Clinical Evaluation of Language Fundamentals—Preschool*. San Antonio, TX: Psychological Corporation.

Wilkins, J.W., Hamby, S.L., and Thompson, K.L. (1996) Difficulties with Boston Naming norms in individuals with below average WAIS-R vocabulary. *Archives of Clinical Neuropsychology*, 11, 464 (abstract).

Wilkinson, G.S. (1993) *Wide Range Achievement Test—3*. Wilmington, DE: Wide Range.

Willeford, J.A. (1985) Assessment of central auditory disorders in children. In: M.L. Pinheiro and F.E. Musiek (Eds.), *Assessment of central auditory dysfunction: Foundations and clinical correlates*. Los Angeles: Williams & Wilkins.

Williams, A.M., Marks, C.J., and Bialer, I. (1977) Validity of the Peabody Picture Vocabulary Test as a measure of hearing vocabulary in mentally retarded and normal children. *Journal of Speech and Hearing Research*, 20, 205–211.

Williams, B.W., Mack, W., and Henderson, V.W. (1989) Boston Naming Test in Alzheimer's disease. *Neuropsychologia*, 27, 1073–1079.

Williams, J.M. and Shane, B. (1986) The Reitan-Indiana Aphasia Screening Test: Scoring and factor analysis. *Journal of Clinical Psychology*, 42, 156–160.

Williams, M. (1965) *Mental testing in clinical practice*. London: Pergamon.

Williams, S.E. (1996) Psychological adjustment following stroke. In: G.L. Wallace (Ed.), *Adult aphasia rehabilitation* (pp. 303–323). Boston: Butterworth-Heinemann.

Willmes, K., Poeck, K., Weniger, D., and Huber, W. (1983) Facet theory applied to the construction and validation of the Aachen Aphasia Test. *Brain and Language*, 18, 259–276.

Willmes, K. and Ratajczak, K. (1962) The design and application of a data- and method-based system for the Aachen Aphasia Test. *Neuropsychologia*, 25, 725–733.

Wilson, R.S., Sullivan, M., Toledo-Morrell, L.D., et al. (1996) Association of memory and cognition in Alzheimer's disease with volumetric estimates of temporal lobe structures. *Neuropsychology*, 10, 459–463.

Wirz, S.L., Skinner, C., and Dean, E. (1990) *Revised Edinburgh Functional Communication Profile*. Tucson, AZ: Communication Skill Builders.

Wolters, P.L., Brouwers, P., Moss, H.A., and Pizzo, P.A. (1995) Differential receptive and expressive language functioning of children with symptomatic HIV disease and relation to CT scan brain abnormalities. *Pediatrics*, 95, 112–119.

Worrall, L.E. (1992) Functional communication assessment: An Australian perspective. *Aphasiology*, 6, 105–110.

Worrall, L.E. and Frattali, C.M. (Eds.) (2000) *Neurogenic communication disorders: A functional approach.* New York: Thieme.

Worrall, L.E., Yiu, E.M.L., Hickson, L.M.H., and Barnett, H.M. (1995) Normative data for the Boston Naming Test for Australian elderly. *Aphasiology, 9,* 541–551.

Yeudall, L.T., Fromm, D., Reddon, J.R., and Stefanyk, W.O. (1986) Normative data stratified by age and sex for 12 neuropsychological tests. *Journal of Clinical Psychology, 42,* 918–946.

Yiu, E.M.L. (1992) Linguistic assessment of Chinese-speaking aphasics: Development of a Cantonese aphasia battery. *Journal of Neurolinguistics, 7,* 379–424.

Ylvisaker, M., Szekeres, S.F., and Feeney, T. (2001) Communication disorders associated with traumatic brain injury. In: R. Chapey (Ed.), *Language intervention strategies in aphasia and related neurogenic communication disorders,* 4th ed. (pp. 745–794). Philadelphia: Lippincott Williams & Wilkins.

Young, F. and Gibbon, F. (1998) Normative Scottish data on the CELF-RUK: A pilot study. *International Journal of Language and Communication Disorders, 33* Suppl., 345–350.

Zagar, R. (1983) Analysis of short test batteries for children. *Journal of Clinical Psychology, 39,* 590–597.

Zaidel, E., Kasher, A., Soroker, N., Batori, G., Giora, R., and Graves, D. (2000) Hemispheric contributions to pragmatics. *Brain and Cognition, 43,* 438–443.

Zarit, S.H., Reever, K.E., and Bach-Peterson, J. (1980) Relatives of the impaired elderly: Correlates of feeling of burden. *Gerontologist, 20,* 649–655.

Zec, R.F., Vicari, S. Kocis, M., and Reynolds, T. (1992) Sensitivity of different neuropsychological tests to very mild DAT. *The Clinical Neuropsychologist, 6,* 327 (abstract).

Zimmerman, I.L., Steiner, V.G., and Pond, R.E. (1992a) *Preschool Language Scale–3.* San Antonio, TX: Psychological Corporation.

Zimmerman, I.L., Steiner, V.G., and Pond, R.E. (1992b) *Preschool Language Scale–3–Spanish.* San Antonio, TX: Psychological Corporation.

Zink, I. and Schaerlaekens, A. (2000) Measuring young children's language abilities. *Acta Oto-Rhino-Laryngologica Belgica, 54,* 7–12.

Zubrick, A. and Smith, A. (1979) Minnesota Test for Differential Diagnosis of Aphasia. In: F.C. Darley (Ed.), *Evaluation of appraisal techniques in speech and language pathology.* Reading, MA: Addison-Wesley.

Zucker, S. and Riordan, J. (1988) Concurrent validity of new and revised conceptual language measures. *Psychology in the Schools, 25,* 252–256.

Zucker, S. and Riordan, J. (1990) One-year predictive validity of new and revised conceptual language measurements. *Journal of Psychoeducational Assessment, 8,* 4–8.

Name Index

Page numbers followed by *f* and *t* indicate figures and tables, respectively.

Test and Subject Index

Page numbers followed by *f* and *t* indicate figures and tables, respectively.